Supervising Individual Psychotherapy

The Guide to "Good Enough"

Supervising Individual Psychotherapy

The Guide to "Good Enough"

Edited by
Katherine G. Kennedy, M.D.
Randon S. Welton, M.D.
Frank E. Yeomans, M.D., Ph.D.

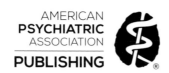

AMERICAN
PSYCHIATRIC
ASSOCIATION
PUBLISHING

First Edition

Manufactured in the United States of America on acid-free paper
27 26 25 24 23   5 4 3 2 1
ISBN 978-1-61537-424-3 (print), 978-1-61537-425-0 (ebook)

American Psychiatric Association Publishing
800 Maine Avenue SW, Suite 900
Washington, DC 20024-2812
www.appi.org

Library of Congress Cataloging-in-Publication Data
Names: Kennedy, Katherine G., editor. | Welton, Randon S., editor. |
    Yeomans, Frank E., 1949– editor. | American Psychiatric Association,
    issuing body.
Title: Supervising individual psychotherapy : the guide to "good enough" /
    edited by Katherine G. Kennedy, Randon S. Welton, Frank E. Yeomans.
Description: First edition. | Washington, DC : American Psychiatric
    Association Publishing, [2023] | Includes bibliographical references and index.
Identifiers: LCCN 2022049309 (print) | LCCN 2022049310 (ebook) | ISBN
    9781615374243 (print) | ISBN 9781615374250 (ebook)
Subjects: MESH: Psychotherapy—education | Preceptorship—methods |
    Internship and Residency—organization & administration |
    Psychiatry—education | Mentors
Classification: LCC RC480.5 (print) | LCC RC480.5 (ebook) | NLM WM 420 |
    DDC 616.89/14—dc23/eng/20221230
LC record available at https://lccn.loc.gov/2022049309
LC ebook record available at https://lccn.loc.gov/2022049310

British Library Cataloguing in Publication Data
A CIP record is available from the British Library.

Contents

Katherine G. Kennedy, M.D.
Randon S. Welton, M.D.
Frank E. Yeomans, M.D., Ph.D.

Part I
Becoming a "Good Enough" Supervisor

Randon S. Welton, M.D.
Katherine G. Kennedy, M.D.

Clifford Arnold, M.D., M.A.
Daniel Knoepflmacher, M.D., M.F.A.

Katherine G. Kennedy, M.D.
Randon S. Welton, M.D.

Katherine G. Kennedy, M.D.
Randon S. Welton, M.D.
David A. Adler, M.D.

Kevin V. Kelly, M.D.

Part IV
Challenges in Psychotherapy Supervision

Contributors

Stewart Adelson, M.D.
Clinical Associate Professor, Weill Medical College of Cornell University, New York, New York; Adjunct Assistant Clinical Professor, Columbia University Vagelos College of Physicians & Surgeons, New York, New York; Senior Visiting Fellow, Yale Law School, New Haven, Connecticut

David A. Adler, M.D.
Professor of Psychiatry and Medicine, Tufts University School of Medicine; Senior Psychiatrist, Department of Psychiatry, Tufts Medical Center, Boston, Massachusetts

Clifford Arnold, M.D., M.A.
Child and Adolescent Psychiatrist, COMCARE of Sedgwick County, Wichita, Kansas

Rosemary H. Balsam, FRCPsych (Lond), MRCP (Edinburgh)
Associate Clinical Professor of Psychiatry, Yale Medical School; Staff Psychiatrist, Department of Mental Health & Counseling, Yale University; Training and Supervising Analyst, Western New England Institute for Psychoanalysis, New Haven, Connecticut

Marina Bayeva, M.D., Ph.D.
Fellow in Hospital-Based Psychotherapy and Psychoanalytic Studies, Austen Riggs Center, Stockbridge, Massachusetts

Annabel C. Boeke, M.D.
PGY4 Psychiatry Resident, Columbia University Department of Psychiatry/New York State Psychiatric Institute, New York, New York

Adam Brenner, M.D.
Professor of Psychiatry and Distinguished Teaching Professor, and Vice Chair for Education and Residency Training Director in Psychiatry, University of Texas Southwestern Medical Center, Dallas, Texas

Deborah L. Cabaniss, M.D.
Associate Director of Residency Training and Professor of Clinical Psychiatry, Columbia University Department of Psychiatry/New York State Psychiatric Institute, New York, New York

Monica Carsky, Ph.D.
Clinical Assistant Professor of Psychology in Psychiatry and Senior Fellow, Personality Disorders Institute, Weill Medical College of Cornell University; Adjunct Assistant Professor, New York University Postdoctoral Program in Psychoanalysis and Psychotherapy; Faculty, Institute for Psychoanalytic Training and Research, New York, New York

Natasha Chriss, M.D.
Clinical Assistant Professor of Psychiatry, Weill Cornell Medicine, New York, New York

Allison Cowan, M.D., DFAPA
Associate Professor and Deputy Training Director, Department of Psychiatry, Boonshoft School of Medicine, Wright State University, Dayton, Ohio

Erin M. Crocker, M.D.
Clinical Associate Professor and Residency Training Director, Department of Psychiatry, University of Iowa Hospitals and Clinics, Iowa City, Iowa

Theunis O. de Boer, B.A.
Medical Student, Northeast Ohio Medical University, Rootstown, Ohio

June Elgudin, M.D.
Resident Physician, Department of Psychiatry, Weill Cornell Medical College, New York, New York

Alyson Gorun, M.D.
Assistant Professor of Clinical Psychiatry, Weill Cornell Medical College; Assistant Attending Psychiatrist, New York–Presbyterian Hospital, New York, New York

Sindhu A. Idicula, M.D.
Associate Professor of Psychiatry and Pediatrics, Associate Program Director, and Director of Psychotherapy Education, Menninger Department of Psychiatry, Baylor College of Medicine, Houston, Texas

Tina Kaviani, M.D.
Assistant Professor of Psychiatry, University of Texas Southwestern Medical Center, Dallas, Texas

Jack R. Keefe, Ph.D.
Research Fellow and Clinical Supervisor, Psychiatry Research Institute at Montefiore Einstein, Albert Einstein College of Medicine, Bronx, New York

Kevin V. Kelly, M.D.
Clinical Professor of Psychiatry and of Ethics in Medicine, Weill Cornell Medicine; Medical Officer, New York City Fire Department, New York, New York

Katherine G. Kennedy, M.D.
Assistant Clinical Professor of Psychiatry, Yale University, New Haven, Connecticut

Daniel Knoepflmacher, M.D., M.F.A.
Vice Chair of Education, Director of Residency Training in Psychiatry; Assistant Professor of Psychiatry, Weill Cornell Medicine/New York–Presbyterian, New York, New York

Alison E. Lenet, M.D.
Assistant Clinical Professor of Psychiatry, Columbia University Department of Psychiatry/New York State Psychiatric Institute, New York, New York

Seamus Bhatt-Mackin, M.D., C.G.P.
Director, Program for Clinical Group Work, VA Mid-Atlantic Mental Illness Research, Education and Clinical Center (MIRECC); Staff Psychiatrist, Operation Enduring Freedom (OEF), Operation Iraqi Freedom (OIF), and Operation New Dawn (OND) Veterans Clinic, Durham Veterans Affairs (VA) Medical Center; Consulting Associate, Duke University Department of Psychiatry and Behavioral Sciences, Durham, North Carolina

David Mintz, M.D.
Director of Psychiatric Education, Associate Director of Training, and Team Leader, Austen Riggs Center, Stockbridge, Massachusetts

Aimee Murray, Psy.D., L.P.
Assistant Professor, Department of Psychiatry and Behavioral Sciences, University of Minnesota, Minneapolis, Minnesota

Michael F. Myers, M.D.
Professor of Clinical Psychiatry, Department of Psychiatry & Behavioral Sciences, SUNY Downstate Health Sciences University, Brooklyn, New York

Rebecca Nejat, M.D.
Clinical Assistant Professor of Psychiatry, Weill Cornell Medicine, New York, New York

Dionne R. Powell, M.D.
Clinical Assistant Professor of Psychiatry, Weill Cornell Medical College; Assistant Attending Psychiatrist, New York–Presbyterian Hospital, New York, New York; Training and Supervising Analyst, Psychoanalytic Association of New York and the Columbia University Center for Psychoanalytic Training & Research

Maya G. Prabhu, M.D., LL.B.
Chief Consulting Forensic Psychiatrist, Connecticut Department of Mental Health and Addiction Services, Division of Forensic Services; Associate Professor, Division of Law and Psychiatry, Department of Psychiatry, Yale School of Medicine; Clinical Associate Professor of Law, Yale Law School, New Haven, Connecticut

Magdalena Romanowicz, M.D.
Associate Professor, Department of Psychiatry and Psychology, Mayo Clinic, Rochester, Minnesota

Evgenia Royter, D.O.
Psychiatry Resident, Tower Health-Phoenixville Hospital, Phoenixville, Pennsylvania

Anne E. Ruble, M.D., M.P.H.
Director of Psychotherapy Training and Associate Program Director, Adult Psychiatry Residency, Johns Hopkins University School of Medicine, Department of Psychiatry and Behavioral Sciences, Baltimore, Maryland

Kimberly R. Stubbs, M.D.
Volunteer Faculty, Department of Psychiatry, Boonshoft School of Medicine, Wright State University, Dayton, Ohio

Donna M. Sudak, M.D.
Professor of Psychiatry, Drexel University; Program Director, General Psychiatry Residency, Tower Health-Phoenixville Hospital, Phoenixville, Pennsylvania

Yi-lang Tang, M.D., Ph.D.
Associate Professor, Department of Psychiatry and Behavioral Sciences, Emory University; Substance Abuse Treatment Program, Atlanta VA Medical Center, Decatur, Georgia

David R. Topor, Ph.D., M.S.-H.P.Ed.
Deputy Associate Chief of Staff for Education, Veterans Affairs Boston Healthcare System; Associate Professor, Department of Psychiatry, Harvard Medical School, Boston, Massachusetts

Christian Umfrid, M.D.
Assistant Professor of Clinical Psychiatry, Weill Cornell Medical College; Assistant Attending Psychiatrist, New York–Presbyterian Hospital, New York, New York

Mary C. Vance, M.D., M.Sc.
Director of Behavioral Health, Pacific Area, United States Coast Guard, Alameda, California; Assistant Professor of Psychiatry and Scientist, Center for the Study of Traumatic Stress, Uniformed Services University of the Health Sciences, Bethesda, Maryland

David Veith, M.D.
Chief Psychiatry Resident, Columbia University Department of Psychiatry/New York State Psychiatric Institute, New York, New York

Cecil R. Webster Jr., M.D.
Lecturer in Psychiatry, Harvard Medical School McLean Hospital, Boston, Massachusetts

Randon S. Welton, M.D.
The Margaret Clark Morgan Professor and Chair of Psychiatry, Northeast Ohio Medical University, Rootstown, Ohio

Frank E. Yeomans, M.D., Ph.D.
Clinical Associate Professor of Psychiatry and Director of Training at the Personality Disorders Institute, Weill Medical College of Cornell University, New York, New York; Adjunct Associate Clinical Professor of Psychiatry, Columbia University Vagelos College of Physicians & Surgeons Center for Psychoanalytic Training and Research, New York, New York; President, International Society of Transference-Focused Psychotherapy, Vienna, Austria

Acknowledgments

Editing this collection of chapters by so many brilliant and thoughtful authors has been an honor and a privilege. Thank you to my co-editors and to all of the contributors—some of whom are my past supervisors and supervisees—for indulging my questions, accepting my feedback, and, at times, using your better judgment to override my edits. I am also deeply grateful to every one of my former supervisors, from whom I have learned so much, and to my former supervisees, from whom I have learned even more. Finally, I could never have accomplished this effort without the love, support, and dinner-making skills of my family—Ted, Kiley, and Teddy. My wish for this book is that new supervisory discussions are sparked and new supervisors inspired.—KGK

As we complete this book, my gratitude is more than I can express. I want to thank my parents—David and Deanna—for always believing in me; my wife—Michelle—for always being by my side; and my kids—Sean and Shannon—for the joy and purpose they bring to my life. I am unbelievably honored to have worked with my co-editors on this project and am still surprised that they let me tag along with them on this journey. To all of our contributors: Thank you for putting up with me. Lastly, I want to thank my former supervisors and supervisees: You have taught me more than I can remember and have inspired me more than I can say.—RSW

First, I would like to thank my co-editors, who initiated this volume and did the heavy lifting, and the talented group of authors, who have made the book what it is. Because supervision never ends, the list of the supervisors who have inspired me gets longer as the years go on. Among these, I would especially like to acknowledge Otto Kernberg, Paulina Kernberg, Ann Appelbaum, Herb Schlesinger, Richard Munich, Michael Stone, Michael Selzer, my colleagues in our ongoing weekly co-supervision, and especially Carlos, my longest and most reliable supervisor. Finally, my thanks go to the many patients who have taught me to better appreciate the far reaches of the heart and mind and have helped me to try to bring that knowledge to those I teach.—FEY

PART I

Becoming a "Good Enough" Supervisor

Introduction

Am I Qualified to Supervise?

Randon S. Welton, M.D.
Katherine G. Kennedy, M.D.

A third-year psychiatry resident working the emergency department has just evaluated a patient who was brought in after an overdose, her third in the past 2 years. Later in the day, he and his psychotherapy supervisor discuss this patient's case.

> SUPERVISOR: What led to her overdose attempt?
> RESIDENT: She and her girlfriend had a fight. That seems to be the pattern. She recently got a new job at a factory. The money was good, but she worked second shift. That led to suspicion and jealousy, so she impulsively quit her job. That led to a fight with her girlfriend, and that led to the overdose.
> SUPERVISOR: What would you like to do for her?
> RESIDENT: I can follow up with her in the outpatient clinic. And maybe start a mood stabilizer or antidepressant.
> SUPERVISOR: What about psychotherapy? Would that be helpful for her?
> RESIDENT: I don't know...I suppose it would. We can certainly send her for a therapy referral.
> SUPERVISOR: It sounds like you were going to follow her for medications. Could you see her for psychotherapy as well?
> RESIDENT: Oh, no...I wouldn't know where to begin, plus I don't think I would be very effective in that role. We need to get her to a professional for help.
> SUPERVISOR: You're probably right. Besides, I wouldn't know how to supervise you in the psychotherapy part anyway.

THROUGHOUT MOST of the last century, psychotherapy was at the core of what it meant to be a psychiatrist. Psychiatry training and practice was steeped in psychodynamic principles. A psychodynamic understanding of patients contributed to all phases of psychiatrist–patient interactions as it permitted a comprehensive perspective of our patients and their lives. With our growing appreciation of epigenetic modification, we could even connect those factors to neurobiological changes (Kay 2017; Ravitz 2017). Abundant evidence existed for the efficacy of psychodynamic psychotherapy in a broad array of common and complex mental disorders, including personality disorders (Abbass et al. 2017; Fonagy 2015; Leichsenring and Rabung 2008, 2011; Ravitz 2017). Psychodynamic psychotherapy informed our understanding of the mind and formed the basis for effective psychiatric treatment. Learning how to provide psychotherapy was viewed as an essential element in training to be a psychiatrist.

Today, this is no longer the case. Beginning in the late twentieth century, a decline in provision of psychotherapy by psychiatrists began to occur. In the 1980s, approximately half of all psychiatric appointments involved psychotherapy (Dorwart et al. 1992). By 2004, the percentage of psychiatric visits involving psychotherapy had decreased to only 29% (Mojtabai and Olfson 2008). Many factors contributed to this drop, including the introduction of novel psychotropic medications, the emergence of managed care, and shifting payment schemes for psychiatric care that discouraged reimbursement for psychotherapy. Additionally, an increase in educational debt has led many early-career psychiatrists to seek more lucrative practices within organizations that discourage the provision of psychotherapy by psychiatrists (Clemens et al. 2014; Kay 2017). A vicious cycle was set in motion: as early-career psychiatrists observed fewer psychiatric attending physicians practicing psychotherapy, the assumption that "psychotherapy is not something that psychiatrists do" became more widespread.

Despite these gloomy trends, hope continues for reviving the practice of psychotherapy by psychiatrists. In a survey study of Canadian psychiatrists ($N=423$), nearly 81% reported practicing psychotherapy, with the most common theoretical orientation being psychodynamic psychotherapy (Hadjipavlou et al. 2015). Percentages of psychiatrists practicing psychotherapy were highest (>85%) among more experienced psychiatrists (>20 years of experience) and early-career psychiatrists (<5 years of experience) (Hadjipavlou et al. 2015). The American Academy of Psychoanalysis and Dynamic Psychiatry reported that the preferred type of psychotherapy among its members was weekly individual therapy and that nearly 95% of members reported psychotherapy session durations of

45–60 minutes (Alfonso and Olarte 2011). In an online survey of applicants to a Canadian psychiatry residency program, 55% of medical students endorsed "emphasis on psychotherapy" as a motivator for them to enter psychiatry; this was the second-highest motivator behind "favorable job market for psychiatry" (Wiesenfeld et al. 2014). Finally, in another online survey examining psychiatry residents' perceptions of and experiences in training, residents expressed a desire for more training in psychotherapy and more hours of psychotherapy practice, and they described supervision as being the most important training modality for psychotherapy (Kovach et al. 2015).

Psychotherapy training continues to be an essential part of psychiatric residencies. The Accreditation Council for Graduate Medical Education (ACGME), which governs the standards for psychiatry residency training, still requires that all graduating residents demonstrate competence in "managing and treating patients using both brief and long-term supportive, psychodynamic, and cognitive-behavioral psychotherapies" (Accreditation Council for Graduate Medical Education 2020, p. 21). Supervision is considered a central component of the psychotherapy education process. Learning to deal with the complex situations and emotional challenges engendered during psychotherapy cannot be done by reading articles and attending lectures alone. Supervision offers the safe space that residents need to express themselves more freely (Kennedy 2016).

We believe that psychotherapy remains a critical skill for all psychiatrists. A psychodynamic understanding allows us to comprehend the combination of genetic vulnerabilities, social/cultural realities, early-childhood experiences, unique circumstances, and personal decisions that contribute to how our patients experience their lives and engage in the world. Gaining competence as a psychotherapist requires a knowledge of theory mixed with experience in clinical work and thoughtful clinical supervision. Psychotherapy supervisors play a critical role in forming the next generation of psychiatric psychotherapists.

With this renewed interest, there is a growing call for more psychotherapy supervision and an expanding need for additional psychotherapy supervisors. Unfortunately, the events of the past 30 years have left the field of psychiatry with a profound shortage of psychotherapy supervisors. Waving the proverbial wand will not make a fresh crop of psychotherapy supervisors magically appear. Becoming a psychotherapy supervisor is a developmental process. Many psychiatry training programs lack the personnel and other key resources required to train new psychotherapy supervisors, despite the ongoing need for a steady supply of new supervisors to replace those who are retiring. Some early- and mid-career psychiatrists are hesitant to take on the mantle of psychotherapy supervisor. They may feel daunted either by memories of their esteemed supervisors or by a lack of any role models at all. This book addresses issues raised when a psychiatrist or psychotherapist wonders "Am I qualified to be a psychotherapy supervisor?"

Although the evidence base is still evolving, psychotherapy supervision is a skill that can be developed, just like any other skill. We put this book together to help. The main prerequisites for becoming a psychotherapy supervisor are a basic understanding of psychotherapeutic principles, a sincere desire to become a "good enough" psychotherapy supervisor, and an opportunity to supervise someone. But prospective supervisors may have a range of other concerns, such as the following:

- *I haven't supervised psychotherapy before.* Experience is a good thing, but every supervisor starts as a novice supervisor. Experience is gained by practice.
- *I don't know enough theory to be a supervisor.* Most of supervision addresses the clinical material from therapy sessions. The trainee has other sources for theoretical knowledge. While possessing a solid foundation of theory is helpful, additional knowledge will be gained along the way.
- *I wouldn't know how to conduct supervision.* There is not one "right" way to supervise. Good supervisors are as varied as good therapists. This book will teach you approaches and priorities to help you provide "good enough" supervision.
- *No one would take me seriously as a supervisor.* Supervisors don't have to have all of the answers at their fingertips. They will have more knowledge and experience than their supervisees, and that is all that is required. Helping trainees to recognize what is going on in their sessions with patients and to think through their options for responding is enough.
- *Being a supervisor is a gift that I just don't have.* Excellent supervisors are made, not born.
- *I can't supervise psychotherapy. I am an inpatient (or addiction/geriatric/forensic/consultation-liaison) psychiatrist. I don't work in an outpatient clinic.* Psychotherapy skills are found in all excellent psychiatrists, and all excellent psychiatrists can provide psychotherapy supervision. In fact, it is often helpful to have supervisors who practice outside of outpatient clinics, because they bring a novel and interesting perspective to the work.

- *I don't have enough experience as a therapist to be a supervisor.* While some personal experience as a therapist is necessary for the supervisor to be credible, their experiences during residency and their clinical careers, combined with a commitment to continue providing therapy in the future, should be enough for them to start supervising.
- *There are better and smarter people out there.* Perhaps…but we don't have enough psychiatrists who supervise psychotherapy. We need you.

Trainees do not need supervisors who are perfect. They need supervisors who are engaged, knowledgeable, and humble, and who provide supervision in a deliberate and thoughtful manner. Mistakes will be made, but as is the case in parenting, making a consistent effort, being willing to acknowledge and correct mistakes, and sincerely desiring to do the right thing will more than make up for a variety of innocent errors. Our goal in compiling this book was to help encourage the growth of the "good enough" supervisor. Just as Winnicott described the "good enough" mother as one who adapts to her child's needs and supports their growth and eventual autonomy (Winnicott 1953/1971), it is our hope that you will recognize that the process of becoming a supervisor is a lifelong journey, that every supervisor will make missteps, and that there is always, always, more to learn.

Although we hope that you will read this book from cover to cover, we realize that many will pick those chapters that seem most immediately relevant to their situation. That is fine. Do what works best for you. To help your efforts, we next explain the organization of the book.

Part I: Becoming a "Good Enough" Supervisor: Chapters in this portion of the book are designed to introduce you to the work of supervision. There is a focus on the supervisory relationship, ethics, and practical considerations. We also have included personal vignettes from recent supervisees to help orient you to their perspectives and to how your words and actions may affect their experience of supervision.

Part II: How to Supervise Psychodynamic Psychotherapy: Chapters in this part focus on the "nuts and bolts" of supervision. We discuss the process and aims of supervision and the benefits of setting goals for supervision and using process notes and/or audiovisual recordings. We look at the complexity surrounding terminating supervision. We examine how all of these elements have been affected by the sudden explosion of teletherapy and telesupervision.

Part III: Factors That Affect Psychotherapy Supervision: Whereas chapters in Part II discuss aspects of supervision that are ubiquitous, chapters in this part focus on specific issues that are commonly encountered but not universal. There are chapters on how issues related to race, gender, and lesbian, gay, bisexual, and transgender (LGBT) identities might affect supervision. We also broaden our focus and look briefly at the supervision of cognitive-behavioral therapy, supportive therapy, and therapy for patients with substance use disorders.

Part IV: Challenges in Psychotherapy Supervision: Chapters in the last section deal with specific situations that occasionally arise that can challenge even the most experienced supervisor. Such situations can involve concerns about burnout and microaggressions, trainees who are perceived as "difficult," or major transitions occurring in the life of the therapist or supervisor. We also review complications from unconscious sexual issues that can arise in supervision and the impact of death and dying on supervision. Finally, we offer a chapter on legal concerns that may arise in supervision.

As a last recommendation, we would suggest that you not read this book alone. If you are supervising trainees, get together with other psychotherapy supervisors and discuss the topics in this book and other pertinent supervision topics. Peer support can be extremely important, as psychotherapy supervision can sometimes feel like a lonely endeavor. Based on our experiences, though, it can also be one of the most rewarding aspects of your career.

"Am I qualified to be a 'good enough' psychotherapy supervisor?"

It is our hope that after you read this book, your answer will be a resounding "Yes!"

References

Abbass A, Luyten P, Steinert C, Leichsenring F: Bias toward psychodynamic therapy: framing the problem and working toward a solution. J Psychiatr Pract 23(5):361–365, 2017 28961665

Accreditation Council for Graduate Medical Education: ACGME Program Requirements for Graduate Medical Education in Psychiatry. Chicago, IL, Accreditation Council for Graduate Medical Education, 2020. Available at: www.acgme.org/Portals/0/PFAssets/ProgramRequirements/400_Psychiatry_2020.pdf. Accessed January 1, 2021.

Alfonso CA, Olarte SW: Contemporary practice patterns of dynamic psychiatrists—survey results. J Am Acad Psychoanal Dyn Psychiatry 39(1):7–26, 2011 21434740

Clemens NA, Plakun EM, Lazar SG, Mellman L: Obstacles to early career psychiatrists practicing psychotherapy. Psychodyn Psychiatry 42(3):479–495, 2014 25211434

Dorwart RA, Chartock LR, Dial T, et al: A national study of psychiatrists' professional activities. Am J Psychiatry 149(11):1499–1505, 1992 1357992

Fonagy P: The effectiveness of psychodynamic psychotherapies: an update. World Psychiatry 14(2):137–150, 2015 26043322

Hadjipavlou G, Hernandez CAS, Ogrodniczuk JS: Psychotherapy in contemporary psychiatric practice. Can J Psychiatry 60(6):294–300, 2015 26175328

Kay J: Psychotherapy by psychiatrists: why choose a bugle when you can play a trumpet? Acad Psychiatry 41(1):24–29, 2017 27943128

Kennedy KG: Residents want to learn more psychotherapy: thoughts on supervision. Psychiatric News 51(14), July 12, 2016. Available at: https://psychnews.psychiatryonline.org/doi/10.1176/appi.pn.2016.7b9. Accessed January 1, 2021.

Kovach JG, Dubin WR, Combs CJ: Psychotherapy training: residents' perceptions and experiences. Acad Psychiatry 39(5):567–574, 2015 25008313

Leichsenring F, Rabung S: Effectiveness of long-term psychodynamic psychotherapy: a meta-analysis. JAMA 300(13):1551–1565, 2008 18827212

Leichsenring F, Rabung S: Long-term psychodynamic psychotherapy in complex mental disorders: update of a meta-analysis. Br J Psychiatry 199(1):15–22, 2011 21719877

Mojtabai R, Olfson M: National trends in psychotherapy by office-based psychiatrists. Arch Gen Psychiatry 65(8):962–970, 2008 18678801

Ravitz P: Contemporary psychiatry, psychoanalysis, and psychotherapy. Can J Psychiatry 62(5):304–307, 2017 28525733

Wiesenfeld L, Abbey S, Takahashi SG, Abrahams C: Choosing psychiatry as a career: motivators and deterrents at a critical decision-making juncture. Can J Psychiatry 59(8):450–454, 2014 25161070

Winnicott DW: Transitional objects and transitional phenomena (1953), in Playing and Reality. London, Tavistock, 1971

2

Psychotherapy Supervision in Context

Historical and Theoretical Perspectives

Clifford Arnold, M.D., M.A.
Daniel Knoepflmacher, M.D., M.F.A.

KEY LEARNING GOALS

- Identify historical precedents for contemporary psychotherapy supervision.
- Describe and compare different theoretical models of psychotherapy supervision.
- Use a historical and theoretical framework to evaluate and refine one's own approach to psychotherapy supervision.

IN THIS CHAPTER we explore the historical development of psychotherapy supervision and highlight three key theoretical models. We describe how psychotherapy supervision grew out of the psychoanalytic tradition, diversified with the proliferation of psychotherapies, gave rise to a variety of theoretical models, and has recently undergone a process aimed at greater theoretical coherence and standardization.

Brief Historical Overview

As with psychotherapy generally, it is difficult to pinpoint a specific historical origin of psychotherapy supervision. Freud's 1909 case of Little Hans is widely cited as the first recorded psychoanalytic supervision, although this designation is imperfect (Milne 2009). The account of Freud's advising Max Graf on psychotherapeutic interventions to treat his son's phobia of horses seems to be more of a consultative relationship between clinician and layperson than a supervision between two professionals. Nevertheless, this case, along with the scheduled didactic discussion groups held at Freud's home beginning in 1902, provided the foundation for a more formalized practice of psychoanalytic supervision (Watkins 2011).

Whereas early supervision emerged in a psychoanalytic tradition and was relatively uniform in its conceptual basis, as the twentieth century wore on, new schools of psychotherapy proliferated and new models for supervision multiplied along with them. The history of psychotherapy supervision can be seen, in broad strokes, as a trajectory beginning with 1) early psychoanalytic supervision uniformity and coherence; progressing to 2) diversity among proliferating modes of psychotherapy and their corresponding modes of supervision and 3) diversity among theoretical models of supervision; and finally leading to 4) efforts at integration. This trajectory will be elucidated and explored in the following sections.

Therapy-Based Model of Psychotherapy Supervision

The earliest and most intuitive model of psychotherapy supervision is arguably the therapy-based model, which applies the basic concepts and practices of psychotherapy to the process of supervision; in other words, supervision is seen as parallel or analogous to therapy and as operating according to similar principles. The earliest examples of this model can be seen in the psychoanalytic tradition, where supervision shared key concepts with psychoanalysis itself, such as the need in the supervisory relationship for alliance, safety, and comfort, and the recognition of transference and countertransference. A supervisee's own psychoanalysis was seen as a sine qua non of the analyst's development exactly because analytic principles pertain across all relationships—in therapy, in supervision, and otherwise. Although psychoanalysis remained the main modality of both practice and supervision throughout more than half of the twentieth century (Mohl et al. 1990), additional psychotherapies gradually gained ground, with the well-known emergence of cognitive-behavioral therapy (CBT) as the most widely practiced of therapies. Although the different, newer psychotherapies vary greatly in their approaches, the analogy between therapy and supervision has been observed consistently across them, and the therapy-based model of supervision has been utilized throughout these diverse approaches. For example, one CBT supervision theorist wrote that "cognitive therapy supervision parallels the therapy itself" (Padesky 1996, p. 281), and that "the same processes and methods that characterize the therapy can be used to teach and supervise therapists" (p. 289).

Strengths of the therapy-based model of supervision are immediately apparent: the principles of therapy can be demonstrated and affirmed in the supervisory relationship, the skills that the supervisor has honed as a therapist are directly applicable to the supervisory task, and these skills are on display for the supervisee to assimilate in both a conceptual and experiential manner. However, this model has been criticized for overemphasizing the similarities between therapy and supervision and blurring the distinctions between them; while they may be complementary, supervision and therapy are distinct practices that require distinct sets of skills (Holloway 2014). Milne gave a balanced consideration of the therapy-based model: "Overall,...there is much to commend the reasoned, cautious transfer of therapy to supervision, and it is perhaps because of the extensive and highly plausible parallels between the two professional activities that using therapeutic thinking is one of the two most popular models of supervision (competing with that of supervising as one was supervised)" (Milne 2009, p. 41).

Developmental Model of Psychotherapy Supervision

Late in the twentieth century, there emerged a recognition that, as one author wrote, "a purely clinical model of training is inadequate in explaining the supervisory phenomenon" (Holloway 1987, p. 209). The developmental model of psychotherapy supervision arose from this awareness. In reaction to the therapy-based model, which merely extrapolated psychotherapeutic principles to construct a theory of supervision, the developmental model brought in theories from a wide range of fields, such as cognitive and emotion processing theory, schema theory, development of expertise theory, social psychology, and motivation theory (Stoltenberg et al. 2014), and applied these theories to the specific process of development as a psychotherapist. Numerous articulations of the model emerged in the early 1980s, including those by Stoltenberg in 1981, Loganbill et al. in 1982, and Blocher in 1983 (Holloway 1987).

One specific and prominent iteration of the model, the integrative developmental model (IDM) (Stoltenberg et al. 2014), elaborated a three-level developmental progression and identified three "structures" that attend each level; these structures are motivation, autonomy, and self- and other-awareness. For example, if we were to follow the *autonomy* structure through the three progressive levels, we would observe that a supervisee at level 1 exhibits a significant degree of dependence on the supervisor and a correspondent external locus of causality, which by level 3 develops into a high degree of independence and an internal locus of causality. Likewise, the model analyzes the supervisee's corresponding progress in terms of motivation and self-awareness through each of these three levels of development. Notably, the model also describes the "supervision environment" that is most conducive to promoting the supervisee's progression forward to the next level of development. For example, the level 1 environment focuses on basic skills; a wide, introductory range of theories; and a predominantly supportive stance, whereas the level 2 environment offers more challenges by focusing on advanced skill development, self-directed literature searches, and mild confrontation with alternative viewpoints (Stoltenberg et al. 2014).

One key strength of the developmental model, and of the IDM in particular, is that it utilizes an intuitive and coherent conceptual framework; many educators already consider the training process from a developmental perspective, and have little trouble applying general developmental theories to the supervision sphere. One critique of the developmental model is that the insights gained from general developmental theory do not fully mirror the process of development in supervision. This conceptual mismatch is primarily related to the incongruence between the progress of the supervisee toward competency and the development of the individual human being across the life span (Holloway 1987).

Social-Role Model of Psychotherapy Supervision

The social-role model of psychotherapy supervision emerged in the 1990s and follows the historical trend of increasing theoretical diversity. Whereas the therapy-based approach conceptualizes the supervisory role merely as parallel to the therapeutic role, the social-role model identifies several potential roles for the supervisor. One theorist wrote, "The most frequently recognized roles are teacher, counselor, and consultant; however, the roles of evaluator, lecturer, and role model of professional practice have also been used to describe supervisor behaviors and attitudes" (Holloway 2014, p. 599). And in contrast to seeing supervision through the singular lens of developmental theory, the social-role model marshals theoretical contributions from a multitude of social science fields, including, for example, insights from symbolic interactionism, social-role theory, and relational cultural theory (Holloway 2014).

Here is an illustrative discussion where a theorist thinks in social theory terms about two key issues in supervision, role conflict and power dynamics:

> Clinical supervision of therapists in training requires a formal relationship in which the supervisor has responsibility for imparting expert knowledge, making judgments of trainees' performance, and acting as a gatekeeper to the profession. These aspects of the role create a hierarchical relational structure that depends on *power over*. Yet the creation of a learning alliance that encourages transparency, vulnerability, and trust requires a *power with* orientation in the relationship. The existence of both *power over* and *power with* has caused considerable consternation for clinical supervisors because of the tension created by having to monitor the trainee's competency to ensure client safety and, at the same time, support the trainee's growing autonomy. (Holloway 2014, pp. 604–605)

This sort of tension can also be seen in the roles of teacher on the one hand and consultant on the other; the supervisor actively imparts insight, but at the same time, supervisees are fully responsible for their own process of discovery. Socrates put this paradox best when he likened himself to a midwife and his students to women giving birth: "It is quite clear that they never learned anything from me; the many fine discoveries to which they cling are of their own making. But to me and the god they owe their delivery" (Plato 1892).

An important strength of the social-role model is that it is comprehensive in scope; it accounts for the many and diverse roles and behaviors that a supervisor might be required to take on. A possible weakness is that it can be seen to involve a multiplicity of theories that risk failing to cohere; in other words, in its efforts at comprehensiveness, it can be seen to fail at maintaining a consistent idea or concept at its center and instead can be seen to consist in a multifarious collection of ideas or perhaps of multiple distinct models. In this way, the social-role model can be seen as an example of the trajectory toward theoretical diversity and multiplicity, and away from the earlier unity and simplicity of the therapy-based model.

Integrative Models of Psychotherapy Supervision

By the early 1990s, the viability of psychotherapy in psychiatry had come into question, and the fate of supervision along with it. Advancements in neuroscientific research, the advent of novel psychopharmacological treatments, and increased concerns about the relative cost of psychiatric services caused many to ask questions such as the following, in a 1990 issue of the *American Journal of Psychiatry*: "Do we think that the remarkable new knowledge in neurobiology…will render psychotherapy obsolete?" (Mohl et al. 1990, p. 7). In the face of new pressures, the article's authors and many others rallied for the preservation of psychotherapy practice and supervision in psychiatric training. In recognition of this need, the ACGME Residency Review Committee for Psychiatry in 2001 introduced new regulations requiring that psychiatry residency programs provide training and ensure competency in five specific psychotherapies: psychodynamic, cognitive-behavioral, supportive, brief, and combined psychotherapy–psychopharmacology (Plakun et al. 2009). A few years later, in 2007, the number of therapy modalities was reduced to three— namely, psychodynamic, cognitive-behavioral, and supportive (Plakun et al. 2009). The trend toward focus and consolidation can be seen as a re- action to the increasing theoretical diversity noted above; as psychother- apy and supervision theory became less unified and cohesive throughout the twentieth century, they became more difficult to implement in the training context, especially in the face of neurobiological hegemony in psychiatry and debates about the relative costs of psychotherapy and psy- chopharmacology. Narrowing the scope of therapy training, while limit- ing in some ways, can be seen as a necessary measure in order to solidify a tradition under duress.

Various integrative models of psychotherapy and supervision emerged in response to the need for coherence and practical efficacy; in the face of the complex differences and competition among various theoretical orien- tations, it was necessary to articulate models that could be easily standard- ized and implemented across a wide range of situations. These integrative models sought to identify the essential commonalities among different schools of psychotherapy and to use these as a conceptual starting point in order to achieve some manner of unity in diversity. One specific exam- ple is the work done by the American Psychiatric Association's Commis- sion on Psychotherapy by Psychiatrists. In 2009, members of this group designed a "Y model," which consists of a single "stem" of fundamental concepts shared by different schools of psychotherapy—setting the frame, building a therapeutic alliance, and establishing goals of treatment—that branches out into specific techniques associated with different psycho- therapeutic modalities and corresponding modes of psychotherapy super- vision (Plakun et al. 2009). Against the backdrop of the recent pressures listed above, one can see how efforts like this are essential for the survival and flourishing of therapy and its supervision in the future.

A few data points might serve to underscore the need for establishing more standardized approaches to psychotherapy supervision. A survey of residency programs in 2001 (Mellman and Beresin 2003), the same year as the ACGME consolidation mentioned above, showed that there had been a vast decrease in psychotherapy training since the 1940s; the total number of psychotherapy supervision hours over the course of a psychiatry resident's training ranged from 50 hours in some programs to 400 hours in others. These numbers present a stark contrast to the 3,000 hours of supervision that the average resident received in the years just after World War II (Mellman and Beresin 2003). In addition, regional disparities persist across the country, with some programs struggling to offer supervision in the three required psychotherapy competencies and others providing direct supervision in numerous modalities, including group therapy, couples therapy, dialectical behavioral therapy, interpersonal therapy, transference-focused psychotherapy, and mentalization-based therapy.

The Path Forward for Psychotherapy Supervision

Although much of psychotherapy supervision takes place outside of psychiatry residency programs, resident training remains an essential and large-scale venue for psychotherapist development, and its success or failure has wide-ranging effects on therapy patient outcomes and the status of psychotherapy. There exists a great need to buttress supervision theory and practices within psychiatry training programs. One difficulty has been the lack of empirically derived models for psychotherapy supervision, given that empirical evidence is the currency of medicine in general and of psychiatry in particular. In response to this need, there has been an emergence, largely since the turn of the century, of empirical studies and empirically grounded models of supervision, most notably by Milne (2009). Another glaring gap has been a dearth of professional standards for supervisors; for example, there exist numerous ways of evaluating trainees, in the form of the ACGME's milestone-based system for example, but there are currently no widely accepted professional standards for supervisors themselves.

In 2017, the Wright State University Psychiatry Program addressed this lack by creating a development program for psychotherapy supervision and studying its efficacy (Welton et al. 2019). The program's curriculum includes integrative approaches to therapy and supervision (e.g., the Y-model discussed above), introduces various supervisor assessment scales, engages learners in discussions about common issues arising in supervision, and implements various psychotherapy tools developed by the American Association of Directors of Psychiatry Residency Training (AADPRT). Of the supervisors who attended the training sessions, 86% found them to be either "very useful" or "extremely useful" (Welton et al. 2019). Efforts at grounding supervision in empirical evidence and widely applied standards are part of the recent trend toward unity and coherence. These unifying influences, along with efforts like this book, act as a bulwark against the fracturing historical forces that only a few decades ago seemed like mortal threats to psychotherapy practice and supervision in psychiatry.

Other essential measures in improving psychotherapy supervision are to recognize and rectify approaches that create and perpetuate systemic inequities, and to actively include perspectives that historically have been absent from the conversation. The history and theory of supervision have involved mainly white European and American males. In an effort to address historical imbalances and biases, the 2020 ACGME Program Requirements for Graduate Medical Education in Psychiatry emphasized multiculturalism and equity: "Residents must demonstrate a competence in forging a therapeutic alliance with patients and their families of all ages and genders, from diverse backgrounds, and from a variety of ethnic, racial, sociocultural, and economic backgrounds" (Accreditation Council for Graduate Medical Education 2020, pp. 20–21). The ability of a resident to form a therapeutic alliance with people whose backgrounds are unfamiliar depends, in turn, on the resident's developing his, her, or their own cultural self-awareness, acquiring knowledge of diverse world views, and learning culturally appropriate interventions in treatment (Hook et al. 2016). Any full-bodied theoretical model for psychotherapy supervision should, therefore, incorporate a pervasive element of self- and other-awareness regarding race, ethnicity, gender, and sexuality in the treatment alliance, and should demand of supervisors that they model this same awareness in their engagement with supervisees. This awareness can bear additional fruit beyond the therapy context by fostering training environments in which a diversity of trainees can flourish, thus furthering the mission of recruiting people from underrepresented minority groups into the field.

Conclusion

It is our hope that this brief summary of historical trends and theoretical models of psychotherapy supervision has helped the reader feel like a welcomed guest at a lively conversation that has long been under way. One can follow the references to a deeper and more comprehensive understanding of what has transpired in the exchange. By delving into the history and theory of supervision, practitioners can gain a deeper awareness of their own theoretical starting points and can evaluate and refine them with reference to the wide-ranging and profound theoretical tradition.

References

Accreditation Council for Graduate Medical Education: ACGME Program Requirements for Graduate Medical Education in Psychiatry. Chicago, IL, Accreditation Council for Graduate Medical Education, 2020. Available at: www.acgme.org/Portals/0/PFAssets/ProgramRequirements/400_Psychiatry_2020.pdf. Accessed August 28, 2021.

Blocher DH: Toward a cognitive developmental approach to counseling supervision. The Counseling Psychologist 11(1):27–34, 1983

Holloway EL: Developmental models of supervision: is it development? Professional Psychology: Research and Practice 18(3):209–216, 1987

Holloway EL: Supervisory roles within systems of practice, in The Wiley International Handbook of Clinical Supervision. Edited by Watkins CE Jr, Milne DL. Chichester, West Sussex, Wiley-Blackwell, 2014, pp 598–621

Hook JN, Watkins CE Jr, Davis DE, et al: Cultural humility in psychotherapy supervision. Am J Psychother 70(2):149–166, 2016 27329404

Loganbill C, Hardy E, Delworth U: Supervision: a conceptual model. The Counseling Psychologist 10(1):3–42, 1982

Mellman LA, Beresin E: Psychotherapy competencies: development and implementation. Acad Psychiatry 27(3):149–153, 2003 12969837

Milne DL: Evidence-Based Clinical Supervision: Principles and Practice. Chichester, West Sussex, UK, Wiley-Blackwell, 2009, pp 1–20, 29, 41

Mohl PC, Lomax J, Tasman A, et al: Psychotherapy training for the psychiatrist of the future. Am J Psychiatry 147(1):7–13, 1990 2242103

Padesky CA: Developing cognitive therapist competency: teaching and supervision models, in Frontiers of Cognitive Therapy. Edited by Salkovskis PM. London, Guilford, 1996, pp 266–292

Plakun EM, Sudak DM, Goldberg D: The Y model: an integrated, evidence-based approach to teaching psychotherapy competencies. J Psychiatr Pract 15(1):5–11, 2009 19182560

Plato: Theaetetus. Translated by Jowett B. Oxford, UK, Clarendon Press, 1892. The Internet Classics Archive. Available at: http://classics.mit.edu/Plato/theatu.html. Accessed August 30, 2021.

Stoltenberg C: Approaching supervision from a developmental perspective: the counselor complexity model. Journal of Counseling Psychology 28(1):59–65, 1981

Stoltenberg CD, Bailey KC, Cruzan CB, et al: The integrative developmental model of supervision, in The Wiley International Handbook of Clinical Supervision. Edited by Watkins CE Jr, Milne DL. Chichester, West Sussex, UK, Wiley-Blackwell, 2014, pp 576–597

Watkins CE Jr: Psychotherapy supervision since 1909: some friendly observations about its first century. Journal of Contemporary Psychotherapy 41(2):57–67, 2011

Welton R, Nelson S, Cowan A, Correll T: Supporting and training psychotherapy supervisors. Acad Psychiatry 43(4):464–465, 2019 31161573

3

The Supervisee's Experience

Katherine G. Kennedy, M.D.
Randon S. Welton, M.D.

As SUPERVISORS, we believe that we can learn a lot from listening to the experiences of supervisees. In the spring of 2021, we decided to solicit personal stories from supervisees who were currently residents or fellows or who had recently graduated from training. We used our professional contacts to solicit these vignettes, and we also posted a message on the listserv of the American Association of Directors of Psychiatric Residency Training (AADPRT). Here is the gist of our listserv post:

> We are asking for your contribution to a chapter about the supervisee's perspective on the experience of supervision. Please share a story from your experience as a supervisee. Your story may take a variety of forms: a single experience in supervision that helped, hurt, or strongly affected you; a contrast/comparison between the styles of different supervisors and what that meant for you; or simply a general overview of what the experience of supervision was like for you. Your submission should be between 150 and 250 words. In order to maintain some degree of privacy for all involved, please de-identify your supervisor(s) and your training institution as much as possible without compromising your narrative. Including relevant demographic information about yourself would be helpful.

We received many, many wonderful and touching contributions. Here we share our favorites. All vignettes have been de-identified. We gratefully acknowledge the following contributors (listed alphabetically): Priyanka Badhwar, D.O.; Jessica Chaffkin, M.D.; Vivian Chan, M.D.; Rachel Cuenot, M.D.; Flavia DeSouza, M.D., M.H.S.; Falisha Gilman, M.D.; Zachary Kelm, D.O.; Richard Krysiak, M.D.; Smita Lahoti, M.B.B.S., H.S.; Csilla Nani Lippert, M.D., Ph.D.; Danielle Patterson, M.D.; Seema Shukla, D.O., M.P.H.; George Teaford III, M.D.; Mary Vance, M.D., M.Sc.; Jason Witmer, M.D.; and Brian Wu, M.D., Ph.D.

The stories that follow are beautiful, moving, and, at times, upsetting. We are deeply grateful for the honesty, courage, and generosity of each contributor in sharing their story in order to help us all, as supervisors, become more aware and thoughtful about the privilege and the power of our supervisory work. There is much to learn.

Supervisee Vignettes

Encouraging Curiosity

When I started residency, I didn't even know what psychodynamic psychotherapy meant. My initial supervision sessions were filled with awkward silences, but over time I learned how to use these valuable hours.

Supervision encouraged me to be inquisitive about my patients' lives. I remember telling my supervisor that I wanted to ask my patient more about a topic but I felt nosy, to which she replied, "You're her therapist. It's your job to be nosy." My supervisor's prompts guided me to develop a deeper sense of self-reflection, monitor my own responses to my patients, and incorporate these into formulations.

I'm grateful for the hours my supervisor dedicated to me and my patients. Psychodynamic psychotherapy supervision is one of my most valuable residency experiences. It helped me gain confidence in myself as a therapist and has made me a better psychiatrist. I recall advocating to take on a new psychotherapy patient I had triaged, telling my supervisor that I had an urge to help her into treatment—but I wasn't sure why. With a sly smile, she looked at me and said, "because you know you have something to offer her."

Redress

As a second-year resident, I couldn't wait to meet my long-term supervisor, who I imagined would be a sort of "therapy guru." However, my excitement quickly evaporated when I heard my supposed guru's first words of wisdom: "You might want to step it up a notch in how you dress, so you feel like a doctor."

I was shocked. I asked for clarification, and she went on to say that I might want to consider wearing pearls. Despite my shock, I decided to share that I did in fact feel like a doctor in my Banana Republic slacks and royal blue blouse. I also shared my disappointment that her comment seemed to assume a certain level of self-doubt on my part and supported sexist ideas about how a woman should dress. We made it through the first session, but the scar it left was hard to ignore.

I worked with this supervisor for the next full year. I recognize now that her comments were intended to alert me to things that may affect therapy even without the patient's awareness—things like the physical space of the office or my physical appearance. While I consider that year valuable, I was never fully able to trust my supervisor during our time together. There was always a concern that maybe I wasn't reacting, dressing, or communicating in a way that was "doctor enough" for her. After a year, I transitioned to a new supervisor and have greatly benefited from having a nonjudgmental supervisory space.

The Path Unknown

My program's postgraduate year 3 (PGY3) outpatient training starts with a 2-day whirlwind of information and is a stark change from performing inpatient work. We are tasked with conducting both cognitive-behavioral therapy (CBT) and psychodynamic psychotherapy as the foundation of our learning in this new environment. We are given a supervisor for each.

The supervision was a welcome chance to spend time each week getting to know an experienced clinician in the field. Yet, it was a blind path and one full of unknowns. Where do we start? I don't have patients yet. What is psychodynamic therapy again? How can I actually make a difference in patients' lives? There is so much uncertainty as the journey begins to unfold.

As I reflect on my journey now, I am thankful to have had these opportunities. I realize that my clinical practice and style contains elements of my CBT supervisor's ability to relate to patients and make them comfortable with uncertainty (and my own uncertainty as a therapist), and also elements of my psychodynamic psychotherapy supervisor's focus on how certain defenses result in predictable outcomes. This experience has helped me to become more confident in forging forward on my own unknown path. I hope that I can continue this two-pronged journey of being both supervisee and supervisor throughout my career. Both of these roles yield invaluable lessons and experiences.

Supervising the Supervisor

My co-resident, Lily, started crying, but our shared psychotherapy supervisor, Dr. W, did not notice. I knew that Dr. W's feedback had hit Lily the same way it hit me. Lily stood up and left the room. "I think it was something I said," Dr. W muttered. "Yes," I thought, but held back from saying.

The following week, in our group supervision, Lily shared that Dr. W had asked her to debrief after hours. "After hours—really?" I nearly blurted out; instead I said, "It seems to me that it would be more helpful to process what happens in shared supervision as a group." Lily agreed.

"I was afraid of facing both of you," Dr. W said. "I needed to talk to Lily alone first."

"Supervision from last week affected me too," I said. "Now I'm struggling to sort through what it means that your needs trump our supervision needs. If you had asked me to meet after hours, I would have struggled to say no."

"I wanted to say no…," Lily said. "Dr. W, when we discuss our therapy cases, please pad your feedback instead of interrupting with an authoritative 'I would not do that!'"

"My saying 'I would not do that' does not preclude your making that choice," Dr. W stated.

"That is helpful for us to know," I added. "It would further help if you were to say, 'This is one approach you can take. Other approaches you may want to consider are…'"

"I can try," Dr. W responded. And he did. He succeeded such that therapy tears stayed with our clients in therapy instead of spilling over into supervision.

Finding the Words

In my experience, the ground traversed within psychotherapy is often murky, subtle, and seemingly ineffable for both the patient and the therapist. Intuitions, affects, and somatic sensations carry deep meaning but can pass by quickly and faintly within sessions. Supervision has given me the satisfying opportunity to more deeply explore these experiences, articulating and reifying what was initially confusing and invisible.

In my presentation of the session to my supervisor, I am able to place into words, explore, and organize my experience. This can, at times, elicit anxiety and a sense of vulnerability in myself as I share my inner world. Yet, I have found that my supervisors have consistently met me with warm reassurance. My experience has been enriched by their enlightening anecdotes and clarifications about the subtle interpersonal dance of psychotherapy. They have provided a safe and open space, containing my anxieties, uncertainties, frustrations, and discomforts as a beginning therapist.

As a result, when I next encounter my patient, I feel solidified and reoriented, equipped with a refined attunement and insight that facilitates further deepening of the therapy. To me, my supervisors have been more than just teachers or instructors; they have also been mentors. I continue to embody and expand upon their wisdom, discernment, support, and connection in both my personal life and my work as a psychotherapist.

Power Dynamics

Being an immigrant woman resident in a largely white department has been a journey of discoveries. Along the way have been mentors who have guided me through the darkest of days and supervisors who viewed themselves as my "boss."

My first supervisor at the beginning of outpatient work (Dr. X) took the job of supervising quite literally. She helped me create templates for psychotherapy by providing her own, and she would send back my notes if she found even a single spelling mistake. If I so much as thought outside the box, she would subject me to a cross-examination.

There is the good and the bad—but here comes the ugly. Dr. X told another supervisor (Ms. Q) that she believed I would not graduate. It is to

Ms. Q's credit that she apologized to me for how this communication had influenced her view of me. We have become lifelong friends, and she continues to mentor me even after our supervisory relationship ended. Fortunately, I have had many other supervisors who have mentored me in clinical and personal life. Their engagement with me and faith in my abilities have helped me grow tremendously. One supervisor even told me that I was "an attending masquerading as a resident."

Modeling Vulnerability

In one of my first sessions of supervision in my third year of psychiatric residency, my supervisor asked about my patient's sexual history. I soon realized that this was an area I needed to become more comfortable thinking and talking about. I had many questions—including just exactly what questions I should be asking.

To model how one might talk about such things, my supervisor shared one of his own early sexual experiences—finding his father's pornographic magazines at a young age. He talked about this with humor and acceptance. At times he also shared personal stories, even discussing his regret about his last exchange with a former patient who committed suicide. He felt he had fumbled awkwardly when she asked him if he liked her dress.

My supervisor's vulnerability helped create a space in which I could acknowledge my discomfort in discussing sexuality with patients and experiment with broaching the topic in more depth. When I was able to do so, I gained valuable information about my patients. I began to more fully appreciate the significance of shame in the life of my patients. Talking about sex also seemed to increase trust in the room. One patient began to open up about previously withheld details in other areas, including marital difficulties.

My supervisor's willingness to share his own experiences helped create an environment in which I could discuss discomfort in other areas as well, including feeling devalued by a patient who repeatedly canceled sessions. Discussing countertransference allowed me to learn from past mistakes and grow in my ability to address challenging situations in therapy. My supervisor's willingness to model vulnerability was key to this process.

Reading the Room

I remember my first psychotherapy supervision vividly. It was in an intensive outpatient program for personality disorders at the start of my second year of residency. I was sitting in front of my psychotherapy supervisor, Dr. S, who warmly welcomed my thoughts on my first week. I shared with him that I was pleasantly surprised at how smoothly the transition had gone. I had expected to immediately experience intense countertransference or to elicit strong transference from my new patient caseload.

As I shared with Dr. S my sessions of the week, his eyes seemed to dance as I described my session with Ms. V, a 20-year-old woman with a Cluster B personality disorder diagnosis. He asked me what I made of her calling herself antisocial, and I shared my initial impressions of how I thought she had more predominantly borderline personality traits masked by an antisocial appearance. He asked me how I felt in the room with her, and I said I quite enjoyed my time with her and found her quite forthcoming and charming. He nodded along, then calmly remarked, "Oh yes, Ms. V told me she hated you." He smiled at me as he asked me what I made of that, closely observing my jaw dropping at his declaration. "She hates me?" I was bewildered. While I felt surprise, I also found myself amused by her response to me, imagining her in a session with Dr. S, revealing her distaste for me, and rolling her eyes about me and my naiveté.

Dr. S and I spent the rest of the session talking about how, as a child, I didn't understand half of what the adults were saying to each other as I sat at the dinner table during large family gatherings; they would speak in a dialect in which I was not fluent. I would try to stay engaged through body language and respond reciprocally, waiting for my mom to translate when she could, satisfied when the body language matched the translation. I reflected back to Dr. S that I didn't feel hate in the room with Ms. V, so I couldn't feel her words landing on me and carrying substantial weight. Dr. S's translation was unexpected, but didn't feel right, which I found jarring.

In the next few months, that dissonance would reveal itself with more clarity, with Ms. V ending each session early by looking outside my office door to see if Dr. S's door was open, so that she could dash out of my room to his. I realized in my short time with Ms. V that it was not so much about her hatred of me as it was about the other side of the coin—her love for Dr. S, and the ways that she was communicating this to us. I was made to bear witness to her desire to connect with others. Dr. S's supervising me during this period also became a mutual observation between supervisee and supervisor; his supervising my relationship with Ms. V was also me contemplating his relationship with our shared patient. It took some time for me to realize how the puzzle pieces from my first supervision would fit together. I had to wait to understand.

Embracing Uncertainty

My psychotherapy supervisor sat back slowly in his chair, turning his head toward the sun-filled window. He rested his head against a half-closed hand and shifted his gaze gently upward, as if searching for an answer from above. For a moment, he looked like a statue, but as his eyes continued to welcome the beaming light rays, it began to appear that the much-anticipated answer was imminent. "I don't know," he said. He shifted in his seat and faced us directly. His lips curled softly with hints of a subtle smile, now looking armed with a more confident answer. Again, but with a more curious tone, he said, "I don't know."

Uncertainty in psychiatry, and in medicine more broadly, is often perceived as an enemy. As residents, we are trained to use protocols, lab results, and careful review of symptomatology in pursuing diagnostic clarity—and, ultimately, more precise and effective treatment. During the early days of my psychotherapy training experience, I found myself striving to apply some of these same principles to the therapeutic framework. I frequently generated hypotheses about my patients, often allowing these beliefs to drive my responses and interactions.

The scene captured in the opening vignette was an important and impactful event during my psychotherapy training. My psychotherapy supervisor conveyed to us that uncertainty is not to be shunned, but rather to be embraced, particularly in a psychotherapeutic context. In my experience, embracing uncertainty can cultivate a more curious, open-minded, empathic, and nonjudgmental experience for both the provider and the patient—one that may lead to further insight and an enhanced therapeutic alliance. As my therapy supervisor affirmed, it is okay to say "I don't know."

Finding My Feelings

One of my most memorable supervisors had an interesting way of conducting supervision. The bulk of our time together was spent reflecting not only on my interpretations but also on my emotions experienced during therapy. I distinctly recall feeling that our sessions felt more like psychodynamic therapy for myself than like a distanced intellectual analysis of my patients. This style of supervision helped me to access particularly challenging topics of countertransference.

During one session, I remember my supervisor stopping my presentation and saying, "You sound frustrated today." That simple observation helped generate a discussion about the irritation I felt toward my patient and helped me to understand how others may view my patient outside of therapy. I used to think supervision was a time to "crack the case" or generate deeper interpretations of the content discussed in therapy. After my year with my supervisor, I learned to appreciate the emotions we, as therapists, feel working with patients and how our use of that human connection can guide our patients to a better understanding of themselves.

The Good Trainee

I determined early on in my medical training that to optimize my learning and to advance, I had to be liked. Without family members in the medical field or connections to institutions of higher learning, I was not part of this coveted old boys' club. Worse, as an underrepresented minority in medicine, I could not, on the surface, pass. My supervisors did not look like me, sound like me, or share my history. How could I ensure their early and earnest investment in my education? I resolved to be the good trainee. I channeled enthusiasm, professionalism, and collegiality. I trained myself to be exquisitely attuned to my supervisors' anxieties, knowing when a shift in their gaze or a change in their tone meant I would need to maneuver myself back into their good graces.

This labor of the good trainee became psychologically challenging when BIPOC (Black, indigenous, and people of color) patients were invited to indicate their preferences for their prospective providers during the clinic's intake process. They overwhelmingly requested BIPOC providers. Clinic directors, wanting to appease patients, assumed that I had expertise with this population because of the color of my skin and the origin of my name. They facilitated patient preferences.

My supervisors, who all happened to be white, seemed totally unaware. Racial identity development, racial bias, and racial trauma were never introduced as topics during our supervision hours. I conspired with their blind spots. The result: I quietly became the clinic's dumping ground. Bombarded with a litany of patients' racial woundings, what was not desired in other providers' backyards was piled up in my mind and nonexistent in everyone else's. As a trainee, I was placed in an unenviable position—should I seek supervision about this seemingly taboo issue of how to process my patients' racialized experiences both during sessions and in the clinic at large, thereby disrupting the silence of the status quo? Or should I remain quiet and hold onto the "safe" role of the good trainee?

After a Latinx patient described depression and disconnection from the majority culture, I tried to speak. During my weekly supervision, I ventured the observation that my patient's experiences could be viewed through a racial lens. Almost immediately, my supervisor deftly introduced different material. Operating from the position of the good trainee, I colluded in this erasure of my thoughts, and my comment disappeared as though I had never spoken it. I felt struck down.

There are dynamics in which the good trainee becomes a repository for material that should not be carried alone and cannot be processed alone. The good trainee needs good supervisors—those who model a willingness to broach difficult yet crucial conversations, keep their attention on the here and now, and honor the humanity of both persons in the supervisory dyad.

Late to the Game

Seven months into my third year of psychiatry training, I finally confronted my dissatisfaction with my CBT supervisor, Dr. D. Until then, my feelings had been communicated by actions: arriving late, canceling sessions, failing to complete worksheets. It started innocently at first, with my miscalculating the time required to commute to her office. After I explained this, we easily rescheduled our weekly meeting time. After a month, however, my lateness resurfaced. How else might I convey my discomfort with and dread of our meetings: "I detest your teaching style. Your rigidity reminds me of grade school."

Months later, I again requested to reschedule a session—another sign of my resistance. Dr. D refused. If her supervision was important enough, then I would make it work. "And anyway," she added dryly, "I don't have any other availability." She intuited my undervaluing of our time. She printed out two copies of pages with definitions of CBT terminology and read them aloud to me as if I spoke a different language. I made no objection, remembering what my immigrant parents taught me—there is something to learn from every situation. I had yet to learn how to name my discomfort to authoritarian figures.

The catalyst for change came when Dr. D threatened to report me for poor compliance with supervision. I immediately reported myself and told program leadership about the issues between Dr. D and me. It turned out that supervisors aren't supposed to feel authoritarian. I wish I had sought guidance sooner, and had found language for my discomfort rather than acting it out. I was assigned a different supervisor, and thereafter, I was never late again.

A Misstep

Compared with the rest of training, my third year of psychiatric residency followed a predictable routine, and psychotherapy supervision with Dr. M was no exception. Hop from the morning outpatient clinic to the afternoon outpatient clinic, park behind the building, cut through the grass, circle around to the main door, and text Dr. M ("Hi, I'm just out front"), at which point Dr. M would promptly open his door and we would begin our session. But on one snowy February afternoon, instead of cutting through the grass, I took the sidewalk to avoid trudging through the muddy snow. As if the one divergence wasn't clue enough, Dr. M never opened the door that day.

Later that week, Dr. M texted me that he had taken the day off and had forgotten to tell me. At our next meeting, he presented me with a book called *Why Good People Do Bad Things*. Lightheartedly, he explained that the book was a gift that would help me to understand why he makes mistakes. We both chuckled and settled back into our old routine—except for one thing. In that moment, I truly understood the purpose of supervision—"this isn't a place to get scrutinized or shamed, this is a place *to share*." As a supervisor, he created a safe environment in which everyone was human and could explore their shadows. This was the true gift, a reminder to me that we are here to learn by sharing and making mistakes. So thank you, Dr. M, for showing me how to embrace myself as a physician more fully, mistakes and all.

Being Seen

Midway through my final year of residency, before I realized how overcommitted I was, I found myself rescheduling or canceling appointments with patients and supervisors more frequently than I used to, in an effort to balance multiple demands on my time. After a few weeks of this, my supervisor quipped, "I've been missing you! We haven't been meeting as often as we used to."

The comment gave me pause. I reflected and began explaining back to her that yes, in fact, things had been very hectic for me recently. "I didn't think anyone noticed," I added.

She replied, kindly, "Some of us want to believe that people don't notice it when we're missing. But people do notice. And if I'm feeling this way, I wonder if your patients are too."

It was then that I began to understand my magical thinking around "time management": that somehow, quality can make up for an extreme lack of quantity; that I could just disappear and fly under the radar; that I wasn't important enough for my absence to be noted.

Shortly thereafter, I backed out of the project that was causing me to be overcommitted. And since then, that lesson—"you are noticed"—has stuck with me and benefited both my personal and my professional life.

Limitations of Supervisors

As I near the end of my training to become a psychiatrist, I often reflect on each unique component of education in this long journey. My psychotherapy supervision experience remains the one I continue to have the most ambivalent feelings about.

Every year during my residency and fellowship training, I was paired with a different clinician, each with a different set of skills and educational background. In retrospect, I see their diverse backgrounds and areas of expertise as an asset in my training, giving me a wide range of therapeutic tools to use. I also always enjoyed the analysis of each case, and how my supervisors' perspectives often led to case conceptualizations I would not have come up with on my own.

However, while going through the experience, I was frequently frustrated by some of its limitations. Take the narrow scope of expertise my supervisors often had. On many occasions, my supervisor was not experienced in the psychopathology of the patient I was seeing or had limited knowledge of the modalities I was interested in employing. As a result, I was forced to rely on self-teaching, often via several-hours-long YouTube searches, to prepare for sessions with patients. I was also bothered by the fact that my supervisors never actually witnessed my therapy sessions with patients. This often led me to wonder "Am I really doing this right?" However, overall, my time in psychotherapy supervision was enriching, and I am grateful to have had the opportunity to take part in this experience.

In Translation

Psychotherapy supervision has been a crucial component of my psychiatry training, a field of inexact science. It was useful to have multiple psychotherapy supervisors over the course of my training, thus allowing me to compare styles and methodologies when constructing patient formulations.

One supervisor in particular encouraged me to bring to my supervision meetings transcriptions of my sessions with a challenging patient. At each supervision, he listened to what I had said and offered alternatives. He suggested that I was "working too hard" in my responses to patients, and he floated the idea that "as psychotherapists, we are not problem solvers." Instead, he said, "we are translators." We give language to what is acted out, to the unnamed subtexts. My patient persistently missed our weekly therapy sessions, and when I called her, she would apologize sincerely for forgetting to let me know that something had come up. I shared my irritation with my supervisor. In response, he challenged me to contemplate who I might be representing to this patient that might cause her to not show up for sessions. I was able to imagine myself as my patient's abusive mother and father, who had emigrated from Jamaica when she was 5 years old and left her behind in the care of her aunt. For my patient, no-showing seemed to be a defense mechanism to reaffirm her agency.

At the next appointment, I gently confronted my patient about what it meant to her to not show up. A few weeks later, she missed an appointment; however, this time she left me a voicemail.

Becoming a Supervisor

The experience of supervision has been especially interesting because of my new roles this year. I've transitioned from being a fellow to being an attending psychiatrist. I'm now leading the psychodynamic psychiatry course for our psychiatry residency, where I teach theory and supervise psychotherapy cases. At the same time, I'm completing my own 2-year training in advanced psychodynamic psychotherapy. Also within this year, I have started my own psychotherapy.

Many times I've had the thought, "How can I be an effective teacher while I am still so early in my training?" Supervision is where I tend to experience all of these new roles at once. This collision is most salient when my supervisor is telling me things that I have just told my residents in supervision or in class a few days ago. I find myself thinking "Why can't I practice what I preach?" Then I find myself remembering how I tell my residents that this is the purpose of supervision. With practice, we can more quickly recognize certain dynamics and intervene. Because of their experience and more objective position, supervisors can almost always recognize these dynamics more rapidly than we can.

Just this week, during my own supervision, as I again was hearing words that I had recently told others, I was able to pause for a moment and recognize my own growth this year as a therapist, patient, teacher, supervisor, and supervisee.

Coda From the Editors

As you read the rest of the chapters in this book, we encourage you to keep these stories in mind. We hope these stories will help to center you on your supervisees' feelings and needs, and remind you of how vulnerable our supervisees are at every stage of supervision.

We also hope these stories help you to reflect on your own experience as a supervisee. Can you recall your first supervisory encounter? Was there a supervisory session that left a lasting mark on you? Who was your favorite supervisor? Did you have a supervisor who challenged you? Which supervisor most influenced your own supervisory style?

We hope these stories prompted questions like these, and more, and that the answers you discover will serve to deepen your own supervisory work.

4

The Supervisor–
Supervisee Relationship

Katherine G. Kennedy, M.D.
Randon S. Welton, M.D.
David A. Adler, M.D.

KEY LEARNING GOALS

- Recognize that a positive supervisor–supervisee relationship is necessary for the work of supervision.
- Describe the essential components of the supervisory relationship.
- Understand that trust is fundamental to a healthy supervisory alliance.
- Discuss how to maintain a healthy supervisory relationship over time.

THE SUPERVISORY relationship is a complex of personal and professional identities that interact and change over time. Foundational for all supervisory work, the supervisory alliance is a crucial aspect of supervision (Wilson et al. 2016). This relationship also may play a critical role toward developing the supervisee's identity as a psychiatrist and psychotherapist.

Each supervisory dyad constructs its own unique relationship, but its success is based on a mutual sense of trust and safety. The asymmetrical power dynamic contributes challenges to the intensely collaborative nature of this alliance and requires ongoing consideration. In this chapter we discuss the importance of the alliance; the multidimensionality of the supervisory relationship; practices that help build mutual trust, including how to manage the unequal supervisory power dynamic; and the evolution of the supervisory relationship over time.

Fostering a Positive Supervisory Relationship

> *Our worst fault is our preoccupation with the faults of others.*
>
> Kahlil Gibran

The quality of the supervisory relationship can foster or deter supervisee learning and growth (Karpenko and Gidycz 2012). Especially for psychiatric trainees learning to conduct outpatient psychotherapy, supervision may do more to foster their identity as a psychotherapist than actually doing psychotherapy (Geller et al. 2010). Historically, an overemphasis on the didactic and instructional function of supervision, and the conceptualization of supervision as an apprenticeship (e.g., "see one, do one") neglected the supervisory relationship as a key growth factor for professional identity (Watkins 2011a, 2011b). Supervisors do more than monitor and provide feedback on the direction and content of treatment; they also function as experienced mentors, sharing their meta-perspectives on the purpose of treatment and theories of change (Wilson and Sperber 2012).

Supervision provides an opportunity for supervisors to model an approach to listening, observing, thinking, judging, and speaking with patients. Supervisees can identify with the internalized representations of the roles, qualities, and abilities that they ascribe to their supervisors. Trainees have reported how enduring and emotionally charged communications between supervisors and supervisees have played a significant role in shaping their work with patients (Geller et al. 2010). Supervisors who are perceived as judgmental, ignore the personal or developmental needs of the supervisee, mishandle conflict, or provide ineffective feedback weaken the supervisory alliance (Karpenko and Gidycz 2012). A negative supervisory relationship may constrain supervisees' confidence, affective range, and openness to their patients' experiences and ideas.

A positive supervisory experience helps supervisees to be more reflective, receptive, creative, and tolerant of ambiguity. One gauge of the success of a supervisory relationship is whether supervisees feel safe enough to try out new skills, communicate their feelings and ideas to their supervisors, and reflect on potential clinical mistakes. From the supervisor's vantage point, it is essential that trainees feel secure enough to bring in their perspectives and question the supervisor's views.

The Power Differential in the Supervisory Relationship

Many factors contribute to the asymmetrical power dynamic in the supervisory relationship. A major factor is the context in which supervision is conducted, which may determine many aspects of the supervisory relationship's frame, boundaries, and duration, including the specifics around the role of the supervisor as evaluator. For example, supervision may be a requirement of training, or a benefit offered to a postgraduate early-career psychiatrist. It may be conducted by peers or more senior faculty. Supervision may be offered at market, reduced, or zero financial cost to supervisees. The supervisor may also be the attending of record and bear clinical responsibility for the supervisee's panel of patients or may have no direct responsibility for their care. These settings and their contingencies help shape the hierarchy of the supervisory power dynamic.

The most common supervisory relationship involves a trainee who is in a psychiatric residency, fellowship, or psychoanalytic training program. Within a training program, the expectations and rules surrounding the relationship between the supervisor and the trainee are defined by outside agencies such as the Accreditation Council for Graduate Medical Education. Often, these relationships are highly structured and are usually based around the academic year. Trainees often have little say in who becomes their supervisor. Additionally, supervisees early in training might be functioning under a supervisor's license, a circumstance that might increase the scrutiny and control exerted by the supervisor.

When a supervisor provides a formal evaluation of a supervisee to a training program, the quality of the evaluation may significantly affect a trainee's future career. Supervisors should understand that the hierarchical nature of the supervisory relationship may contribute to supervisees' distortions or inaccurate depictions of the therapy they are providing (Coburn 1997). For example, trainees may intentionally minimize or omit aspects of therapeutic encounters out of concern that certain details may reflect negatively on them in an evaluation, or they may exaggerate or fabricate episodes in therapy to present their work in a more positive light.

Differences in social identity may also affect the power dynamic. Race, gender identity, sexual orientation, ability/disability, socioeconomic status, culture/ethnicity, religion, academic degree, and the ways in which these identities intersect, together with their perceived social value, can affect the power differential. For example, in some settings, the social value of an educational degree, such as M.D., Ph.D., or M.S.W., may be hierarchically organized, and which educational degree a member of the supervisory dyad holds may increase or lessen some measure of privilege or power.

Finally, perhaps the largest contributor to the asymmetrical power dynamic, regardless of the setting, is enfolded in the primary task of supervision: supervisees are expected to expose the specifics of their clinical work, especially their feelings, challenges, and missteps, for the purpose of focused critique and comment. In undertaking this difficult task, supervisees take far greater personal risks than do supervisors, who, although they may communicate their own feelings and associations, are far less vulnerable to feeling shamed and/or criticized than are supervisees.

The Complex Nature of the Supervisory Relationship

Within a therapeutic relationship, therapist and patient interact along multiple planes. These encompass the working alliance, the real relationship, and the unconscious relationship, which includes the dynamics of transference and countertransference. The supervisory relationship mirrors this tripartite composition. How these three components emerge, engage together, and develop throughout the relationship will determine the quality and outcomes of the supervisory experience.

The Working (Therapeutic) Alliance

The *working alliance* between a patient and a therapist, also called the *therapeutic alliance*, has been defined as a combination of 1) an emotional bond involving trust and mutual respect, 2) collaboratively chosen goals, and 3) mutually agreed-upon expectations about tasks, roles, and boundaries (Bordin 1983). Other vital components of this alliance are its interactive nature and the shared belief that the patient can benefit from the therapeutic process.

A successful supervisory working alliance has the same elements as any working alliance (Bordin 1983; Karpenko and Gidycz 2012). Ideally, over time, a positive emotional bond forms between the supervisor and the supervisee. This affective connection can be facilitated when each member of the dyad demonstrates trustworthiness, expresses empathy, and offers understanding, acceptance, and validation to the other. Perceptions by either party of being judged, criticized, or dismissed—even unintentionally—by the other may impair or fracture this bond. Additionally, the dyad will want to acknowledge that each can safely disagree with the other. Finally, while an intentional effort to establish a positive working alliance must be mutually made by both parties, the greater burden rests with the supervisor, given the asymmetrical power dynamic.

Although the supervisor and the supervisee may have different expectations about the form and the content of the supervision, ideally they will work together to identify collaboratively determined goals. Such work contributes to an intentional examination of the range of tasks, roles, and boundaries involved in the supervisory process. For example, should the supervision session focus on one or a few cases at length each week, or should it touch briefly on all of the patients being seen by the supervisee? Can the supervisor ask about the supervisee's personal life, and vice versa? What proportion of the supervision session should be spent on clinical material versus theoretical discussions of psychodynamic concepts? If the supervisor and the supervisee answer these questions differently, it is crucial that time and effort be spent on exploring, understanding, and clarifying differences and working to reach mutually agreed-upon alignments (see Chapter 8, "Setting Goals for Psychotherapy Supervision").

The Real Relationship

The *real relationship* is the personal relationship that is experienced and perceived by two people. It is considered the cornerstone of communication between supervisor and supervisee, as it is between clinician and patient. Historically often overlooked or neglected, the real relationship exists as the social interaction between two people, who potentially have very different backgrounds and experiences, who are endeavoring to communicate with and be understood by each other in order to work toward common goals. The real relationship involves the interplay of personalities, cultural backgrounds, and social identities, including race, gender identity and expression, sexual orientation, religion, ability/disability, and other social characteristics, and the ways these qualities intersect and influence each other. The relationship is further modulated by each participant's attachment, engagement, and communication styles. Because the real relationship involves the thoughts, affects, biases, and behaviors of two people who share a space together, both participants will need to discover ways to work with one another toward an honest, safe, and authentic style of relating, while simultaneously respecting each other's personal boundaries (Watkins 2011a).

This paradoxical tension—of being open yet constrained by boundaries—can be challenging. How personal can questions be? How much of one's social identity can be revealed? How can personal information be shared in a professional manner? How can each person express curiosity about the other and yet not cross an invisible, unidentified line? What may seem like "fair game" for one person may cause discomfort, or even harm, for the other. For example, a supervisor may offer personal information without assessing the comfort level of the supervisee. A supervisor may inquire about a supervisee's life, unaware that (for example) the supervisee is a refugee who fled an authoritarian dictatorship, who may find it too painful to share details about her harrowing childhood, particularly at the outset of a new supervisory relationship.

Negotiating the real relationship requires tact, courage, humility, and time. Ideally, the supervisor and the supervisee will discuss the specific ways they feel comfortable sharing information about themselves, how they will question each other, and how they will handle the inevitable misunderstandings and mishaps that occur in all relationships. The supervisor is encouraged to maintain a respectful, open, curious, and humble stance toward the supervisee's cultural background, social identity, and personal experiences. Making assumptions based on a trainee's name, attire, hairstyle, accent, demeanor, or any other characteristics may cause confusion and misunderstanding. For example, making an assumption about gender identity based on an individual's appearance should be avoided. Supervisors should be open to sharing their own social identities to help trainees understand more about themselves and their backgrounds, while paying close attention to supervisees' responses and taking care to not overshare. When offering this kind of information, supervisors can make it clear that they do not expect supervisees to reciprocate with similar material unless they feel comfortable doing so. When differences are identified, supervisors need to pay close attention to supervisees' reactions. If any level of supervisee discomfort is detected, supervisors will want to acknowledge and inquire about this. If a supervisee seems upset or withdraws, offering an apology may help. Supervisors should monitor the pace of self-disclosure: what might feel too quick for one supervisee might feel agonizingly slow for another. No hard-and-fast rules for self-disclosure exist. Each dyad will need to discover for themselves what works for them, and what does not.

Supervisors need to understand that exploration of one another's social identities may feel unfamiliar, uncomfortable, or unnecessary to some supervisees. By the same token, some supervisors, especially those who have never engaged in this type of inquiry, will find the notion of discussing social identity to be strange or "boundary violating." Some supervisors may believe that it is not part of their job to be self-revealing and may feel bewildered or upset that reciprocal self-disclosure is an expectation of the supervisory process. For some, avoiding such sharing may feel easier than engaging in it. However, many of today's supervisees trend toward expressing greater openness and social diversity, so it is increasingly important that supervisors be able to foster open, inquisitive, and authentic dialogues with supervisees about various aspects of each other's social identities.

Supervisors can explore their differences simply and directly. For example, a supervisor might say, "We have different cultural backgrounds. How do you see that influencing our supervisory relationship?" (Hook et al. 2016). This approach also models for supervisees how to approach exploration of differences with patients (Wilson et al. 2016). The supervisory relationship provides an opportunity to consider going beyond merely identifying their cultural and social identities. It can help supervisees to recognize how their own social identities and personal experiences function as the lens through which clinical material is viewed and understood. It may also be useful to remind supervisees that despite their importance as sources of self-knowledge, personal identities and lived experiences may potentially contribute to a disregard for or distortion of data. Supervisors may want to point out how their own "social lens" contains potential biases and blind spots.

Another aspect of the real relationship involves monitoring the level of engagement both participants bring to supervision. Engagement, enthusiasm, and focus can be adversely affected by exhaustion experienced by either the supervisor or the supervisee (see Chapter 25, "Addressing Exhaustion and Burnout in Psychotherapy Supervision").

The Unconscious Relationship

Of the three planes of the supervisory relationship, the *unconscious relationship* is the least well characterized in the literature, but our psychodynamic understanding of the mind strongly suggests the existence of an unconscious aspect to this pivotal relationship. In therapy, *transference* involves the patient's unconscious feelings and thoughts directed toward the therapist. Although *countertransference* has been defined in different ways, it basically encompasses the therapist's own unconscious emotional and cognitive responses to the patient. Similarly, unconscious reactions occur in both directions in supervision. The supervisory relationship can be an intimate one in which both the supervisor and the supervisee are expected to disclose the workings of their mind and share their emotional responses to patients. It can be difficult to create and maintain such intimacy in a dyad in which one member will ultimately be responsible for evaluating the performance of the other. Previous complications in relationships can adversely affect supervision when compliance, inhibition, mistrust, fear, or interpersonal sensitivity are central aspects of a trainee's personality (Baudry 1993). Both the supervisor's and the supervisee's pre-existing biases and interpersonal relationship patterns can affect supervision. Supervisors may be perceived as authority figures who must be deferred to, misled, or resisted, or they may be viewed as a nurturing parent, a bumbling uncle, or a cold-hearted stepmother. The supervisor may regard a supervisee in a maternal or paternal way. These perceived role expectations might be met, gratified, or frustrated within the supervisory dyad. Just as in the therapist–patient dyad, these factors are independent but mutually interactive.

Historically, a supervisor's emotional response toward a supervisee was considered to be either incidental or an impediment to the work of supervision. However, today, supervisors are encouraged to pay careful attention to their own emotional responses toward supervisees and the process material, as this additional focus can yield enriching and helpful insights. These responses may initially be outside the awareness of the supervisor, but paying close attention to associations and feelings can lead to a deepening of the supervisory relationship. Supervisors can also model for supervisees how to use countertransference as a tool in therapy (Kay 2015).

Trust and Trustworthiness in the Supervisory Relationship

It is essential to address the importance of mutual trust as a critical aspect of the therapeutic alliance (Nelson et al. 2008). When a trusting supervisory relationship is fostered, the difficult, and perhaps painful, work of supervision can proceed effectively. Supervisors may overestimate a supervisee's level of trust or may fail to demonstrate trustworthiness themselves. Without a foundation of trust, the supervisory alliance risks compromise and may falter when stressed.

An alliance built on trust requires both members of the supervisory dyad to manifest 1) *trustworthiness* and 2) *the capacity to trust*. Elements of trustworthiness include being seen as competent and demonstrating that one is dependable. The capacity to trust develops over a lifetime of experience with relationships and varies according to an individual's biology (nature) and experiences (nurture). This capacity may be understood as encompassing three levels (Wilson and Sperber 2012). The first level, *basic trust*, is rooted in our biological makeup and our feelings, when in relationship, and evolves from our earliest relationship experiences, laying the groundwork for our attachment style. The second level, *epistemic trust*, develops from our experiences with multiple relationships. This type of trust involves an individual's willingness to consider new knowledge as trustworthy and relevant to their life. Epistemic trust depends on acceptance of the authenticity of interpersonally transmitted information and an openness to believing the new information to be credible and personally useful (Wilson and Sperber 2012). The third level type of trust, *societal trust*, is the belief that the actions of others in society are, in general, honest, principled, and reliable. An absence or lack of any form of trust is termed *mistrust*, whereas an individual may develop *distrust* after a harm has occurred.

Although an intentional effort to establish trust in the supervisory dyad must be mutually made by both participants, the onus is on the supervisor, who holds more power in the dyad. It is reasonable for supervisors to expect that all new supervisees will enter the office with some level of mistrust. This mistrust may stem from the asymmetrical power dynamic and/or from perceived differences in social identities, attachment styles, and culturally influenced communication styles. There is no one right way to foster trust within the dyad; however, we offer a few general principles for earning a supervisee's trust:

- *Strive to be reliable.* Show up on time; don't cancel supervisory sessions at the last minute; don't be distracted by devices; be available for emergencies.
- *Practice humility.* Say "I don't know"; apologize when you make an error; be respectful.
- *Foster a culture of openness and personal revelation* while respecting personal boundaries. Offer personal musings; speak about your own feelings and responses; find words to convey your nuanced and complex thoughts. Be open, transparent, and authentic.
- *Model integrity* by protecting confidentiality, honoring privacy, being honest, and respecting personal boundaries.
- *Validate the supervisee.* Be present and listen attentively. Strive to be accepting and nonjudgmental, especially about the supervisee's physical presentation and communication style. Model empathy.
- *Demonstrate clinical competence.* Are you knowledgeable about psychotherapeutic theories and approaches? Is what you say helpful? Do your suggestions work?

As with any effort, there is always the risk of going too far, of being rigidly constrained by guidelines, or of acting in the service of an ideal at the expense of a relationship. Table 4–1 provides examples of ways to earn trust, as well as some of the unintended consequences of overuse of these approaches.

Trust in the supervisory relationship, as in all relationships, goes both ways. At the most basic level, both participants will want to agree that discussions throughout the course of the relationship will be kept confidential (except as required to complete the evaluation of the trainee). Each will be given the benefit of the doubt when concerns arise. Supervisors want to be able to assume that trainees are being honest, describing clinical material to the best of their ability, refraining from intentionally distorting or omitting clinical material, and sharing when they feel hurt, upset, or angry—either with the cases they are discussing or with the supervisor. In a safe supervisory environment, the supervisor provides a balance of support and constructive feedback, and the supervisee is able to accept suggestions and experience growth (Karpenko and Gidycz 2012).

How do supervisors "know" that an environment of trust has been established in the supervision? Supervisors may note that supervisees seem increasingly able to express emotions, acknowledge missteps, explore biases, offer jokes, and even critique their supervisors. Supervisors may also find that supervisees are sharing a broader range of material from clinical encounters, including feelings, thoughts, musings, mistakes, and questions.

The Supervisory Relationship Over Time

> People change and forget to tell each other.
>
> Lillian Hellman

Like all relationships, the supervisor–supervisee relationship evolves over time. While each supervisory relationship has its own unique trajectory, certain characteristic changes and stages typically unfold. Intentional efforts to develop and maintain trust and trustworthiness are key to preserving an ongoing relationship. When supervisors are stymied over how to proceed in a situation, using an approach of open and empathic inquiry will often work. One supervisory goal might be to maintain enough openness in the supervisory space for either member to feel free enough to offer "what comes to mind."

Beginning Supervision

Unless there is a previously established relationship, naming and understanding the real relationship will be an important focus when starting supervision. Differences in training, experience, expectations, and social

Table 4–1. Ways of earning trust and unintended consequences of overuse

Ways of earning trust	Example	Unintended consequence of overuse
Be reliable; be able to be "counted upon"	Set a regular day and time for supervision	Overly rigid adherence to a set supervisory time
Be humble	Acknowledge your own failings and mistakes	Excessive apologizing may lead supervisees to feel burdened to reassure or take care of you
Be honest, transparent, and open	Share your ideas, musings, impressions	Unfettered openness on the part of supervisors may lead to inadvertent commission of microaggressions
Be tactful and respectful of boundaries	Explore a supervisee's affect only in the context of the treatment of the patient (e.g., don't pry or be intrusive)	Supervisees may feel that supervisors are withholding or uninterested in how their life experiences intersect with their clinical work
Communicate empathy	Validate the feelings and experiences of supervisees	Supervisors may fail to address potential unprofessional behavior on the part of supervisees; supervisees may feel intruded upon by excessive concern
Demonstrate clinical competence; be a credible clinician	The supervisor's clinical judgment is validated (e.g., when the supervisor says something may happen, it actually happens)	Supervisors may overdirect the treatment and leave no room for supervisees to offer input
Validate the life experiences of supervisees and what they bring to the clinical encounter	Make positive, affirming remarks to show that you "see" or "recognize" supervisees for who they are and value their perspectives on the clinical material	Overfocus on the needs of supervisees may lead supervisors to neglect adequate review of the clinical material
Be an active, engaged listener	Attend closely and respond to supervisees' presentations	Supervisees may have difficulty tolerating times when supervisors are perceived as too quiet

identities will need to be shared and examined as the two individuals learn about each other. Given the inherent power differential in the dyad, supervisors should take the lead in introducing themselves, describing their social identity, summarizing their professional background, and discussing their approach to psychotherapy. In turn, supervisors will want to learn about their supervisees' social identity (to the level that they are comfortable sharing), academic background, experience as a clinician, interests in various approaches to psychotherapy, and previous experiences in supervision (both good and bad). Each will learn about how the other communicates and expresses themself and will get to know the other's manner and personal style, sense of humor, and ability to focus on the content at hand. At the beginning of supervision, supervisors should provide education regarding their view of the interpersonal nature of supervision (similar to a therapist educating a patient about the therapeutic process) and should encourage feedback from supervisees. Supervisors will want to lead discussions about their approach to supervision and be attentive for feedback about concerns or suggestions for potential changes. Supervisors' openness to feedback will be a model for supervisees (Karpenko and Gidycz 2012).

Beginning the supervisory conversation with humor and openness can help to foster a safe supervisory environment.

> At the initial meeting between a supervisor and a supervisee, the supervisor welcomes the supervisee and begins the conversation with "I'm a PGY48." This disclosure draws a broad smile from the supervisee, whose shoulders visibly relax.

Such preliminary exchanges set the stage for forging the supervisory working alliance. Displaying an interest in the supervisee and providing a welcoming environment will help create a warm emotional bond. This is also a time to elicit what the supervisee would like to learn over the course of supervision. (See Chapter 8 for a more detailed discussion of setting goals for supervision.) To make the best use of this time, the supervisor should lead the supervisee in a discussion of the boundaries and expectations of supervision. Topics should include the following:

- Where and how often will the supervisor and supervisee meet? If via an online platform, who will send the invitation?
- How long will each supervision session last (30 minutes, 45 minutes, 60 minutes)?
- What will be the process of and approach to supervision?
- How many patients will the dyad discuss during each supervisory session?

- Will the supervisee be reviewing the entire course of a specific patient's therapy or focusing on a single therapy session?
- Is the supervisee expected to bring audio or visual recordings or process notes to each supervisory session?
- Is the supervisee expected to bring to each session a specific question to be discussed?
- How active will the supervisor be in offering direction for the supervisee's clinical work? For example, will the supervisor role-play potential supervisee–patient interchanges?
- How much can the supervisor ask about the supervisee's personal life?
- How much will the supervisor be available to the supervisee between supervisory sessions, and what is the best way for the supervisee to contact the supervisor (e.g., phone, text, email)? If there is an urgent need, is this contact method still the best way?
- What are the supervisor's obligations in regard to medical record documentation (e.g., signing progress notes, reviewing patient charts)?

These topics will help establish the boundaries of supervision and also clarify the roles and expectations of each participant, strengthening the supervisory working alliance. As is true in all of our relationships, the unconscious aspects of the early supervisory relationship will likely stem from previous relationships. At this early stage, overtly focusing on structure and mutually acceptable collaboration, while also acknowledging that other feelings may be engendered, helps in the "getting to know you" process.

> At the first supervisory session with a second-year resident, the supervisor shared details about her personal life, including that she had a daughter who was 26 years old. The supervisee said with a smile, "I am 27 years old. I wonder if there may be times that you will treat me like a daughter in our supervision." The supervisor laughed and said, "What a wonderful observation! Let's be on the lookout for that, and also for any other relationships that we may unconsciously displace on each other."

The beginning phase may last several weeks, or even months, before the supervisor and the supervisee find their way to mutually agreed-upon goals, routines, and practices and understand what to expect from each other, so that each can speak and comprehend what the other is trying to say. There will inevitably be confusion and misunderstandings, but if they can be discussed openly and honestly, without fear of repercussions, the supervisory relationship can lead to growth. Supervisors can help strengthen this relationship by focusing on nonjudgmental acceptance of supervisees and their efforts. Modeling by supervisors helps supervisees learn how to calm themselves and also how to tolerate the intensity of the emotions they experience both in their clinical work and in supervision. A study examining resident supervisees' perspectives found that residents were most likely to rate their supervision as excellent when there was a trusting relationship that allowed them to present their problems in a nondefensive manner (Shanfield et al. 2001). As the supervisor increasingly learns to listen in an accepting, nonjudgmental fashion, the bond with the supervisee should strengthen.

It is inevitable that the supervisory dyad will have highs and lows, successes and perceived failures. The supervisor and the supervisee may go through times when one or the other seems distracted or uninvolved. These are potentially growth experiences and can foster the development of an even stronger dyadic bond. As trust grows, the supervisor will gradually introduce more challenging and conflictual material. Ideally, the supervisory space should provide opportunities to reflect on misunderstandings and mistakes, on both sides of the dyad, as well as to discuss difficult issues with openness and thoughtfulness.

Middle Phase of Supervision

Just as it is in therapy, the middle phase of supervision is often the period in which most of the progress is made toward meeting mutually acceptable goals. Supervisees are given opportunities to explore, practice, and demonstrate the competencies selected as their goals. Supervisors should intentionally and overtly monitor progress toward those goals. As original goals are mastered, new goals can be formulated around the circumstances of the treatment the supervisee is providing. For early goals, the supervisor may take a more active role in directing the supervisee's clinical work. The novice therapist may desire a step-by-step guide to providing treatment, including therapy. In time, however, most trainees will take a more active role in directing the course of their own clinical work and will become increasingly assertive and self-activated. Supervisors can then step back and encourage greater autonomy in supervisees. As trainees develop their own style as clinicians and therapists, supervisors may alternate between more actively trying to direct treatment and stepping back to observe and comment on the work. Ideally, as a trainee's clinical skill increases, the supervisor and the trainee will find themselves interacting as "co-clinicians," with each valuing the other for their knowledge and experience (Brown et al. 2020).

As the relationship matures, supervisors may introduce a number of new techniques, including modeling for supervisees how the use of fantasy and imagery can open up the therapist's mind to new perspectives in their work with patients. For example, sharing personal associations and daydreams and using words such as "wish," "imagine," and "fear" can foster acquisition of these new skills. Table 4–2 provides suggestions for ways that supervisors can help supervisees to more deeply access their own internal life and—by extension—the internal life of their patients.

The middle of supervision can also be a time of competing demands as well as a more open exchange on differences in expectations, goals, and approaches. Acknowledging and managing the competing tensions becomes critical. Awareness of the reality of the evaluation component of supervision and concerns about productivity and documentation are inherent in the supervisory process. In a formal training environment such as a psychiatric residency, evaluation is part of the supervisory experience. How does the supervisor balance the responsibilities of the evaluation process with other needs of the supervisory relationship (e.g., education, support)? Supervisors can model humility, transparency, and openness to feedback from supervisees, but they need to be aware of and avoid the potential pitfalls of extremes (e.g., being hypercritical of vs. trying to be "pals" with supervisees). Issues related to differences in, and assumptions about, social identities may also arise. Disagreements about goals and expectations may surface. Far from being a sign of failure, the presence of such conflicts reveals the empowerment of supervisees to express themselves more freely. As long as supervision is experienced as a "safe-enough" environment, working through these conflicts can lead to growth for both supervisor and supervisee and can foster a more collaborative environment equipped to address whatever issues may arise (Nelson et al. 2008).

Supervisors should be alert for signs of *parallel process*, defined as a state in which the dynamics of the supervisory relationship are mirroring some aspects of the dynamics of the therapeutic relationship (McNeill and Worthen 1989). This phenomenon arises when a supervisee unconsciously brings elements of the therapeutic relationship into the transference–countertransference dynamic of the supervisory relationship. On both the supervisor's and the supervisee's part, these dynamics may reflect elements that have gone unrecognized in their own lives or in the therapeutic work. When the supervisory dyad is able to recognize these elements as enactments of processes playing out in therapy, there are benefits for both the work of therapy and the work of supervision.

Termination of Supervision

As their time together is coming to an end (just as in therapy), supervisors and supervisees will need to plan for how to say good-bye. It can be

Table 4–2.   Modeling in supervision how to access the internal life
                   of patients

Supervisor's stance	Thoughts	Feelings	Fantasies
Maintain openness in the supervisory dialogue	Ask "What comes to mind?"	Ask "How does this make you feel?"	Ask "What do you imagine?" or "What images come to mind?"
Foster safety in the supervisory space	Be curious about the supervisee's associations	Validate the supervisee's feelings	Encourage the supervisee to share
Make connections to clinical material	Provide theoretical explanations for clinical material	Ask "How do your emotional responses echo the patient's expressed feelings?"	Model ways to "play" with clinical material (e.g., by story-telling, sharing of reveries)

growth promoting to discuss what they have been through along the supervisory experience and journey, including which goals and expectations have been fulfilled and what potentially lies ahead as supervisees continue their training. Supervisees will benefit from truthful, specific feedback that is immediately and directly useful. As the supervisory working alliance enters this ending phase, new issues may become more prominent. Continuation of a real relationship between supervisor and supervisee may be possible but is not mandatory. For both members of the dyad, unconscious aspects of supervision may arise. How previous significant relationships have ended may affect how the supervisor and the supervisee terminate this relationship. As in any meaningful long-term relationship, discussion of the termination of supervision should begin long before it is time to terminate (see also Chapter 12, "Termination of Psychotherapy Supervision").

Conclusion

As humans, we learn about relationships through our relationships with others. The supervisory relationship has components analogous to the therapeutic relationship. Negotiating and navigating the supervisory relationship will help supervisees grow as clinicians and therapists. Supervision requires an embrace of the complexity of relationships. Maintaining trust is fundamental to a healthy supervisory alliance. Using empathic inquiry will strengthen the supervisory relationship so that the work of supervision can take place and evolve over time.

References

Baudry FD: The personal dimension and management of the supervisory situation with a special note on the parallel process. Psychoanal Q 62(4):588–614, 1993 8284333

Bordin ES: A working alliance based model of supervision. The Counseling Psychologist 11(1):35–42, 1983

Brown J, Reid H, Dornan T, Nestel D: Becoming a clinician: trainee identity formation within the general practice supervisory relationship. Med Educ 54(11):993–1005, 2020 32350873

Coburn WJ: The vision in supervision: transference-countertransference dynamics and disclosure in the supervision relationship. Bull Menninger Clin 61(4):481–494, 1997 9401152

Geller JD, Farber BA, Schaffer CE: Representations of the supervisory dialogue and the development of psychotherapists. Psychotherapy (Chic) 47(2):211–220, 2010 22402048

Hook JN, Watkins CE Jr, Davis DE, et al: Cultural humility in psychotherapy supervision. Am J Psychother 70(2):149–166, 2016 27329404

Karpenko V, Gidycz CA: The supervisory relationship and the process of evaluation: recommendations for supervisors. The Clinical Supervisor 31(2):138–158, 2012

Kay J: Without parallel in human relations: the mirror between treatment and supervision. Psychiatry 78(3):231–235, 2015 26391828

McNeill BW, Worthen V: The parallel process in psychotherapy supervision. Professional Psychology: Research and Practice 20(5):329–333, 1989

Nelson ML, Barnes KL, Evans AL, Triggiano PJ: Working with conflict in clinical supervision: wise supervisors' perspectives. Journal of Counseling Psychology 55(2):172–184, 2008

Shanfield SB, Hetherly VV, Matthews KL: Excellent supervision: the residents' perspective. J Psychother Pract Res 10(1):23–27, 2001 11121004

Watkins CE Jr: The real relationship in psychotherapy supervision. Am J Psychother 65(2):99–116, 2011a 21847889

Watkins CE Jr: Toward a tripartite vision of supervision for psychoanalysis and psychoanalytic psychotherapies: alliance, transference-countertransference configuration, and real relationship. Psychoanal Rev 98(4):557–590, 2011b 21864147

Wilson DB, Sperber D: Meaning and Relevance. Cambridge, UK, Cambridge University Press, 2012

Wilson HMN, Davies JS, Weatherhead S: Trainee therapists' experiences in supervision during training: a meta-synthesis. Clin Psychol Psychother 23(4):340–351, 2016 25917244

5

Ethical Issues in Psychotherapy Supervision

Kevin V. Kelly, M.D.

KEY LEARNING GOALS

- Recognize that some trainees need to limit their focus to the case at hand, while others are able to consider broader issues.

- Understand how an ethical dilemma differs from a moral problem or a clinical problem.

- Appreciate the importance of attending to the trainee's management of transference and countertransference.

- Recognize potential boundary problems that occur in the supervisory relationship.

PSYCHOTHERAPY SUPERVISORS play multiple roles in supervisees' lives: teacher, mentor, role model, consultant, colleague, and sometimes administrative superior, evaluator, critic, cheerleader, supportive therapist, and/ or friend. Each of these roles carries ethical implications, but the ethical issues that arise in the supervisory situation have not been as fully examined as those in the treatment situation. In this chapter I attempt to articulate and to systematize both the issues that arise from the supervisor's responsibility to impart ethical values and principles to the trainee (i.e., the supervision of ethics) and the ethical questions and pitfalls that attend the supervisory relationship itself (i.e., the ethics of supervision). These separable aspects of the topic are merged in the supervisor's modeling function; supervisors' management of the supervisory situation provides trainees with an immediate and powerful example of how to create and maintain a professional relationship in a setting that often involves uncertainty, ambiguity, and emotional intensity.

The Supervision of Ethics

Psychotherapy supervision usually takes place as a component of a larger training program that provides didactic instruction in the theory and practice of psychotherapy and may also include personal psychotherapy for the trainee. Graduates of such programs sometimes choose to engage supervisors privately, outside the context of a training institution, in order to hone their skills further. In any of these cases, the supervisor is challenged to perform two different functions simultaneously: 1) attending to the specifics of the case being supervised, and 2) using the clinical material of the case to exemplify broader theoretical and technical principles. The balance between these two functions will depend on the trainee's level of skill and experience; with a less experienced trainee, the supervisor will need to attend more closely to the safe and effective conduct of the particular patient's treatment, while a more experienced trainee will require less attention to the case at hand, freeing the supervisor to focus on the more general issues raised by the clinical material.

Similarly, the teaching of ethics, whether in the classroom or in clinical supervision, involves two related but distinct activities:

1. Teaching students the "rules" of professional ethics, as summarized in the ethical codes and statements of various governmental and professional bodies.
2. Teaching students the theory and practice of ethical reasoning to equip them to make ethical decisions independently and to contribute to the ethical discourse of their chosen profession.

Again, the balance of these activities varies according to the stage of training; beginning students need to have the "rules" presented clearly, while more advanced students can be engaged in discussion about why these rules exist, what alternative rules might be considered, and how the rules are applied in clinical practice.

An *ethical dilemma* can be usefully defined as a situation in which an individual (in this case, a psychotherapist or a supervisor) has to choose between two or more courses of action, each of which has some "good" attached to it, and the "goods" come from different realms (Michels and Kelly 1999). An ethical dilemma is thus distinguished from a moral dilemma, in which an individual must choose between doing good and doing evil, or a clinical dilemma, in which an individual must choose between alternative paths to the same good, such as choosing between types of psychotherapy and/or psychopharmacology for a specific mental condition.

Theorists and practitioners of psychotherapy often blur the distinction between *issues of ethics* and *issues of technique*, and a supervisor can perform a useful service by teaching the trainee how to make this distinction. For example, in psychoanalytic therapies, the principle of *anonymity*—that the analytic therapist should withhold personal information—is often treated as an ethical injunction that must be upheld at all times, but it is better understood as a matter of technique. Anonymity is thought to be useful because it allows the patient to have a free range of transference fantasies, which can then be used to therapeutic advantage, but if this turns out not to be the case, the principle can be abridged with no ethical harm done. By contrast, the principle of *confidentiality* can be seen either as a matter of technique (because the treatment can work only if the patient feels free to reveal confidences) or as a matter of ethics (because in most cases, the good of protecting the patient's privacy outweighs the good that might be done by revealing information to a third party). Both perspectives are supportable, and both may be true, but there are important differences between them, and the trainee should be taught to distinguish between ethical imperatives and points of technique.

The principle of *neutrality*, also derived from the psychoanalytic tradition, presents a problem for many psychotherapy trainees (Zaslavsky et al. 2005). In its pure form, this principle holds that therapists should not seek to promote any particular social, political, or moral value in patients' lives, but rather should seek only to facilitate the discovery and enactment of those values that are most authentic to patients. Many psychotherapists, and many supervisors, disagree with this principle, holding that a legitimate goal of psychotherapy is to promote values such as psychological-mindedness, integrity, social justice, and respect for persons. The advocacy of such values, and the use of psychotherapy to promote them, can be appropriate, provided that the practitioner recognizes that these are ethical choices that should be made explicit, rather than self-evident desiderata, and that the effort to inculcate these values in one's patients constitutes a deviation from neutrality.

Management of transference and (especially) countertransference is another common area of difficulty for trainees. Strong feelings toward the patient can lead to a variety of ethical missteps. These might include positive feelings such as admiration, sympathy, or romantic attraction or negative feelings such as disgust, boredom, or condemnation. The trainee must be taught to recognize such feelings, be curious about their origins, and try to understand them as fully as possible rather than simply acting on them. Boundary violations between the therapist and the patient are unfortunately a common result of the failure to recognize and manage countertransference feelings. The supervisor should be alert to the development of such feelings in the therapist, should call attention to them early in the treatment, and should educate the therapist to understand these feelings as a source of data about the patient, and possibly also about the therapist, but not as a reason to violate a therapeutic boundary (Walker and Clark 1999).

> Ms. A, a psychotherapy trainee who was unmarried and childless, was treating Mr. B, a widower with two small children. Ms. A's supervisor noticed that Ms. A often spoke with a great deal of admiration and sympathy about Mr. B's struggles to raise his children alone. On one such occasion, the supervisor asked Ms. A whether she might have had the thought that she could fill the void in Mr. B's life. Ms. A, surprised and embarrassed, said that she had not, but on further reflection realized that she had entertained the fantasy of accidentally meeting Mr. B outside the office. This awareness allowed Ms. A to recognize her countertransference, and to use it to understand the therapeutic process more fully.

The question of whether and how explicitly the patient's *informed consent* should be required for psychotherapy has been extensively debated (Furlong 2020; Sherry 1991). Some institutions require written informed consent for psychotherapy, usually in order to protect the institution against medicolegal liability. Some ethicists hold that, as with any other medical procedure, the patient should be informed about the potential benefits and risks of psychotherapy, and the alternative courses of action, before beginning the treatment. Others maintain that a patient with no previous experience in psychotherapy cannot appreciate the possible benefits or the possible dangers involved, and that consent to psychotherapy is an ongoing process that evolves over the course of the treatment. A supervisor can responsibly advocate either of these positions but should discuss the question of consent with the trainee early in the course of supervision.

The ethical category of *dual agency* refers to situations in which the therapist's responsibility to promote the patient's best interests may be in tension with other responsibilities, such as those to other patients, to an institution, to the profession, to the public, or to prospective future patients. Beginning psychotherapists often bristle at the suggestion that they should consider anything apart from the welfare of the particular patient. The supervisor can point to common examples—such as limiting the time one spends with a particular patient in order to make time for other patients, or using confidential material about a patient to educate other therapists—to illustrate that the individual therapist is always striking an ethical balance between the patient's treatment and other concerns.

The tension between an individual patient's needs and other concerns becomes particularly vivid and fraught when insurance plans or clinic policies dictate a limit to the number of psychotherapy sessions a patient can receive. In this situation, the supervisor's task is to help the trainee to recognize and accept these imposed limits, to understand (although not necessarily endorse) the reasoning behind them, and to think creatively about how to maximize the therapeutic benefit to the patient under these circumstances.

Involuntary hospitalization or treatment, when undertaken to protect the public from a potentially dangerous patient, offers a vivid example of the need to respect the interests of entities other than the patient, even at the cost of curtailing an individual patient's freedom. Ideally, such situations will be rare, but trainees need to be taught how to recognize them and how to feel ethically comfortable taking the required action.

Protection of the patient's *confidentiality* in psychotherapy requires explicit education, some of which may be best undertaken in supervision. The therapist's didactic training should cover the general principle that information communicated in psychotherapy must not be disclosed to others, as well as the circumstances in which this principle can or must be overridden (e.g., avoiding harm to the patient or others, promoting scientific and educational activities). However, the application of this principle to specific situations arising with patients can be most profitably discussed in the course of supervision. The supervisor should be aware of the relevant legal requirements for documentation and should educate the trainee about what material belongs in the official treatment record, including the electronic medical record, and what material should be kept in the more protected psychotherapy notes.

Dr. C, a psychiatry resident, was seeing a patient, Mr. E, for twice-weekly individual psychotherapy at a hospital's outpatient clinic. One day, Mr. E, who was normally mild-mannered, described feeling "so angry I could shoot somebody." Alarmed, Dr. C asked the patient whom he might shoot. Mr. E replied, "Anybody who gets in my way." Dr. C was aware of the *Tarasoff* decision, which he understood to impose a "duty to warn," but because he was unsure about how to discharge this duty, he asked his supervisor whom he should warn about Mr. E's outburst. The supervisor, who was familiar with the legal and ethical arguments surrounding *Tarasoff*, was able to explain to Dr. C that in this situation, the "duty to warn" was replaced by a "duty to protect" intended victims by any of a number of means. Because no potential victim had been identified, Dr. C's challenge was to determine whether Mr. E's situation met criteria for involuntary hospitalization, a decision with which he was familiar and comfortable.

The supervisor's role-modeling function can also be used to educate the trainee about the importance of *self-care* for the psychotherapist. Beginning trainees are likely to err on the side of overinvolvement with patients and their problems, often mulling over patients' issues during nonwork hours and/or encouraging telephone contact by patients between sessions, at the expense of both the patient's development of autonomy and the therapist's own mental health. Supervisors should help trainees cultivate a stance that balances commitment to patients with maintenance of boundaries that protect the therapist's privacy and ability to avoid burnout. Trainees need to feel comfortable taking time away from work for activities such as family time, recreation, and vacations without succumbing to the self-serving generalization that "anything that's good for me is good for my patients." The trainee's observation of how the supervisor handles such issues will provide a powerful lesson.

On rare occasions, a supervisor will become aware of behavior on the part of the trainee that the supervisor considers frankly *unethical*, and will feel obligated to report such behavior to the training institution or a professional body. Ideally, the supervisor will recognize situations that carry such risks before they escalate to the point of unethical conduct, and will warn the trainee about the risk. Early-warning signs of possible boundary violations in three areas are presented in Table 5–1. (It should be noted that "time-related" and "nonsexual" boundary violations can also lead to sexual boundary violations.) If such behavior has already occurred and the supervisor feels obliged to report it, the trainee should be informed of the supervisor's concerns and plans before the report is made.

The Ethics of Supervision

The most obvious responsibility of a psychotherapy supervisor is to supervise well. Doing so requires having a knowledge of the theory and practice of psychotherapy, including the ability to judge when another form of psychotherapy, or another mode of treatment, is indicated; gaining a knowledge of the supervisee's level of training and skill, learning style, and personality factors that might affect the course of treatment or supervision; gaining a sufficient knowledge of the patient to judge

Table 5–1. Range of possible boundary violations

Category/ Type	Minor level	Intermediate level	Severe level
Time-related	Routinely extending sessions beyond the agreed ending time	Scheduling sessions outside regular work hours	Being available 24/7, without time boundaries
Nonsexual	Sharing food with patient	Giving patient a ride in therapist's car	Becoming involved in patient's financial life
Sexual	Commenting favorably on patient's appearance	Discussing therapist's romantic life with patient	Frank sexual involvement with patient

whether the treatment being given is appropriate, safe, and effective; and having or acquiring a familiarity with the art and practice of supervision, including how to optimize the trainee's autonomous functioning without endangering the patient's welfare. However, these responsibilities are unexceptionable, and are therefore better understood as matters of supervisory technique than as ethical dilemmas.

The supervisory situation involves the addition of a third party to the dyadic relationship of therapist and patient, and thereby introduces a host of new ethical considerations (Brodsky 2017). When the "third party" includes not only a supervisor but also a training institution, the supervisor's ethical responsibilities are more extensive and more complicated than they would be in the case of private supervision. In the institutional setting, the supervisor has a *responsibility to the institution and to the public* to judge when or whether the trainee is ready to practice without supervision. Thus, the interests of the trainee's future patients are at stake, along with the interests of the patient whose treatment is being supervised. The supervisor also has the responsibility of determining whether the supervisee's functioning has been impaired by exhaustion, burnout, or depression. In such instances, the supervisor will want to discuss the issue with the training director (see Chapter 25, "Addressing Exhaustion and Burnout in Psychotherapy Supervision").

Administrators of training institutions, as well as supervisors and ethicists, have debated the question of *whether the patient must be informed that the therapist is under supervision* (Thomas 2014). The ethical considerations at stake in this question involve both professional honesty (because the patient has a right to know about the therapist's level of expertise) and confidentiality (because the patient's private information is being shared with a third party). Patients who are being treated in a clinic or training facility, and who are not familiar with how such institutions operate, may be unaware that the therapist is a trainee, or that the patient's treatment is being discussed with a psychotherapy supervisor. In many cases, institutional policies require that patients be informed of these facts, that patients give written consent to being treated by a supervisee, and/or that the supervisor see patients in person periodically. Even in institutions where no such policy exists, patients should be informed that their therapist is in training and that their therapy is being discussed with a psychotherapy supervisor.

> Dr. G was waiting outside the clinic office of Dr. V, his supervisee, when Ms. I emerged from the office. Dr. G and Ms. I were both surprised, because they knew each other socially, but they exchanged smiles, and Ms. I left quickly. At that point, Dr. G realized that Ms. I was the patient whom his supervisee had been discussing for several weeks. Dr. G explained the situation to Dr. V, and they agreed to terminate their discussions of Ms. I and to arrange for a different supervisor to be appointed. Ms. I had known that her therapy was being supervised, but she was distressed to learn that the supervisor was Dr. G, whom she knew personally. However, she was satisfied with Dr. V's explanation that neither she nor Dr. G had known of the connection before that occasion, and that a new supervisor would take over from Dr. G.

In the case of private supervision, the supervisee may be already fully licensed and credentialed to function independently, and the patient may have no reason to anticipate that his or her therapy is being discussed with a supervisor. In this situation, there is no requirement to inform the patient that the therapist is pursuing further professional education, although the ethical concern about confidentiality remains.

Regardless of whether supervision is being conducted under institutional auspices or privately, the issue of *sharing confidential material with a supervisor* is best handled by invoking the same principles that apply to the publication of clinical material—those of *disguise* and *consent* (Gabbard 2000). *Disguise* refers to the practice of altering or omitting data from the patient's story that could render the patient identifiable to a third party, such as the supervisor, and *consent*, in this case, refers to the practice of requesting the patient's agreement to the therapist's discussing confidential material for the purpose of supervision. Using disguise may be problematic in supervision because some details of a patient's story will be essential to include, because the trainee may not be in a position to judge reliably which details can safely be altered, and/or because the supervisor has legal or administrative responsibilities that require knowing the patient's identity. However, it is still a useful practice for the trainee to learn that no confidential information should be shared without the patient's consent, even with a supervisor, unless the sharing of that information is necessary for the patient's treatment. The trainee who chooses to request the patient's consent to use confidential material in supervision should be prepared for the possibility that the patient will refuse. If the treatment is taking place under the umbrella of an institution that requires supervision, the trainee may have to inform the patient that the treatment cannot continue without this consent. In any case, the trainee can and should inform the patient that the supervisor will be bound by the same tenets of confidentiality that bind the therapist.

An issue that often provokes disagreement among administrators and supervisors is the question of *whether and to what extent supervisors are responsible for the clinical outcome* of the patients being treated by their supervisees. Indeed, the term *supervisor* can be misleading, because in the business world it usually describes an administrative superior who has the authority to order a subordinate to perform the work in a certain way, and to penalize or terminate the subordinate who does not comply. The psychotherapy supervisor, by contrast, is usually empowered only to advise the trainee, and in most cases has to rely on the trainee's report of whether the supervisor's advice is being followed. Some institutions have addressed this problem by creating two different supervisory roles for each patient under treatment: an *administrative supervisor* who assumes clinical and legal responsibility for the treatment and its results, and an *educational supervisor* whose job is to use the clinical material of the case to further the trainee's education, but who is not in a position to assume responsibility for the clinical outcome. At a minimum, the extent of the supervisor's authority and responsibility should be made clear at the outset of supervision to both trainee and supervisor.

Some discussions of supervisors' roles and responsibilities include recommendations that supervisors and trainees have a *written contract* governing their work, and/or that all supervisory sessions be documented in a manner similar to the documentation of clinical treatment. These proposals raise important administrative and legal considerations, but they do not present any special ethical dilemmas.

Issues of background and identity inevitably affect both psychotherapy and supervision and present ethical and technical challenges in both. Differences between patient and therapist with respect to gender, race, ethnicity, culture, religion, sexual orientation, ability/disability, and so forth require careful attention but are often ignored or minimized because of the therapist's unawareness or discomfort. Supervisors can perform an important educational function by reminding trainees of the necessity of attending to these issues thoughtfully, respectfully, and explicitly and by pointing out that commonalities between patient and therapist along these dimensions can also present problems, creating blind spots or shared but unspoken assumptions. Similarly, commonalities and differences between supervisor and trainee along these same dimensions should be articulated and examined.

Trainees themselves are often in psychotherapy, and this situation has the potential to create conflict and confusion in the supervision. It is never advisable for a supervisor and a supervisee to engage in both personal psychotherapy and supervision, because the transference distortions arising in this situation are likely to compromise both the therapy and the supervision. When a trainee is seeing one senior clinician for psychotherapy and another senior clinician for supervision, each clinician should be aware of the other's role, and both should be attentive to maintaining the boundaries between their functions. In psychodynamic therapy, such boundaries can be particularly difficult to preserve, because the supervisor's role will include regularly and appropriately calling attention to the influence of the trainee's own psychology on the therapy being provided. A useful approach for this situation might be for the supervisor to point out those psychological tendencies in the trainee that complicate the trainee's work with the patient but to leave it to the trainee's own therapist to explore the reasons for these tendencies and the possibility of changing them (Arlow 1963; Debell 1963).

> Dr. L was supervising a psychoanalytic candidate, Dr. K, who was also seeing a training analyst for his personal analysis. Over the course of supervision, Dr. L noticed that Dr. K rarely, if ever, expressed any negative reactions toward his patient, despite the patient's entitled and provocative behavior, and she suggested that perhaps Dr. K was constrained by an inhibition of his own aggression. Dr. K seemed surprised by this observation, and asked Dr. L why she thought so. Rather than detailing the numerous observations that had led her to this conclusion, Dr. L suggested that Dr. K raise the issue with his treating analyst.

The relationship between supervisor and supervisee may have aspects similar to relationships between employer and employee, teacher and student, or therapist and patient (Haesler 1993). These multiple relational possibilities can complicate the ethical understanding of *boundary issues in supervision*. Such complications are evident in the variety and the vagueness of statements by professional bodies on the topic of boundary violations, and particularly on the issue of sexual contact between therapist and supervisor. These statements usually prohibit sexual activity between a therapist and a current supervisor in institutional settings where the supervisor has the power to affect the trainee's professional future, but avoid commenting on other situations. For example, the American Psychiatric Association's Code of Ethics states that

> Sexual involvement between a faculty member and a trainee or student, in those situations in which an abuse of power can occur, often takes advantage of inequalities in the working relationship and may be unethical…. (American Psychiatric Association 2013, p. 7)

The American Psychological Association states that

> Psychologists do not engage in sexual relationships with students or supervisees who are in their department, agency, or training center or over whom psychologists have or are likely to have evaluative authority. (American Psychological Association 2017, Section 7.07)

The American Psychoanalytic Association states, somewhat more boldly, that

> *Sexual relationships between current supervisors and supervisees are unethical.* (American Psychoanalytic Association 2010)

All of these statements agree, in essence, that to the extent that a supervisory relationship resembles an employment relationship, sexual contact should be prohibited. This conclusion is unsurprising, given that the current general social and legal consensus holds that sexual activity between employer and employee is prohibited in any field.

The more difficult and controversial questions concern those situations in which the supervisor holds no administrative authority over the supervisee, such as in private supervision or after termination of a training supervision. Even when there is no possibility of the supervisor exploiting a power differential, either because the supervision is private or because the supervisory relationship has been terminated, there remains the possibility that sexual attraction could be stimulated by powerful transference feelings arising from the supervision. Thus, to the extent that the supervisory relationship resembles the psychotherapy relationship, there is reason for concern. However, the same can be said of any situation in which sexual attraction arises—that it is likely to be influenced by transference and other unconscious forces. The silence of most professional bodies on the question of sexual contact after the termination of supervision suggests a tacit agreement that, assuming both parties are competent adults, they should be accorded the freedom to use their own judgment about sexual involvement.

Nonsexual boundary violations can also occur in the supervisory relationship, such as a supervisor suggesting that a clinic patient be referred to the supervisor's private practice, or asking a trainee to participate in the supervisor's research project. The first situation should never occur unless 1) there is an explicit agreement with the clinic's administration that such self-referrals are permissible and 2) the referral is clearly in the patient's best interest. An invitation to collaborate on a research project might be advantageous to, and welcomed by, a trainee, but the supervisor should be alert to the risk that the trainee might feel compelled to accept the offer because of the supervisor's position of authority, or because of a transferential distortion arising from the supervisory relationship.

An important aspect of professional education that is sometimes neglected is the provision of honest and usable *feedback* to the trainee. Giving an evaluation of the trainee's performance and suggestions for improvement is more of a technical than an ethical requirement, but supervisors may avoid fulfilling this requirement out of a wish to protect a trainee's sensibilities. Supervisors of psychodynamic therapy may also adopt a stance similar to that of the classical psychoanalyst, who strives to be nonjudgmental and to keep interventions to a minimum. However, a robust back-and-forth exchange between supervisor and supervisee is more effective in fostering the trainee's growth in autonomy, self-confidence, and professionalism.

Conclusion

The supervisory relationship, like the psychotherapy relationship, can generate a variety of ethical questions. By attending in advance to these potential issues, supervisors can create an atmosphere in which supervisees can be helped to develop an attitude of respect for ethical considerations, to recognize and manage ethical issues when they arise in a patient's treatment, and to contribute to the ethical discourse of their chosen profession.

Additional Resources

Barnett JE, Erickson Cornish JA, Goodyear RK, Lichtenberg JW: Commentaries on the ethical and effective practice of clinical supervision. Professional Psychology: Research and Practice 38(3):268–275, 2007
Barnett JE, Molzon CH: Clinical supervision of psychotherapy: essential ethics issues for supervisors and supervisees. J Clin Psychol 70(11):1051–1061, 2014

Blomfield OHD: Psychoanalytic supervision: an overview. International Review of Psychoanalysis 12:401–409, 1985

Ladany N, Lehrman-Waterman D, Molinaro M, Wolgast B: Psychotherapy supervisor ethical practices: adherence to guidelines, the supervisory working alliance, and supervisee satisfaction. The Counseling Psychologist 27(3):443–475, 1999

Newman AS: Ethical issues in the supervision of psychotherapy. Professional Psychology 12(6):690–695, 1981

Watkins CE Jr: The competent psychoanalytic supervisor. International Journal of Psychoanalysis 23:220–228, 2014

References

American Psychiatric Association: The Principles of Medical Ethics With Annotations Especially Applicable to Psychiatry. Washington, DC, American Psychiatric Association 2013

American Psychoanalytic Association: Code of Ethics. Section 14. New York, American Psychoanalytic Association, 2010

American Psychological Association: Ethical Principles of Psychologists and Code of Conduct. Section 7.07 (Sexual Relationships with Students and Supervisees). Washington, DC, American Psychological Association, 2017

Arlow J: The supervisory situation. Journal of the American Psychoanalytic Association 11(3):576–594, 1963

Brodsky H: Supervision triangles and the attempt to turn a blind eye to them. Contemporary Psychoanalysis 53(3):393–413, 2017

Debell DE: A critical digest of the literature on psychoanalytic supervision. Journal of the American Psychoanalytic Association 11(3):546–575, 1963

Furlong A: Consenting and assenting to psychoanalytic work. J Am Psychoanal Assoc 68(4):583–613, 2020 32927986

Gabbard GO: Disguise or consent: problems and recommendations concerning the publication and presentation of clinical material. Int J Psychoanal 81(Pt 6):1071–1086, 2000 11144850

Haesler L: Adequate distance in the relationship between supervisor and supervisee. The position of the supervisor between "teacher" and "analyst." Int J Psychoanal 74(Pt 3):547–555, 1993 8344773

Michels R, Kelly K: Teaching psychiatric ethics, in Psychiatric Ethics, 3rd Edition. Edited by Bloch S, Chodoff P, Green SA. New York, Oxford University Press, 1999, pp 495–509

Sherry P: Ethical issues in the conduct of supervision. The Counseling Psychologist 19(4):566–584, 1991

Thomas J: International ethics for psychotherapy supervisors, in The Wiley International Handbook of Clinical Supervision. Edited by Watkins CE Jr, Milne D. Chichester, West Sussex, UK, Wiley-Blackwell, 2014, pp 141–142

Walker R, Clark JJ: Heading off boundary problems: clinical supervision as risk management. Psychiatr Serv 50(11):1435–1439, 1999 10543852

Zaslavsky J, Nunes MLT, Eizirik CL: Approaching countertransference in psychoanalytical supervision: a qualitative investigation. Int J Psychoanal 86 (Pt 4):1099–1131, 2005 16040312

Practical Methods That Foster Supervisor Growth

Erin M. Crocker, M.D.
Sindhu A. Idicula, M.D.
Randon S. Welton, M.D.

KEY LEARNING GOALS

- Enhance the efficacy of feedback in supervision through trainee self-assessment and review of objective data from recordings and other tools.

- Use structured assessment tools to guide supervision and to generate specific feedback that is directly useful to the trainee.

- Promote formal assessment of patient preferences and outcomes to help identify potential problems in the therapeutic relationship and augment the treatment.

MANY PSYCHOTHERAPY supervisors face supervision with a combination of excitement and trepidation. They want to help but secretly doubt whether they are knowledgeable enough to assist their trainees. Their approach to supervision may be characterized by a lack of direction and intentionality.

The ways of the psychotherapy supervisor may seem mysterious and inaccessible. In this chapter we discuss specific approaches and tools that will help guide supervision. These tools are not intended to take the place of experience, wisdom, insight, or intuition, but rather are intended to provide a framework for the supervisory hour. Whereas other chapters in this book address specific techniques, such as creating goals for supervision (Chapter 8) and using audio or video recordings in supervision (Chapter 9), our objective in this chapter is to illustrate how to provide effective feedback, how to use structured assessment tools, and how to incorporate patient preferences and outcome measures into supervision.

Providing Effective Feedback

Becoming a physician has always included an apprenticeship component. Experienced supervisors direct trainees to gather information effectively, synthesize that information, and create comprehensive treatment plans. Increasing one's capacity to provide and receive direct, practical feedback has always been a part of growing as a medical professional. Providing focused feedback offers one of the most beneficial means of improving performance in any skill (Hattie and Timperley 2007) and is an essential component of psychotherapy supervision. In a literature review ($N=41$ studies), feedback provided to physicians was found to improve their clinical performance in 74% of the reviewed studies (Veloski et al. 2006). Although there are variations in study findings, certain components of feedback have been found to be more consistently helpful than others, as outlined in the following subsections.

Shared Goals

It is important that the trainee and the supervisor are both working toward the same acknowledged goals (Brehaut et al. 2016; Ende 1983). These goals define the standards the trainee is hoping to attain. Having specific, predetermined, collaboratively agreed-upon standards allows a comparison in which both parties can agree on whether or not a particular goal was met (see Chapter 8).

Self-Assessment

Modern medicine promotes the virtue of lifelong learning based on continual self-assessment (Wood 2000). Supervisors can help trainee therapists to develop the ability to assess their own clinical performance and detect knowledge and performance gaps. This skill allows an iterative process of self-assessment, self-feedback, and self-directed learning. For health professionals, self-directed learning seems to be at least as effective as other methods of learning in enhancing knowledge and skills and in changing attitudes (Anderson 2012). Having trainees assess their own performance during supervision can be the starting point for feedback. Although self-assessment is vital, it is often unreliable on its own. A systematic review of studies examining the accuracy of physician self-assessments found that 65% of studies showed either no correlation or an inverse correlation between findings from self-assessment and those from external assessment (Davis et al. 2006). Some of the most marked discrepancies were seen in the lowest performers, who frequently rated their performance as above average (Sargeant et al. 2013). In light of these findings, building the capacity for more accurate self-assessment should be a key aspect of professional development (Stalmeijer et al. 2010). One means of improving the reliability of self-assessments is to repeatedly compare them with external, objective evaluations such as assessments made by supervisors.

Supervisor Response to Trainee Self-Assessments

By reviewing trainees' self-assessments, supervisors demonstrate their interest in the learner's perspective (Wood 2000). Supervisors can highlight areas where there is agreement or discordance between the trainee's self-assessment and the supervisor's assessment of the trainee's performance (Branch and Paranjape 2002). Creating opportunities for open, respectful reflections on supervisee self-assessments can foster trainee engagement with the feedback process, facilitate acceptance of suggestions, and lead to subsequent improvement (Sargeant et al. 2013). Combining self-assessment with external feedback can be a powerful motivator for change (Stalmeijer et al. 2010).

Review of Objective Data

Compared with feedback based on supervisee report, comments based on direct observation and first-hand data will consistently have a greater impact and be less subject to bias and preconceptions. Supervisees cannot recall or discuss what they fail to notice. The capacity to review what actually happened in the therapy session via audiovisual recording can facilitate a more accurate, objective assessment of trainee performance (see also Chapter 9). Feedback can focus on specific decisions and actions taken by the learner rather than generalizations or surmised intentions (Anderson 2012; Brehaut et al. 2016; Ende 1983; Wood 2000). Some trainees may deliberately or unconsciously alter their presentations in ways that they think will please or impress the supervisor (Hoop 2004;

Yourman 2003). While supervisees' reporting of process material from therapy sessions has many training benefits, this method may not provide supervisors with the objective data needed to inform a more accurate assessment of, and generate meaningful feedback about, supervisees and the therapy they are providing (Haggerty and Hilsenroth 2011).

Benefits of Structured Assessment Tools

Trainees tend to ignore or devalue supervision discussions and feedback that do not relate to their clinical case material (Shanfield et al. 2001).

> Dr. J, a trainee therapist, is complaining to her training director about her supervisor, Dr. U: "When I come in to supervision, I am all prepared to discuss my cases, but Dr. U starts talking about psychodynamic theory or journal articles. I don't want to interrupt her, but soon, most of the supervision hour is gone, and she has spent the time talking about psychodynamic concepts, or one of her own cases, instead of mine. I know that she is smart and is a great therapist, but I am afraid that I am wasting this year."

Although the topics addressed in supervision sessions will occasionally roam beyond the mutually identified goals of supervision, use of a well-designed, structured assessment tool can help to focus supervision, document the trainee's improvement, and assist in generating useful feedback. Having this tool reminds both members of the supervisory dyad about the purposes of supervision. The use of structured assessment forms offers additional guidance to trainee therapists who are uncertain about how to approach supervision. The categories highlighted in the assessment form will help trainees organize their observations and comments. As trainees become familiar with these assessment instruments, they develop confidence and are able to approach therapy sessions with a greater sense of what to emphasize.

> Dr. T, a novice therapist, is overwhelmed by his emotions after hearing a patient's history of abuse. He is feeling an urge to rail against the perpetrator but pauses and remembers the assessment form that was used during his supervision sessions. He recalls that it is always safe to emphasize empathy, and he uses that knowledge to guide his subsequent comments to the patient.

Training programs can share structured assessment forms with supervisors and also introduce them during didactic training. Although the more subtle nuances of therapy will not be captured by these forms, such tools provide a helpful starting point for instructors and supervisors. Su-

pervisors will develop an awareness of what has been emphasized in didactic training, and instructors will develop confidence that supervisors
will reinforce what they have taught.

Documenting trainee improvement in supervision can be challenging.
Even if both supervisor and supervisee see growth and maturation, it is
often hard to say specifically what is different by the end of supervision.
The ultimate intent of structured forms is to provide a framework for documenting change and generating specific, immediately useful feedback.
There should be a direct correspondence between what is recorded on the
form and what feedback is given to the learner. For example, supervisors
can point out behaviors that were once absent from a trainee's repertoire
but now are routine. Ideally, the "Areas of Strength" will increase and the
"Areas for Improvement" will diminish, and trainees will gain self-confidence in their therapy skills, just as supervisors may experience a corresponding increase in confidence in their supervisory skills.

Useful Structured Assessment Tools

The stated purpose of the Psychotherapy Committee of the American
Association of Directors of Psychiatry Residency Training (AADPRT) is
"to create and disseminate information, training materials, and assessment tools to support psychotherapy training in residency programs"
(AADPRT 2020). In pursuit of this goal, the AADPRT Psychotherapy
Committee undertook an initiative to develop structured assessment
forms for psychotherapy supervision.

AADPRT Milestone Assessment of Psychotherapy

To begin the development process, the committee decided to focus on
three common elements of psychotherapies: the therapeutic alliance, empathy, and boundaries. The committee created the AADPRT Milestone
Assessment of Psychotherapy (A-MAP) to examine these areas. Each of
the three elements was tethered to a series of anchor points that could be
rated on a scale of 1 to 5.

The A-MAP assessment begins with the supervisor and the resident reviewing the components of the A-MAP. The resident then picks a 15-min-
ute section of a recorded psychotherapy case to review. The supervisor
and the supervisee watch the taped session together, and the supervisor
records their comments along with the resident's score on the "Observed"
section of the A-MAP. After watching the video, the supervisor uses a series of scripted questions to address the three common elements. The supervisor combines the "Observed Score" with the "Discussion Score" to

obtain the "Final Score." A primary benefit of the A-MAP is the discussion that follows the scoring. The supervisor uses the score and their recorded comments to identify what the resident has done well and what could have been better. These focused comments on observed behaviors and answers to related questions provide the foundation for the feedback.

Continued experience with the A-MAP has revealed its potential as a tool for supervisor training and development. Groups of psychotherapy supervisors can observe a portion of a therapy session and then discuss how they would score what they observed and what feedback they would offer. This exercise may improve interrater reliability, but more importantly, it familiarizes supervisors with using the tool and thinking about psychotherapy and psychotherapy feedback in a more structured way. AADPRT hosts on its website a Virtual Training Office (available to nonmembers by special application; see https://www.aadprt.org/training-directors/virtual-training-office) that provides training materials and videos for its structured psychotherapy tools, including the A-MAP.

AADPRT Foundations of Psychodynamic Psychotherapy

The popularity and utility of the A-MAP among members of the AADPRT Psychotherapy Committee led that committee to create similarly themed forms for assessing dimensions of psychodynamic psychotherapy. In undertaking this task, the committee faced several challenges. Such forms would need to be based on observation of trainees providing psychotherapy and not simply a test of the resident's knowledge of psychodynamic principles. The committee also wanted a tool that could be used in a variety of psychodynamic orientations (e.g., ego psychology, object relations, self psychology). This challenge was addressed by identifying common characteristics of psychodynamic psychotherapy, as articulated in the work of Blagys and Hilsenroth (2000) and highlighted by Shedler (2010). The Psychotherapy Committee created two forms that can be filled out as the resident and the supervisor watch a video of a psychodynamic psychotherapy session.

The first, the Foundations of Psychodynamic Psychotherapy—Priorities (Figure 6–1), is a rating scale for evaluating the resident's use of six foundational principles of psychodynamic psychotherapy. The rating scale provides anchor points for rating performance in these foundational areas on a 1 (poor) to 5 (excellent) scale. The supervisor can also provide a global assessment of the supervisee's use of psychodynamic priorities and a rating of 1–5 for overall performance. The second form, Foundations of Psychodynamic Psychotherapy—Interventions (Figure 6–2), is a rating scale for evaluating the resident's use of 15 interventions typically employed in psychodynamic psychotherapy. For each listed intervention, the supervisor can indicate whether the resident used it appropriately, used it especially successfully, or missed an opportunity for using the intervention. The form gives the supervisor a way to rate the resident's overall use of interventions, from poor to excellent, and includes anchor points exemplifying each level on the rating scale. Together, these two forms help the supervisor and the supervisee to assess their approaches and interventions.

> Dr. N, a second-year resident, has scheduled an intake interview with her first "official" psychotherapy patient. However, she is feeling increasingly anxious about spending 45 minutes on a weekly basis with the same patient. Won't the two of them run out of things to talk about? Won't she already have most of the patient's information after the intake process? While reviewing the A-MAP with her supervisor, Dr. N notices the prominence given to building the alliance, using empathic intervention, and allowing patients to explore their own stories and the emotions they evoke.

Trainees can use these forms as part of their self-assessments. Observing their own performance in light of the principles and interventions highlighted in the form often uncovers facets of trainees' responses that might have been difficult for them to notice while engaging in psychotherapy.

> Dr. P has noticed that her supervisee, Dr. O, a third-year resident, implements problem-solving strategies every time her psychotherapy patient has an intense display of affect. Dr. P rewinds the video and asks Dr. O to score herself with the AADPRT Foundations of Psychodynamic Psychotherapy–Interventions form during a portion of therapy in which her patient starts crying. Dr. O recognizes that she finds it difficult to sit in silence and allow her patient to talk about her emotions. She hypothesizes that she feels guilty for not doing something to help this person in obvious distress. She acknowledges that although she feels like a competent problem-solver, she feels like an impostor as a therapist. Dr. P empathically validates Dr. O's urge to "fix" the patient and takes this opportunity to role-play other ways to respond to the patient's distress.

The use of structured forms creates opportunities to praise trainees for specific things they have done well. Although generalized praise can leave residents feeling proud that they have done a good job, they may be unable to identify exactly what they did well.

> Dr. H, a fourth-year resident, has always received glowing reviews in psychotherapy and other clinical work, but he sometimes wonders whether those good reviews are merely due to his likability as a person and strong work ethic. During supervision, he and Dr. Y, his supervisor, review several minutes of video footage from a therapy session with Ms. R, his patient.

AADPRT Foundations of Psychodynamic Psychotherapy—Priorities

Supervisors: Use this form to evaluate the resident's performance within a patient care encounter

Resident: _____   Supervisor: _____

Global Ratings: Based on your observation, how would you rate the following?

1. **Focusing on affect and expression of emotions**   Not Observed _____

1	2	3	4	5
Obviously not attuned to the patient's emotional expression	Recognizes important emotional cues from the patient	Recognizes important emotional cues from the patient and facilitates the patient's exploration of these emotions	Facilitates the patient's exploration of complex and conflicting emotions	A model of successfully facilitating the patient's exploration of emotional content and its meaning

Comments: _____

2. **Exploring attempts to avoid distressing thoughts and feelings**   Not Observed _____

1	2	3	4	5
Does not recognize the patient's attempt to avoid distress, does not express any awareness of that pattern to the patient	May recognize the pattern to avoid but unable to share that information with the patient in an effort for meaningful exploration	Recognizes and brings to attention some instances of distress-inducing content	Routinely recognizes and shares with patient instances of distress-inducing content	Successfully shares evidence and patterns of the patient's avoidance of distressing thoughts and feelings, including in-the-moment exploration. Able to tie this into interpretations of past relationships or transference

Comments: _____

3. **Identifying recurring themes and patterns in relationships**   Not Observed _____

1	2	3	4	5
Misses opportunities to comment on recurring relational patterns occurring within a single session / Does not explore past or current relationships	Notices and comments on recurring relational patterns occurring within a single session / Explores past and current relationships sporadically	Explores past and current relationships as they pertain to current relationships / Can surmise a theme based on the recurring patterns of relationship	Facilitates the patient's reflection on past and current relationships and their impact on current relationships / Links current relational themes to events from the patient's childhood	Offers interpretations which connect the patient's recurring relational themes to the patient's childhood, their life outside of therapy, and transference experiences within therapy

Comments: _____

4. Discussing past experiences (developmental focus)   Not Observed _____

1	2	3	4	5
Does not explore past experiences which may be contributing to current behaviors and problems	Explores past experience in an unfocused manner, without looking for connections to present problems or behaviors	Explores past experience as it pertains to current problems or behaviors	Facilitates the patient's reflection on past experiences and their impact on current problems or behaviors	A model of successful use of the past to further the patient's insight into current problems

Comments: _____

5. Focusing on the therapy relationship   Not Observed _____

1	2	3	4	5
Does not recognize that therapeutic impasses or strains in the relationship have occurred	Identifies strains in the alliance but does not address them	Recognizes therapeutic impasses and attempts to address them	Successfully manages therapeutic impasses and strains in the alliance	A model of successfully using therapeutic impasses to further the treatment relationship

Comments: _____

6. Exploring fantasy life   Not Observed _____

1	2	3	4	5
Does not acknowledge content brought forth by the patient regarding fantasies	Acknowledges content but does not facilitate the patient's exploration of the meaning of this content	Facilitates the patient's reflection on the meaning of fantasies and wishes	Helps the patient to understand how their fantasies and wishes can be used to inform their treatment goals	A model of successful use of fantasy life to help the patient understand their wishes, desires, and goals

Comments: _____

Overall Comments: _____

_____

_____

Overall Rating of Psychodynamic Priorities:

Poor	Below Average	Average	Above Average	Excellent

Adapted from
Shedler J: The efficacy of psychodynamic psychotherapy. *American Psychologist* 65(2):98–109, 2010
Blagys MD, Hilsenroth MJ: Distinctive features of short-term psychodynamic-interpersonal psychotherapy: a review of the comparative psychotherapy process literature. *Clinical Psychology: Science and Practice* 7(2):167–188, 2000

Figure 6–1. American Association of Directors of Psychiatry Residency Training (AADPRT) Foundations of Psychodynamic Psychotherapy—Priorities.

Source. Reproduced with permission from American Association of Directors of Psychiatry Residency Training.

AADPRT Foundations of Psychodynamic Psychotherapy—
Interventions

While watching the resident work with a patient or watching a video of the resident working with a patient, please indicate which skills were observed. Use the following system:

O   = Missed opportunity (please explain further in the "Comments" section)
?   = Observed
?– = Appropriate intervention but not well timed or executed
*   = Particular area of strength (something the resident did particularly well)

Allows patient to set agenda, pace, and tone of session   _____

Encourages free association   _____

Listens empathically and follows patient's affect cues   _____

Emphasizes uncovering techniques without neglecting supportive
   interventions   _____

Asks patient to discuss their thoughts and experiences without
   offering advice   _____

Tolerates appropriate silences to help patient "say the next thing" _____

Encourages patient to talk about their feelings, even when difficult _____

Promotes patient's reflection, self-observation, and mentalization _____

Gently encourages patient to talk more deeply about feelings,
   memories, and experiences (e.g., open-ended questions, "go on,"   _____
   "tell me more")

Tries to link conscious thoughts, feelings, and behaviors to
   thoughts and feelings that are out of the patient's awareness   _____

Helps patient link current behaviors/emotions to their past
   experiences   _____

Tries to link resistance, defenses, recurring patterns of
   relationships/behaviors, and thoughts/feelings that are out   _____
   of awareness

Connects patient's experience of therapy and especially of the
   therapist with past experiences and expectations from past   _____
   relationships

Uses empathy to better understand the patient   _____

Maintains therapeutic frame and reflects on boundary crossings
   with patient   _____

Overall Use of Psychodynamic Psychotherapy Techniques	
Poor	Neglects to use uncovering techniques Emphasizes techniques from other types of therapy (Does not know the techniques appropriate to psychodynamic psychotherapy) Does not follow the patient's lead during the session Asks predominantly closed-ended questions Cannot identify transference or countertransference
Below Average	Uncovers patient's feelings and experiences through the use of closed-ended questions Sets an agenda for the session Predominance of supportive interventions Does not tolerate silences Follows patient's lead during session Identifies transference but cannot link it to the experience in the session
Average	Lets patient set the agenda Regular use of closed-ended questions, offers advice Emphasizes supportive techniques over uncovering techniques Listens empathically Does not promote uncovering or deepening of understanding Identifies transference and countertransference but cannot use them to deepen the patient's experience
Above Average	Lets patient set the agenda Asks mostly open-ended questions Promotes uncovering and deepening of understanding Tolerates silence Listens empathically Comments on the transference when appropriate Identifies countertransference in supervision
Excellent	Lets patient set the agenda Promotes uncovering and deepening of understanding Tolerates silence Asks mostly open-ended questions Listens empathically Begins to link conscious thoughts and feelings of the patient to past experience and expectations of others Comments on the transference to deepen the patient's experience Deftly uses countertransference for diagnostic purposes and to understand the formulation

Figure 6–2.   American Association of Directors of Psychiatry Residency Training (AADPRT) Foundations of Psychodynamic Psychotherapy—Interventions.

Source.   Reproduced with permission from American Association of Directors of Psychiatry Residency Training.

In the video, she is discussing her difficulty accepting her boyfriend's wishes to spend time with his friends without her, and then shifts into having felt so alone when her father died after she had graduated from college. Dr. H remains silent but engaged while Ms. R discusses her loneliness and feeling left out. After a few minutes, he asks her whether there were similarities between her experience with her father and her feelings with her boyfriend. Dr. Y refers to the AADPRT Foundations of Psychodynamic Psychotherapy—Priorities form and points out that Dr. H's response warrants a "4 or better" rating on areas 1 ("Focusing on affect and expression of emotions") and 3 ("Identifying recurrent themes and patterns in relationships") of the form. Dr. H tolerated his patient's intense affect around loneliness and allowed her to continue speaking, and in supervision identified and reflected on his own feelings of sadness in hearing the patient's story. Finally, at a time that felt appropriate, he asked Ms. R about connections between the two experiences, thereby facilitating further exploration rather than shutting down the affect or subject area. Dr. H leaves the supervision session with increased confidence in his abilities as a therapist.

Structured forms also allow for constructive feedback about concrete ways to improve practice.

A few weeks later, during a session with the same patient, Dr. H abruptly announces an upcoming absence and his need to cancel a future session. Ms. R momentarily looks deflated and catches her breath when Dr. H makes the announcement. Within moments, however, she is smiling and appears recovered. Dr. H does not seem to notice her affect at the time, and they end the session. In supervision, Dr. Y uses the AADPRT Foundations of Psychodynamic Psychotherapy—Priorities form. After the two of them re-watch this discussion, Dr. Y asks Dr. H to rate himself on area 5 ("Focusing on the therapy relationship"). Dr. H immediately identifies the nonverbal cues he had not noticed or addressed during the session. He gives himself a "1." He recalls having felt anxious about discussing his upcoming vacation. Although Ms. R has always handled his absences graciously, Dr. H found himself "feeling weirdly uncomfortable" about announcing it, and he avoided bringing it up until the last minute. After Dr. Y and Dr. H discuss this countertransference material, they role-play different strategies for announcing upcoming absences.

When integrated periodically into regular psychotherapy supervision, these tools may help identify salient areas for improvement or praise and lead to direct conversations about trainees' performance.

The "Priorities" and "Interventions" forms can also be used to develop and train psychotherapy supervisors. One approach might be to introduce the forms in didactics to interested faculty, followed by practice, in small groups, in using the forms with a video of psychotherapy. In a small pilot study in which attendees of a monthly psychotherapy supervisor group received training in the use of structured assessment tools for supervision, these tools were described as "very useful" or "extremely useful" by 85% of attendees, and 100% said that they had used at least one of the tools (Welton et al. 2019). Familiarity with a variety of assessment tools with differing approaches and priorities helps new supervisors develop confidence in their growing skill sets.

In the process of using and educating others in the use of these tools, the forms' authors have encountered skepticism in some colleagues regarding the forms' anticipated utility. Here are some suggested answers to concerns that might arise:

- These forms do not try to capture the expertise and nuance that individual supervisors bring to supervision; rather, they are intended to help provide a consistent structure and ensure that "the basics" are sufficiently covered.
- These forms are not intended to take the place of "regular" supervision; rather, they are used to augment supervision.
- Supervisors might consider trying these forms as an experiment to see whether they lead to a more productive, focused discussion. If they do not, or if they appear to derail supervision, supervisors should stop using them.

Incorporating Patient Preferences and Outcome Measurement Into Supervision

Psychotherapy supervision aims to help both supervisees and the patients they are treating. Optimally, for a fuller perspective on the work of trainees, supervisors would also obtain feedback from trainees' patients. Although discussions between supervisor and patient may be potentially problematic and lead to new complications, depending on the setting, this information can be obtained in other ways. Preferences of patients and measurement of outcomes are crucial sources of information that are often overlooked by psychotherapy supervisors.

Patients usually arrive in the therapist's office with preexisting ideas about how psychotherapy will be conducted that are based on their own previous experiences, on what they have heard from others, or on what they have seen in popular media. Patients might have fixed expectations about the topics that will be covered by the therapist or the style of interactions they expect to experience. Discrepancies between what the patient expects and what the therapist plans on offering can fracture the therapeutic alliance and may lead to early termination. Studies have found that addressing patients' preferences leads to improved patient outcomes and reduces the likelihood that patients will prematurely leave treatment (Swift et al. 2011). The Cooper-Norcross Inventory of Preferences (Cooper and Norcross 2016) is one example of a form developed to help therapists discuss these issues with their patients. Supervisors can recommend that supervisees use this form when starting therapy with a new patient. The form may help supervisors and supervisees identify and label patient preferences that, if undisclosed, might threaten therapy (Cooper and Norcross 2016).

Supervisors can also recommend periodic use of outcome measures designed to document patient progress. Although therapists may view the benefits of psychodynamic psychotherapy as being less amenable to measurement via standardized tools, patients may appreciate the opportunity to report on their symptoms or functioning. Patient-completed questionnaires can provide objective reassurance that therapy is helping. Equally, a lack of progress on these measures may signal a stalled or "stuck" therapy. While therapists often serve as the containers of the hope necessary to advance the difficult work of therapy, therapists may at times hold overly optimistic views of their patients' potential for change. In these instances, routine use of outcome measures can be helpful. One of the best-studied instruments for ongoing outcome measurement is the Outcome Questionnaire–45 (OQ-45) (Lambert et al. 2004), which monitors patient distress, relationships, and social functioning. Use of this type of measure has been found to enhance the impact of psychotherapy and lead to greater posttreatment gains, including higher percentages of patients reporting clinically significant change, and reductions in dropout rates. In a meta-analysis of 24 studies examining the use of routine outcome monitoring (ROM), 73% of the studies using ROM showed improvement in outcomes (Lambert et al. 2018; Whipple and Lambert 2011). ROM seems most helpful in detecting signs that a patient's situation is deteriorating. Use of outcome measures can decrease the rate of deterioration and actually improve outcomes (Tarescavage and Ben-Porath 2014) and can remind supervisees of the importance of patient perspectives within the therapeutic relationship. Two related tools are the Outcome Rating Scale and the Session Rating Scale (Campbell and Hemsley 2009). These brief visual analog scales take only seconds to complete. The Outcome Rating Scale asks patients to indicate how they are doing individually, interpersonally, socially, and overall, while the Session Rating Scale measures aspects of the therapeutic alliance. Both scales have good psychometric properties (Campbell and Hemsley 2009) and offer an objective way to access patients' perspectives.

Conclusion

Use of structured tools and approaches may help supervisors and supervisees organize supervision and foster more objectively based feedback. The rating scales developed by the AADPRT Psychotherapy Committee (such as the A-MAP and the Foundations of Psychodynamic Psychotherapy forms) can help supervisors bring more clarity to the assessment of observed patient encounters and offer more detailed and specific feedback. Use of patient preference forms and outcome rating scales can lead to lively discussions in supervision about the therapy process and can improve the trainee's performance and highlight the patient's progress in therapy. These forms can also be used to train psychotherapy supervisors and help them develop their skills.

References

AADPRT: AADPRT (American Association of Directors of Psychiatric Residency Training) Psychotherapy Committee. 2020. Available at: www.aadprt.org/application/files/5115/9119/8671/Compiled_Committee_Charges_on_Letterhead_060120.pdf. Accessed December 30, 2020.

Anderson PAM: Giving feedback on clinical skills: are we starving our young? J Grad Med Educ 4(2):154–158, 2012 23730434

Blagys MD, Hilsenroth MJ: Distinctive features of short-term psychodynamic-interpersonal psychotherapy: a review of the comparative psychotherapy process literature. Clinical Psychology: Science and Practice 7(2):167–188, 2000

Branch WT Jr, Paranjape A: Feedback and reflection: teaching methods for clinical settings. Acad Med 77(12 Pt 1):1185–1188, 2002 12480619

Brehaut JC, Colquhoun HL, Eva KW, et al: Practice feedback interventions: 15 suggestions for optimizing effectiveness. Ann Intern Med 164(6):435–441, 2016 26903136

Campbell A, Hemsley S: Outcome Rating Scale and Session Rating Scale in psychological practice: clinical utility of ultra-brief measures. Clinical Psychologist 13(1):1–9, 2009. Available at: https://www.tandfonline.com/doi/abs/10.1080/13284200802676391?journalCode=rcnp20. Accessed August 12, 2022.

Cooper M, Norcross JC: A brief, multidimensional measure of clients' therapy preferences: the Cooper-Norcross Inventory of Preferences (C-NIP). Int J Clin Health Psychol 16(1):87–98, 2016 30487853

Davis DA, Mazmanian PE, Fordis M, et al: Accuracy of physician self-assessment compared with observed measures of competence: a systematic review. JAMA 296(9):1094–1102, 2006 16954489

Ende J: Feedback in clinical medical education. JAMA 250(6):777–781, 1983 6876333

Haggerty GH, Hilsenroth MJ: The use of video in psychotherapy supervision. British Journal of Psychotherapy 27(2):193–210, 2011

Hattie J, Timperley H: The power of feedback. Review of Educational Research 77(1):81–112, 2007

Hoop JG: Hidden ethical dilemmas in psychiatric residency training: the psychiatry resident as dual agent. Acad Psychiatry 28(3):183–189, 2004 15507552

Lambert MJ, Gregersen AT, Burlingame GM: The Outcome Questionnaire–45, in The Use of Psychological Testing for Treatment Planning and Outcomes Assessment: Instruments for Adults. Edited by Maruish ME. Mahwah, NJ, Lawrence Erlbaum, 2004, pp 191–234

Lambert MJ, Whipple JL, Kleinstäuber M: Collecting and delivering progress feedback: a meta-analysis of routine outcome monitoring. Psychotherapy (Chic) 55(4):520–537, 2018 30335463

Sargeant J, Bruce D, Campbell CM: Practicing physicians' needs for assessment and feedback as part of professional development. J Contin Educ Health Prof 33(1, suppl 1):S54–S62, 2013 24347154

Shanfield SB, Hetherly VV, Matthews KL: Excellent supervision: the residents' perspective. J Psychother Pract Res 10(1):23–27, 2001 11121004

Shedler J: The efficacy of psychodynamic psychotherapy. Am Psychol 65(2):98–109, 2010 20141265

Stalmeijer RE, Dolmans DHJM, Wolfhagen IHAP, et al: Combined student ratings and self-assessment provide useful feedback for clinical teachers. Adv Health Sci Educ Theory Pract 15(3):315–328, 2010 19779976

Swift JK, Callahan JL, Vollmer BM: Preferences. J Clin Psychol 67(2):155–165, 2011 21120917

Tarescavage AM, Ben-Porath YS: Psychotherapeutic outcomes measures: a critical review for practitioners. J Clin Psychol 70(9):808–830, 2014 24652811

Veloski J, Boex JR, Grasberger MJ, et al: Systematic review of the literature on assessment, feedback and physicians' clinical performance: BEME Guide No. 7. Med Teach 28(2):117–128, 2006 16707292

Welton R, Nelson S, Cowan A, Correll T: Supporting and training psychotherapy supervisors. Acad Psychiatry 43(4):464–465, 2019 31161573

Whipple JL, Lambert MJ: Outcome measures for practice. Annu Rev Clin Psychol 7:87–111, 2011 21166536

Wood BP: Feedback: a key feature of medical training. Radiology 215(1):17–19, 2000 10751460

Yourman DB: Trainee disclosure in psychotherapy supervision: the impact of shame. J Clin Psychol 59(5):601–609, 2003 12696135

PART II

How to Supervise Psychodynamic Psychotherapy

7

The Process of Psychotherapy Supervision

Monica Carsky, Ph.D.
Frank E. Yeomans, M.D., Ph.D.

KEY LEARNING GOALS

- The process of supervision requires clarification of roles, boundaries, and expectations for supervisors and therapists.

- Supervisors can help therapists create appropriate boundaries and expectations with patients.

- Supervision plays a crucial role in enabling therapists to accept, identify, and use countertransference to identify otherwise hidden aspects of the patient that, when understood, may help advance the therapy.

- Supervision can help therapists develop a way to balance intellectual and emotional processing of therapy session material.

PSYCHOTHERAPY SUPERVISION has dual goals: to improve the skills of the trainee therapist being supervised, and to improve the quality of therapy received by the supervisee's patient so as to maximize that patient's progress. In some cases, supervision is part of a formal training program for a not-yet-licensed clinician, and the supervisor may be taking legal responsibility for the treatment. Beyond this, therapists at all stages in their careers who seek to increase their sensitivity and knowledge may pursue supervision or consultation, either on a regular basis or for specific cases. Indeed, regular sharing of one's work is recommended to avoid chronic blind spots or stalemates that may be more easily recognized by an outside observer. Supervision requires addressing both the intellectual and the emotional learning of the supervisee.

Within psychodynamic thinking, varying theoretical positions interpret session material differently and therefore may favor different techniques or recommend alternative approaches, influencing what is conveyed in supervisory meetings. In general, psychodynamic psychotherapies use techniques organized around free association. The overall goal is to help patients become aware of elements within their minds that have an impact on what they feel, think, and do that they have previously resisted awareness of. Material from the patient's past and present life, fantasies, dreams, and transference developments, are seen as windows into the patient's current psychological functioning, which can be understood and interpreted. Communication between patient and therapist may take place via nonverbal as well as verbal avenues, including the emotions each one experiences in the session. How patients interact with their therapists can illuminate unconscious assumptions about the self and other people that have caused or significantly contributed to patients' emotional and behavioral problems. Therapists try to show patients how their thoughts and actions, especially those in the session, are colored by perceptions and assumptions that may not fully apply to the present situation.

Establishing the Supervisory Frame

Supervisors have the primary responsibility for introducing and managing important concrete aspects of the supervisory frame to facilitate the intellectual and emotional learning of supervisees. These aspects include both the boundaries and the details of the supervisory process.

Boundaries

The supervisor is primarily responsible for clarifying and managing the boundaries of the supervisory setting (McWilliams 2021). The specific situation of the supervisee, whether in training, an employee, or a colleague, will determine the responsibilities to any outside systems, such as a health care organization (records, policies), a training program (documentation of material learned, evaluations), and/or a governmental/administrative entity (licensing, legal notifications or reporting). For example, there may be specific requirements pertaining to what information about the patient or supervisee will be shared, and with whom; how evaluations, if any, will be handled; who will receive the trainee's feedback about the supervisor; how often the supervisor and supervisee will meet, and for how long; and how communications between sessions will be handled. These details, as well as how the supervisor plans to translate the institution's expectations into practice, should be clearly established at the outset of supervision. These discussions with supervisees will help them to understand the frame and also will model how to create and maintain adaptive boundaries with patients and other systems.

Goals and Details of the Supervision Process

What will be taught in supervision? Is any specific material (e.g., types of interventions, disclosure of staff training levels, name of supervisor) required by the program or setting? Does the therapist have a specific area that he or she wishes to work on? Will the therapist in training be learning one "brand" of psychodynamic thinking or learning several? What will be presented, and how? What additional material (e.g., readings, counter-transference issues, theoretical questions) should the supervisee expect to discuss? In a study of "best" and "worst" psychotherapy supervision experiences, Allen et al. (1986) found that graduate students gave higher ratings to supervisors who clearly communicated their expectations and feedback. How will feedback about the supervisee's strengths and weaknesses be provided during the course of supervision? How will supervisory goals (see Chapter 8) be set?

It is the supervisor's responsibility to create and maintain a setting that facilitates the work of supervision. This task requires fostering a foundation of mutual trust, so that the therapist can trust the supervisor enough to talk about countertransference, and the supervisor can trust that the therapist is reporting honestly. Discussion, understanding, and (hopefully) agreement between the supervisor and supervisee set the framework for the supervision, so that each knows how to prepare and what to expect. This discussion models for the therapist the importance of introducing a frame to provide structure, as will be necessary in the psychotherapy. The resulting supervision and therapy structures support containment of anxieties in the participants so that these can be addressed.

Supervisors can encourage therapists to think about their recent therapy sessions ahead of supervisory meetings by asking themselves the following questions:

- How did this session feel? What was my/the patient's strongest emotion?
- How was the patient relating to me?
- What types of transference/countertransference did I notice or experience?
- How might recent therapy session interactions or events in the patient's life be affecting the patient's current situation? Was one of us absent recently, or is a break planned?
- Does the patient have a recent personal situation affecting him or her? Has the patient called me since the last session?

Facilitating Learning in Supervision

The supervisor's role is to encourage the supervisee's learning in four key areas:

1. Mastery of theory and technique
2. Emotional learning
3. Connection of emotional learning with intellectual learning
4. Development of a personal identity as a therapist

Teaching Theory and Technique

Traditionally, learning psychotherapy techniques requires a combination of didactics and apprenticeship. The supervisee presents a description and an account of the patient and of the therapy sessions. The supervisor fills in gaps in the supervisee's cognitive knowledge, particularly regarding how to think about a given patient, and helps the supervisee to understand their emotional reactions to the patient and to transform intellectual understanding of theory and technique into interventions.

In supervision, as in therapy, a clear set of issues and priorities needs to be kept in mind (Yeomans et al. 2015). At the beginning of supervising a case, the supervisor will want an accurate diagnosis to assess the appropriateness of the therapy being provided and whether the structure of the therapy is adequate for this patient. One aspect of the evaluation prior to beginning therapy is clarification of the patient's reasons for seeking treatment and goals for therapy. This task often requires helping patients to describe how they hope their lives will be different as a result of therapy, regardless of whether these hopes are realistic. The therapist may try to tactfully add any problems that the patient has omitted but that are evident in the patient's interactions. As both the therapy and the supervision proceed, the supervisor monitors the therapist's attention to both the process in the sessions and developments in the patient's life, including the emergence of new and/or urgent issues (O.F. Kernberg, personal communication, September 2021). This is in contrast to a purely psychoanalytic approach that strictly follows the material the patient provides without the therapist ever inquiring about the patient's current life.

Teaching supervisees to think about their work requires helping them to identify a patient's communications (both verbal and nonverbal) in terms of their function and meaning in the therapy. For example, does the patient's way of communicating express wishes or fears? A need to control the therapist? A need to either push away or cling to the therapist? An attempt to compete or attack? A wish to care for, or to elicit care from, the therapist? A starting point in understanding a patient is to understand the patient's attitude toward the therapy and the therapist, which might be implicit in his or her way of communicating.

It is helpful for the supervisor to label interventions—for example, clarification; confrontation; interpretation of defenses, wishes, and fears and hypotheses about what might motivate these. Supervision helps the therapist to identify and interpret defenses that are played out in the therapeutic field, such as splitting or projective identification. Supervision then proceeds to help the therapist develop hypotheses regarding the internal conflicts underlying these defenses, ideally while keeping in mind the patient's reality and the overall goals of the therapy. We add the latter consideration because of the risk that a dynamic therapy can become an exercise in intellectualization, separate from the patient's life problems. Supervisors can help therapists identify their own actions and emotions in and around the session in order to understand the dynamics underlying the therapy.

> SUPERVISEE: Today Mr. Z (the supervisee's patient) told me that I was clueless. I was already feeling that way, and decided that he was right. He went on to say that I could never understand him because I never get drunk, so I have no idea what it's like to feel out of control and therefore all I do is criticize him! And then he said that just because he can't talk to me doesn't mean I'm special, because he can't talk to his friends either. I felt his devaluation, but I held off commenting on it because I thought he looked sad.
>
> SUPERVISOR: I think it would be fine for you to point out how important it is to him to make sure you will not think you are special, as if this would somehow, in his mind, diminish him. Your feeling may be a good example of projective identification—you end up feeling stupid, while the patient feels superior and, in effect, has managed to transpose all of his weak, stupid, undesirable feelings to you, where he can look at them with contempt. We can see how Mr. Z accom-

plishes this; he drops hints and discourages you from asking questions by making it seem as if he is about to tell you more. Then he takes pleasure in telling you that you are stupid, for not knowing something he has not told you!

When supervisors help trainees to identify potential meanings behind the processes in the patient–therapist pair, a more thoughtful consideration of potential responses and interventions may ensue.

In addition to reviewing process material, an essential role of supervisors is to assist supervisees in setting and maintaining the frame in the treatment. Attention to the treatment frame can help therapists feel comfortable with their emotional reactions. For example, a supervisee might say, "I'm feeling guilty that I don't extend the sessions for this patient when he is so upset. Is that a reasonable way for me to feel, given the severity of his problems? Or is it something evoked in me from something in the patient's internal world, maybe his intense neediness or entitlement?" The supervisor can remind the supervisee of the treatment frame that was initially set ("You and the patient agreed that sessions would be 45 minutes") to help the therapist distinguish between the reality of the situation and the evoked emotions that correspond to a part of the patient's internal experience. This needs to be elaborated and discussed to further the process of understanding. Failure to maintain time and other boundaries and to make sure that all participants are informed is likely to represent a maladaptive acting out or a collusion with some level of pathology in the system or the individual. Often it is the supervisor, as an outsider, who first notices challenges to or breaks in the frame. Sometimes a boundary problem in the therapy parallels a dynamic in the patient's life. For example, patients engaged in outpatient therapy who also see a separate coach or counselor can create systems based on splits in their internal world, dividing others into "the good" and "the bad," the idealized and the devalued.

The treatment frame is also an important tool for containing intense and unsymbolized affects (i.e., affects that are experienced but not yet captured in words). These split-off affects may be at the core of many patients' difficulties and thus need to be reflected upon and integrated into patients' conscious experience (Yeomans et al. 1992, 2015). In some cases, a supervisee's difficulties in dealing with emotions evoked in therapy sessions may lead the supervisor to discuss the advisability of the supervisee engaging in personal therapy to work on what may be his or her own unresolved issues (Kernberg 2023).

Supervisors can facilitate supervisees' recognition of how the patient's level of functioning affects the treatment frame and how interventions are understood and managed. Traditionally, psychodynamic psychotherapy has been conducted with patients who are in the higher-functioning category of personality disorders. In the therapy of patients who are generally functional (if conflicted), standard aspects of the therapeutic frame, such as expectations regarding attendance and payment, are less likely to be used by patients to express defended-against wishes and fears or to enact maladaptive relationship paradigms. With patients who are prone to impulsive behavior and acting out, or who simply have difficulty being aware of and communicating their emotions verbally, negotiation of frame expectations and treatment requirements is very important at the beginning of therapy, as is attention to these issues as the therapy progresses (Carsky 2020; Yeomans et al. 2017). Usually it is necessary for the supervisor to help the therapist explore and interpret patients' inevitable challenges to these agreed-upon conditions of treatment. For example, a patient who keeps talking after the therapist points out that it is time to end the session may be communicating an intense neediness, a sense of entitlement, or a need to control the other. Attention to the deviation from the frame provides a window into these issues.

Offering theoretical constructs can help orient therapists to interventions necessary for a particular patient. Reviewing these at the beginning of a case helps supervisees integrate their clinical assessments with theory. For example, to what extent does a patient's level of pathology dictate how much structure is required in the therapy and the supervision? Does the supervisor's preferred theory, or assessment of a particular patient, focus on conflict or deficit as the core of the patient's difficulties? Subsequent to that, will the therapy be focused on the internal and external manifestations of psychic conflict, or will it include some support regarding life issues, along with interpretation of psychological conflict? Will the therapy focus more on antecedents of current problems, or on how problems are manifested in the present? To operationalize this: should the therapist be sensitive to and listen primarily to the content of what the patient is saying, to the interpersonal process in the session, or to both?

Some therapeutic approaches emphasize work in the "here and now," using patients' references to the past to help describe how patients relate to the therapist and other important people in their current lives. These approaches focus on how patients enact their internal relationship paradigms interpersonally. Therapists using these approaches learn to identify a relationship that a patient seems to be enacting or activating with the therapist, who may initially sense this only through countertransference. Here, the supervisor serves the crucial role of "observer of the relationship," a third party who is free to identify with either the therapist or the patient in order to describe how each person seems to be relating, and perhaps why, based on the patient's needs to defend against awareness of certain aspects of the patient's internal world.

Facilitating Emotional Learning

The process of becoming a skilled psychodynamic therapist is an emotional as well as an intellectual journey. Aspects of psychodynamic psychotherapy require therapists to access and make use of their own emotional responses, in contrast to being overwhelmed or disabled by them (Carsky 2021). This entails awareness of countertransference tendencies, blind spots, and urges to "fix" a patient's problems, for example, instead of cultivating an attitude of curiosity and openness to the new components—thoughts, experiences, feelings, associations—in the patient's material. Supervision facilitates the trainee's development of an emotional stance for listening in therapy, with the supervisor simultaneously teaching and modeling how to do this work—accepting, identifying, and dealing with transference and countertransference feelings; determining what enhances the patient's involvement and progress in the therapy; and clarifying the patient's emotional responses to interventions, to name but a few.

Helping therapists to tolerate feelings is a major role for the supervisor (Ungar and de Ahumada 2001). Therapists with a limited view of dynamic therapy may assume that they are supposed to say little and feel little emotion. Supervisors have an important part to play in reducing supervisees' anxious responses to their own and the patient's affects, particularly negative affects. This requires the supervisor to share theoretical knowledge about the use of countertransference in understanding patient dynamics and to show how the therapist's experience and observations in this realm may clarify a patient's internal world of relationship patterns and assumptions about the self and others.

> Following the evaluation, a trainee therapist presented her diagnostic impressions to the patient in lay language and connected this understanding of the patient's problems with a recommendation for psychodynamic therapy. In discussing what was entailed in this therapy, she spoke of how important it was for the patient to share everything that was going through his mind, including any thoughts, even negative ones, about the therapy or the therapist. The patient began to describe episodes of intense rage in his life and how hard he was finding these to control. The therapist felt unsettled and nervously waited for more material. With some anxiety, she brought this interaction up in supervision, saying that she felt as though the patient's comments were particularly directed at her.
>
> The supervisor agreed that patients and therapists are always reacting to one another, and in addition, suggested that the patient might be "testing" to see whether the therapist was serious about her willingness to lis-

ten to all of the patient's thoughts and be exposed to all of his emotional states, even rageful material that could be directed at the therapist. The supervisor proposed that the therapist could usefully share this idea with the patient—that the patient was "checking," in effect, to see whether the therapist really meant what she said. Both the patient and (to some extent) the therapist were "testing the waters" to see what they were able to talk about. This is also an example of *parallel process* (discussed later; see section "Parallel Process and Transference in the Supervisory Relationship").

To carry out effective psychodynamic therapy, therapists must be able to access their own internal world of intense affects—desires, fears, fantasies—in an unconflicted way. Although most supervisees consciously desire to learn how to be good therapists, the need to acquire a complex skill is typically accompanied by unconscious or even conscious wishes that this learning will not be too painful to their self-esteem. Supervisees respond well to supervisors who are trustworthy and supportive, who emphasize personal growth (Allen et al. 1986), and who provide examples of what to say and do (Eubanks et al. 2019). Therapists are grateful for a supervisory atmosphere of support and validation, which makes it easier for them to report confusing and difficult encounters with patients, particularly embarrassing ones, and to share negative transference and countertransference experiences.

Learning how to assess one's own countertransference is a basic task for new psychotherapists. One important potential source of conscious or unconscious countertransference is the social identities of the patient and the therapist, their similarities, and their differences. Do they share cultural, racial, gender, geographic, professional, sexual, or religious identities? What is the patient's social and financial situation? Is therapy paid for by the patient, the family, insurance, disability, or government programs? Therapists may need education, modeling, and practice to become sensitive to the potential effects of these factors on the patient and the therapy, as well as on their own countertransference tendencies.

Supervisors should monitor themselves for their own countertransference responses when listening to trainees describe their encounters with patients. Their countertransference response may match the therapist's countertransference response, or it may differ from what the therapist is feeling, in which case it might reflect a defensive position on the part of the therapist or the supervisor that should be discussed.

A trainee therapist was discussing the case of a 50-year-old patient with a diagnosis of narcissistic personality disorder who spoke angrily in session about the incompetence of the boss who had just fired him. In supervision, the therapist emphasized the need to help the patient deal with his anger.

The supervisor, who was more familiar with the dynamics of narcissistic personality disorder and the risk of the sudden, total collapse of a narcissistic patient's self-esteem after his defensive outrage ceased to contain his despair, experienced anxiety about the possible risk of suicide in the patient after the narcissistic injury of being fired. She was struck by the relative calmness with which the therapist discussed the issue as principally a problem around the patient's angry affects. The supervisor tactfully introduced her concern into the discussion, and the therapist became aware that he was defensively accepting his patient's grandiose devaluation of his boss. He was avoiding, as was the patient, being in touch with the despair that the patient's fragile grandiosity was defending against.

Supervisees can experience fear of negative affects. Many psychiatric conditions, such as anxiety, depression, and personality disorders, involve a patient's difficulties in accepting and successfully managing negative affects. Trainees sometimes do not recognize how aggressive and devaluing some patients can be in the transference (and in their daily lives) and are unaware that this is not obvious to the patients, who feel completely justified in these behaviors (Yeomans et al. 2015). Therapists often need assistance in discussing patients' aggression toward them without appearing aggressive, apologetic, or fearful, and they also need examples of how to analyze a patient's response to such therapist statements. Negative countertransference can be particularly difficult for many supervisees. They may have chosen a field that on a conscious level aligns with their values of helping others but on an unconscious level involves expiation of childhood guilt through a fantasy of being perfectly understanding and all-giving. A therapist with such a self-image would not take well to statements by a patient that challenged the therapist's competence or good intentions. Identifying this tendency in supervision can be helpful, but addressing it fully should be left to the supervisee's personal psychotherapy. Unless negative countertransference feelings are adequately worked through, the psychotherapist will be substantially inhibited by this issue.

A trainee therapist in supervision who was treating an extremely narcissistic, infantile patient, agreed to see the patient for a low fee at an inconvenient time, even though the patient often canceled at the last minute. When the patient told the therapist that his pharmacologist had also agreed to see him for a low fee but had stipulated that when the patient got a raise, he would increase the patient's fee, the therapist was surprised but failed to see any transference reference in the patient's disclosure of this information, and he resisted his supervisor's recommendation that he explore making the same stipulation with the patient. From the supervisor's perspective, the therapist was participating in, rather than exploring, a treatment situation involving both the patient's devaluing and exploit-ative characteristics and perhaps the therapist's own need to adhere to an image of himself as a "good object."

Supervisees may fear primitive (i.e., bizarre sexual or aggressive images), intense, emotional, or irrational material related to unconscious fantasies. Some fear hearing about primitive thoughts, fantasies, or behaviors in patients, and may react, for example, by becoming overly strict in structuring the therapy. Their interventions are more about behavioral control and less likely to encourage patients to think about their internal world and the associated unconscious dynamics motivating their behaviors. This is one reason that supervisors need to know the details of what therapists say to their patients, to recognize when the trainee's anxiety interferes with further psychological exploration and also to have hypotheses as to why. Therapists with a rigid or hypercritical sense of self may find it hard to entertain what might be primitive aggressive and/or erotic countertransference reactions and fantasies. They need to witness supervisors' comfortable acceptance of such feelings in themselves and their supervisees, which reinforces the idea that even bizarre-seeming negative or erotic responses in the therapist may be extremely useful in understanding patients.

Some therapists fear upsetting patients. Although the timing of interpretive comments is important, some therapists may be hampered by a feeling that they should never say anything that will upset a patient. However, in the therapy of acting-out and self-destructive patients, it is necessary to discuss difficult material, such as the patient's aggressive behavior toward self or others, contradictory statements, or lapses in reasoning. The therapist may need to remind the patient of the constraints of reality (for example, stalking an ex-lover could lead to a restraining order). Therapists have trouble with this for many reasons, one of which is fear that the patient may respond to the session with even more distressing activities. Sadly, this can prevent therapists from discussing dangerous behaviors in an open way. The most extreme example is avoiding a potentially suicidal patient's negative transference feelings or self-destructive acting out because the therapist fears that the patient might make a suicide attempt in response to discussion of these feelings. Failure to address a patient's real and fantasized destructiveness with appropriate limits can lead to treatment failures (Gabbard 2003; Maltsberger and Buie 1974; Plakun 2001). The supervisor must be very sensitive in listening for any evidence that the therapist is avoiding material and must help him or her overcome that resistance.

After a careful initial evaluation, a patient with a history of suicidal feelings or self-destructiveness should be asked to engage in planning, with the therapist, for how to address such impulses in the future. Non-psychotic patients should be capable of determining when they are at risk of actually acting on such feelings and can be asked to commit to seeking help by going to the emergency room or calling 911 if they feel unable to control a suicidal or self-destructive impulse. This is clearly differentiated from the possibility that the patient might well continue to have suicidal thoughts and feelings that he or she can control and should bring these into sessions for exploration. With this agreement in place, the therapist should feel less inhibited about presenting and examining challenging material with the patient and freer to notice and address negative transference and countertransference. The careful development of treatment arrangements before therapy proper begins is a way to help both the patient and the therapist feel comfortable exploring these feelings, in contrast to feeling anxious and intimidated by them (Yeomans et al. 2015). Importantly, the therapist and the patient will have agreed on the plan prior to beginning the treatment. The supervisor's care with the frame of the supervision—time, responsibilities, expectations—conveys a similar message about the importance of a setting in which all feelings can be discussed safely.

Connecting Emotional Learning With Intellectual Learning

Experienced therapists are able to alternate smoothly and relatively rapidly between experiencing and conceptualizing, conveying a sense of engaging in these processes simultaneously. The development of this skill is aided by a supervisor who supports the therapist's emotional engagement with the patient while teaching and modeling how to understand such engagement as a possible clue to session dynamics. Over time, this enhances therapists' ability to integrate cognition and affect in themselves and their patients.

Supervisors can help trainees to conceptualize the therapeutic process both cognitively and emotionally. Apart from the risk of therapists enacting their countertransferences, perhaps the greatest single challenge in supervision is helping supervisees translate their understanding of an aspect of the patient's mental functioning into language that is accessible to the patient (i.e., "patient-friendly") rather than abstract and intellectualized. It helps to start by observing a specific aspect of the interaction between patient and therapist and using that to create a hypothesis about patient dynamics, so that patients understand how they came to experience the interaction in a particular way.

> A trainee therapist is treating a patient with borderline personality disorder with depressive moods, superficial cutting, rejection sensitivity, and

conflictual relationships with others. Two months into this treatment, the therapist brings the following material into supervision:

> THERAPIST: This patient's way of communicating is a pressured monologue that leaves me no room to respond. I can understand why she was previously diagnosed as bipolar. Because the nonverbal aspect of communication is important, I pointed out that her way of interacting with me was very controlling and proposed that this might be a reason a lot of people seemed to avoid her.
>
> SUPERVISOR: You're probably right, but your words might be seen as a directly critical confrontation of her behavior, without taking into account its unconscious motivation. Sharing an understanding of possible motivations might be more effective in helping her change.

The supervisor suggested a more gradual approach in which the therapist would engage the patient in a mutually curious reflection on her style of interacting. The next supervision session included the following exchange:

> THERAPIST: When I asked the patient if she had any thoughts about her way of speaking with me, she initially said she's doing what I told her: to say what's on her mind. I accepted that but pointed out that people do that in different ways, and that her way of speaking with me was so energetic and nonstop that it left me little room to reply or respond. I said that was OK, but I wondered if she had any thoughts about why she acts in that particular way. In response, she burst into tears, saying "If I didn't control you, you'd leave me, like everyone else."
>
> SUPERVISOR: It sounds like you started your intervention "from the ground up," with a mutual reflection on the interaction between you. Now you have a great opportunity to help her understand the dynamics of omnipotent control. People with this defense split off any aggressive feelings, not seeing them in themselves but imagining them in others. If their assumption is that others will be hostile to them, they feel that the only safe position is to control others in order to control their anticipated (albeit imagined) hostility. This behavior, of course, annoys others, so interactions become a vicious cycle, often leading to the feared rejection.

In the next session, the therapist used this formulation, which helped the patient see that her assumption that "people will leave me" led her to behave in ways that could be experienced as negative by others. The therapist and patient then proceeded to explore the origins of the patient's assumption that others would be hostile and rejecting of her.

When supervisors enable trainees to feel comfortable reporting difficulties with their therapy patients, trainees may become more aware of the process of therapy and more accepting of their own feelings. Seeing their patients respond positively to interventions recommended by the supervisor as being helpful will also enhance supervisees' learning of therapeutic techniques, particularly if the supervisor explains why an intervention was useful and shows how the patient's response demonstrates this. In general, a useful intervention frees patients to share more of themselves—whether in the form of insight, elaboration of material, or corroborating examples, or even in the form of a clearer example of a defense in process (e.g., a patient who responds to a clarification of reality with "I don't care!" or a similar dramatic denial).

Enabling a Supervisee to Develop an Identity as a Therapist

In a survey of 205 subjects, including 78 supervisor–therapist pairs, Nagell et al. (2014) found that supervision experiences that emphasized "relational competence" as well as knowledge and skill received the highest ratings for identity development (from supervisees) and satisfaction (from both parties). A potential complication in this may be idealization of the supervisor by the supervisee. One way to counter supervisor idealization is to help therapists develop an independent capacity to think about session material, their patients' conflicts and defenses, and their own reactions, defenses, and conflicts in a way that will advance the treatment. A respectful, serious, but relaxed attitude by the supervisor helps (Kernberg 2010). Encouraging supervisees to freely question supervisors about their thinking and decision making also facilitates this goal.

Development of an individual's professional identity may involve the therapist borrowing from different therapy models. Even though supervisors have preferred theories, they should be knowledgeable about other approaches and be open to discussing how these might understand a particular patient differently. Therapists need a balance between dogmatic adherence to a single therapy model and chaotic use of interventions from disparate models. It takes time and supervisory support for therapists to internalize what is learned and establish a personal voice within the application of a model.

Parallel Process and Transference in the Supervisory Relationship

At times during the supervisory process, the trainee therapist or the supervisor may unwittingly take on the role of one of the patient's *internal objects* (an unconscious mental representation of self or other that corresponds to an urge or a defense), so that the supervisory pair enacts the same dynamic that is active in the patient–therapist pair. This "parallelism" phenomenon (Caligor 1981; Gediman and Wolkenfeld 1980) may also be seen as a subtype of the influence of system dynamics.

> A supervisee was reporting on a complex patient who rejected most of what he said to her in therapy sessions. The patient claimed that his questions about her activities were inappropriate and that his interpretations were just wrong, and when he tried to simply reflect back what she said by rephrasing it, the patient criticized him even more. In response to his suggestions, she would explain why this was impossible to do or would not help her situation. The therapist became rather animated as he described this interchange, and the supervisor then suggested several alternative approaches. The therapist shot down each of these suggestions, asserting either that he had already tried that technique or that using that technique with this patient "would go nowhere." After a period of back and forth, the supervisor realized that nothing was being accomplished, except perhaps that he was now feeling like the supervisee had felt with his patient. He asked the supervisee whether the exchange they had just had was similar to the therapist's meetings with the patient, with one person trying hard to help and the other continually rejecting the suggestions; one very negative, and the other feeling increasingly useless. In such an interaction, both felt frustrated.
>
> The supervisor shared his observation that perhaps he was acting as the therapist had, trying to offer something helpful, while the trainee therapist was acting like the patient, rejecting all that was offered, so that the supervisor was rendered useless. The therapist was initially quite embarrassed when he recognized this pattern, but the supervisor explained that parallel process can vividly illuminate what is happening in therapy. Together they decided that the therapist would try pointing out the patient's rejection of whatever the therapist said in a nondefensive way ("You may be absolutely right in everything you say, but it still might be helpful to think about this pattern of interaction"). The supervisor suggested that the patient had a need to make the therapist feel helpless and deficient, perhaps to communicate how the patient herself often felt. In this patient's internal world, she had only two choices: identify with a weak, inferior, submissive self, or identify with a powerful, negative, rejecting internal object. Given these alternatives, the patient might well seek to make the therapist feel weak and useless, and the therapist, in turn, had shown the supervisor what they were struggling with in therapy.

In addition to parallel process situations, supervisee transference to supervisors is common. Frequently the supervisor is seen as either a critical authority or a nurturing caretaker, or the supervisee's transference alternates between the two, as when wishes for care are frustrated. Supervisors are not immune to experiencing transference reactions to their often-younger supervisees, including wishes for gratification of narcissistic needs to be idealized or to have a disciple, feelings of envy or competition, or wishes to continue a positive supervisory relationship when the supervisee is ready to be more independent. Supervisors should watch for any evidence of enactments on their part, such as being excessively critical, being excessively nurturing, or having a tendency to collect a group of admiring students. Of course, supervisors who break ethical or professional boundaries are severely damaging to a supervisee's development. Any of these could interfere with the responsible guidance and facilitation of a colleague's professional and personal growth.

Conclusion

Supervision is an emotionally and intellectually challenging undertaking for both parties, demanding careful thinking but also emotional honesty, openness, and maturity to deal with interpersonally complex and difficult situations. Skill in creating and managing goals, structures, and expectations is necessary, along with the capacity for developing appropriate teaching and mentoring relationships. Supervisors also need the ability to think in terms of systems and their boundaries as these are manifested in both the supervisory relationship and the patient-therapist relationship. Self-analytic ability will help both supervisor and supervisee to manage the interpersonal and internal work involved in a good supervisory experience.

References

Allen G, Szollos S, Williams B: Doctoral students' comparative evaluations of best and worst psychotherapy supervision. Professional Psychology: Research and Practice 17(2):91–99, 1986

Caligor L: Parallel and reciprocal processes in psychoanalytic supervision. Contemporary Psychoanalysis 17(1):1–27, 1981

Carsky M: How treatment arrangements facilitate transference interpretation in transference focused psychotherapy. Psychoanalytic Psychology 37(4):335–343, 2020

Carsky M: Managing countertransference in the treatment of personality disorders. Psychodyn Psychiatry 49(2):339–360, 2021 34061647

Eubanks CF, Muran JC, Dreher D, et al: Trainees' experiences in alliance-focused training: the risks and rewards of learning to negotiate ruptures. Psychoanalytic Psychology 36(2):122–131, 2019

Gabbard GO: Miscarriages of psychoanalytic treatment with suicidal patients. Int J Psychoanal 84(Pt 2):249–261, 2003 12856351

Gediman HK, Wolkenfeld F: The parallelism phenomenon in psychoanalysis and supervision: its reconsideration as a triadic system. Psychoanal Q 49(2):234–255, 1980 7375592

Kernberg OF: Psychoanalytic supervision: the supervisor's tasks. Psychoanal Q 79(3):603–627, 2010 20726178

Kernberg OF: Reflections on supervision, in Hatred, Emptiness, and Hope: Transference-Focused Psychotherapy in Personality Disorders. Washington, DC, American Psychiatric Association Publishing, 2023, pp. 113–130

Maltsberger JT, Buie DH: Countertransference hate in the treatment of suicidal patients. Arch Gen Psychiatry 30(5):625–633, 1974 4824197

McWilliams N: Psychoanalytic Supervision. New York, Guilford, 2021

Nagell W, Steinmetzer L, Fissabre U, Spilski J: Research into the relationship experience in supervision and its influence on the psychoanalytical identity formation of candidate trainees. Psychoanalytic Inquiry 34(6):554–583, 2014

Plakun EM: Making the alliance and taking the transference in work with suicidal patients. J Psychother Pract Res 10(4):269–276, 2001 11696654

Ungar VR, de Ahumada LB: Supervision: a container-contained approach. Int J Psychoanal 82(Pt 1):71–81, 2001 11234115

Yeomans FE, Selzer MA, Clarkin JF: Treating the Borderline Patient: A Contract-Based Approach. New York, Basic Books, 1992

Yeomans FE, Clarkin JF, Kernberg OF: Transference-Focused Psychotherapy for Borderline Personality Disorder: A Clinical Guide. Washington, DC, American Psychiatric Publishing, 2015

Yeomans FE, Delaney JC, Levy KN: Behavioral activation in TFP: the role of the treatment contract in transference-focused psychotherapy. Psychotherapy (Chic) 54(3):260–266, 2017 28922005

8

Setting Goals for Psychotherapy Supervision

Randon S. Welton, M.D.
Katherine G. Kennedy, M.D.
Frank E. Yeomans, M.D., Ph.D.

KEY LEARNING GOALS

- Work with supervisees to establish, maintain, and monitor goals for psychotherapy supervision.

- Recognize that goals in psychotherapy supervision may be chosen for many purposes, including promoting effective therapy, meeting training requirements, or improving specific clinical skills.

- Understand that goals in psychotherapy supervision will shift over time.

JUST AS PURSUING mutually acceptable goals is key for an effective therapeutic alliance, the supervisory alliance also requires both members of the supervisory dyad to work toward consensual goals (Bordin 1983) (see Chapter 4, "The Supervisor–Supervisee Relationship"). In this chapter we discuss how supervisory goals can be set for 1) learning psychotherapy skills, 2) fulfilling external program requirements, and/or 3) identifying developmentally appropriate objectives for self-improvement.

Residents devalue supervision that overlooks their concerns or does not maintain a learner-centered focus (Shanfield et al. 1993). A small pilot study dramatically demonstrated the scope of this problem. In a course evaluation survey of 16 third- and fourth-year psychiatric residents, 9 indicated that they had never discussed potential goals of supervision with their supervisor, and only 8 understood what they were supposed to be learning in psychotherapy supervision. Most of the respondents felt that there was a lack of common educational goals among their various psychotherapy supervisors (Rojas et al. 2010).

Some forms of psychotherapy, such as cognitive-behavioral therapy (CBT), focus on specific goals and objectives. CBT posits that, for both supervision and therapy, positive changes in thought and behavior require working toward consistent goals. The goals of therapy and supervision develop from identified problem areas and weaknesses. Once these deficits are identified, the supervisor and the supervisee decide which CBT-related activities (practice, homework, role-play) will help foster positive change (Sokol and Fox 2016) (see Chapter 18, "Supervision of Cognitive-Behavioral Therapy").

For psychodynamically oriented supervisors, the use of supervisory goals may feel foreign. This may stem from a mistaken view within some psychoanalytic schools that introducing goals in supervision decreases the spontaneity of both the therapy and the supervision. Yet clinical experience has revealed that a lack of clear goals may lead to unfocused, and even interminable, therapies which, in turn, has contributed to unfortunate critiques of the value of psychodynamic therapies. In fact, identifying goals in both supervision and therapy helps trainees and supervisors focus on what is important. For example, some dyads may emphasize the therapeutic frame, while others will attend to transference and countertransference; the emphasis may change as the therapy progresses. When goals are mutually chosen and phase-appropriate, they will naturally guide the supervision process (Cabaniss and Arbuckle 2011).

The Process of Setting Goals for Supervision

Supervisors can begin the goal-setting process by explaining that supervision should help supervisees develop the requisite knowledge, skills, and attitudes to enhance their effectiveness as psychotherapists. Supervisors can help supervisees increase their knowledge (e.g., master the core concepts of psychotherapy), improve their skills (e.g., ability to implement effective interventions), and change their attitudes (e.g., coming to see psychotherapy as an intrinsically collaborative effort and not as a therapist "fixing" the patient) (Cabaniss et al. 2014). Supervisors will want to ask trainees what they hope to accomplish from supervision. Anything that pertains to improvement as a therapist can form the basis of a goal.

> After 10 therapy sessions, a resident is questioning whether her patient is suitable for psychotherapy and is considering referral of the patient for medication management. The supervisor has noted a pattern for this resident of referring patients for a medication evaluation after several months of psychotherapy. The supervisee acknowledges this pattern.
>
> > SUPERVISEE: After a couple of months, I'm beginning to doubt whether therapy is helping.
> > SUPERVISOR: I wonder if the issue is really "Am I able to help?"
> > SUPERVISEE: I know that therapy works, but I'm not sure I'll ever be a good-enough therapist.
> > SUPERVISOR: It's probably not a surprise for you to hear that a lack of self-confidence is common for beginning therapists. Actually, I'd find it hard to trust any therapist who is overly confident *(normalization and validation)*. I certainly wasn't confident at your stage in training *(self-disclosure)*. But let me ask you this: based on what you already know, what are some of the most impactful aspects of therapy?
> > SUPERVISEE: Well, I know that a good therapeutic alliance correlates with improvement in therapy.
> > SUPERVISOR: So, what if we make managing the therapeutic alliance a goal for therapy and monitoring the alliance a goal for supervision? As you focus on the alliance, your patient should become more engaged in treatment. Let's look together at the process material for interactions that touch on the alliance. How does that sound? *(collaboration)*

When potential goals are not obvious, the supervisor can ask questions such as "What aspect of being a therapist seems to be the most difficult for you?" "What would you like to learn while working with me?" "What seems to be holding back your progress as a therapist?" When multiple issues are identified, the supervisor can facilitate a discussion about which goals to pursue; the ultimate choice of goals will be based on what the pair see as being most likely to be helpful. As supervision unfolds, the list of supervisory goals will be fluid and may need frequent reexamination. Met goals can be removed, and new goals added. How goals are prioritized may shift over time, as well. Choosing new goals for supervision is a collaborative and iterative process. While there is no fixed rule for the number of goals, managing more than three or four at a time may be challenging.

Learning Psychotherapy Skills

Learning to conduct any type of psychotherapy involves acquiring a complex set of knowledge, including competency with specific techniques. Developing these skills is a useful goal for supervision. While assessment of goals will structure some of the supervision, the majority of the session will focus on the process material as presented by the supervisee. A clinical crisis, such as a patient threatening self-harm, will always take precedence over process material and predetermined goals of supervision. In most supervisions, when there is no crisis, the supervision goals form the frame through which to observe the process material.

Early supervisory goals assist trainees in developing a clear understanding of the frame of psychotherapy, their role as a psychotherapist, and the conduct of therapy. Supervisors should ensure that supervisees can answer questions such as the following:

- How do I assess and conceptualize patients engaging in psychotherapy?
- How do I assess for safety issues?
- What is the rationale for/what are the goals of the psychotherapy?
- What is the purpose of free association?
- How do I maintain a therapeutic stance and avoid the temptation to engage in a more conversational dialogue?

Supervisors can help supervisees understand that therapy is designed to uncover aspects of the patient's mind, of which the patient is unaware, that greatly affect how the patient feels, thinks, and behaves. Supervisors can help supervisees develop goals for therapy based on symptom change (e.g., anxiety), behavioral change (e.g., inability to finish college), or personality change (e.g., inability to establish deep and stable interpersonal relationships). They also can help supervisees assess whether these treatment goals are shared by the patient and are realistic. Supervisors can remind trainees to maintain a focus on the patient's communication (verbal or nonverbal) in a way that invites reflection on possible deeper levels of the communication. They can assess whether trainees are using technical interventions properly (e.g., maintaining therapeutic neutrality, proposing interpretations) and using "patient-friendly language" while avoiding jargon. Supervisors can assist supervisees in connecting aspects of the patient's life with the patient's associations and generating hypotheses regarding the patient's unconscious motivations and fantasies. Trainees will need help in identifying and managing affects that arise in therapy. As supervision progresses, supervisors can help direct trainees' attention to the process of therapy. Supervisors can also ascertain whether trainees are monitoring the patient's responses to their interventions and using those responses to guide them in their next interventions (O.F. Kernberg, F.E. Yeomans, unpublished manuscript, September 15, 2021).

For the neophyte therapist, these must be among the earliest goals in supervision. As supervisees progress in their training, goals should be reviewed periodically to see if a goal has been met. If, during the course of supervision, a more pressing goal becomes obvious, that goal should become the new supervisory focus.

> SUPERVISOR: Early in the year we decided that one goal would be for you to be able to accurately explain the frame of psychotherapy and the basics of the psychodynamic approach to patients. You've had six new patients over the last several months, and we've watched videos of you discussing these issues with those patients. I think you seem comfortable with these discussions. How do you think you are doing with that goal?
>
> SUPERVISEE: After the first few times, it got easier. Actually, the last time, it just came out without me worrying at all. I feel pretty good.
>
> SUPERVISOR: Great. Let's consider that goal achieved for now. What should we focus on next?

As therapists continue to advance, they will become aware of additional areas where they need to improve. The supervisor should gently encourage this reflection and self-awareness. The supervisor and trainee should work together to establish explicit, personalized goals for learning psychotherapy skills.

> During the previous session, the resident had corrected a factual error made by the patient. In the current session, the resident makes an interpretation, to which the patient responds, "That sounds like a beginner's interpretation. I wonder what an experienced therapist would say." The supervisee is distressed by his own powerful affective response to the patient, and is so distracted by his emotions that he disengages from the session. This has happened before. After discussing this incident, the supervisor and the supervisee identify a need for two new goals in supervision: 1) recognizing and managing countertransference and 2) maintaining the focus of the session when countertransference has been stimulated.

Fulfilling External Program Requirements

The supervisee's training program may impose requirements on both the supervisor and the supervisee. Assessing and fulfilling these program-directed goals will be a necessary part of supervision. Because these goals are external, they can become a focus of resistance from both trainees and supervisors.

> An early-career psychiatrist has been assigned as a psychotherapy supervisor for a third-year resident. This novice supervisor works on an inpatient unit and secretly doubts his competence to supervise psychotherapy.
>
> SUPERVISOR: I know the residency requires you to write out four psychodynamic formulations, but I really don't see the point. I haven't written a formulation since I left residency. How about if we just discuss the patients at length. I will count that as the formulation.

New supervisors will need to work with the training director to understand the rationales for the program's requirements and to ensure that trainees fully comply with the requirements.

Psychotherapy supervision provides a unique opportunity to reinforce psychotherapy concepts stressed in lectures and other training venues. However, one pilot study ($N=16$ third- and fourth-year psychiatric residents) showed that one-third of participants did not feel that what they learned in supervision correlated with what they were learning in classes (Rojas et al. 2010). In fact, lectures should provide a theoretical understanding of what is observed and experienced in therapy and discussed during supervision (Cabaniss and Arbuckle 2011). This is analogous to the lecture and laboratory approach of many college classes, in which didactics are enlivened by a hands-on component. Any disconnect decreases the potential beneficial synergy between supervision and didactics. Supervisors and training directors should work together to facilitate greater awareness of the psychotherapy topics in the didactic schedule.

Although psychotherapy supervisors in training programs are typically appointed for a year, the training process spans several years, allowing training directors to develop a continuum of psychotherapy goals that spans the entire course of training. Considerable variation will occur, depending on the efforts and aptitudes of the residents. Some will progress rapidly, while others will struggle with specific aspects of psychotherapy. Nevertheless, identifying typical goals by stages can be helpful. A review of supervisees' progress on programmatic goals might start a useful conversation among the program, supervisors, and supervisees. At least one program has published a set of psychotherapy-related objectives based on the year of training (Cabaniss and Arbuckle 2011).

Identifying Stage-Appropriate Objectives for Self-Improvement

Beyond meeting external program requirements and fostering psychotherapy skills, supervisors help their supervisees set developmentally appropriate goals for becoming psychotherapists. Having a clear sense of the typical trainee developmental trajectory helps in setting realistic and attainable goals. Although issues of assessment, diagnostic clarity, therapeutic alliance, theoretical understanding, and appropriate use of technique are present from the start in every case, what to emphasize in supervision may shift as the supervisee advances through training. *Early learners* have a limited knowledge of theory. They may struggle to set the therapeutic frame and to tolerate affects. Objectives for these learners might focus on the common elements of psychotherapy and the therapeutic alliance. *Intermediate learners* are becoming more versed in theory and technique, and they are better able to contain increasingly intense and sometimes negative affects—the sign of a solid therapeutic alliance. Objectives for these learners might focus on understanding, identifying, and skillfully applying the most appropriate interventions. *Advanced learners* are developing strong relationships with their patients and can use a wide variety of therapeutic interventions based on their formulation of the patient. These learners have become more skilled in gathering information from all channels of communication in therapy (verbal, nonverbal, and countertransference) and can engage with the therapeutic process in a way that propels the therapy forward. Objectives for these learners might focus on adapting their approach and interventions based on their formulation of the patient or identifying when countertransference is impeding the flow of treatment.

These developmentally based stages also roughly correspond with Goldberg's (1997) progressive categories for structuring training goals for psychodynamic psychotherapy: 1) observation and description, 2) conceptualization, and 3) synthesis. Depending on the supervisee's stage of learning, a typical progression of goals might follow the sequence shown in Table 8–1.

The supervisory dyad can decide to set any mutually agreed-upon goal for supervision. Using the "SMART" mnemonic to formulate these goals may be helpful (Doran 1981). In this mnemonic, *Specific* refers to the need for a goal to be detailed enough for both members of the dyad to describe the goal. If the goal is to create a comprehensive formulation, an understanding of that process would be included in the goal's definition.

Table 8–1.   Examples of stage-appropriate supervisory goals

Knowledge	Skills	Attitudes
Early		
• Assessing the patient's suitability for psychotherapy • Understanding the components of the therapeutic alliance • Identifying common psychological defenses	• Establishing a secure therapy frame • Making empathic statements • Accurately identifying and reporting key moments in therapy sessions • Recognizing and discussing recurrent patterns of behaviors, emotional responses, and relationships with the patient	• Realizing that therapy attempts to understand the patient's feelings and behaviors, both conscious and unconscious • Beginning to tolerate both one's own and the patient's affects • Developing a nonjudgmental acceptance of the patient and practicing cultural humility
Intermediate		
• Understanding potential manifestations of resistance, transference, and countertransference • Understanding the patient's conduct and emotions in terms of a comprehensive formulation	• Creating a comprehensive formulation • Observing their own behavior and its impact on therapy • Providing appropriate interventions and interpretations based on the patient's latent communications	• Increasing tolerance of strong affects • Tolerating ambiguity • Appreciating countertransference
Advanced		
• Comparing and contrasting specific psychodynamic theories and approaches • Constructing a patient formulation from multiple psychodynamic viewpoints	• Allowing the formulation to guide the choice of interventions • Identifying and managing resistance, transference, and countertransference	• Conducting a more precise appraisal of what part of the affect in the session stems from the patient versus the therapist • Understanding how one's own culture and childhood influence one's work

Source.   Adapted from Bordin 1983; Cabaniss and Arbuckle 2011; Goldberg 1997.

Measurable denotes that goals must be easily quantified, observed, or demonstrated. The dyad might choose to create an informal, subjective scale. *Achievable* means that the goals of supervision need to be realistic. Enthusiastic learners may choose too many goals or choose goals that are not appropriate for their stage of training. The supervisor will need to help adjust the goals accordingly. *Relevant* reflects how goals must be related to learning psychotherapy or developing one's identity as a psychotherapist. Learning therapeutic dosage ranges for antidepressants is not an appropriate goal for psychotherapy supervision, but learning the psychodynamics of prescribing medication in psychotherapy is an excellent goal (see Chapter 11, "Supervising Integrated Psychotherapy and Pharmacotherapy"). *Time-limited* references how goals without a definite ending point tend to be postponed indefinitely. The supervisor and the supervisee will want goals that can be attempted within the time frame of supervision. Progress can be noted without the expectation that trainees will have reached their maximum potential.

Notably, some valuable goals are not amenable to the SMART goal formulation (e.g., developing one's identity as a psychotherapist). Nonetheless, developing SMART goals—when practicable—may help focus the supervisor's and supervisee's attention on the goals and increase the likelihood of success.

Conclusion

Choosing goals for psychotherapy supervision creates a focus for the supervision, strengthens the alliance, and helps ensure that time is spent productively. Goals identify areas for improvement and can be used to monitor progress over the course of supervision. When possible, goals should be specific, measurable, achievable, relevant, and time-limited. They should be established early in supervision and evaluated and reassessed over time. Although there might be some initial resistance to goals, once the benefits are experienced, both supervisors and supervisees may become proponents of this approach.

References

Bordin ES: A working alliance based model of supervision. The Counseling Psychologist 11(1):35–42, 1983

Cabaniss DL, Arbuckle MR: Course and lab: a new model for supervision. Acad Psychiatry 35(4):220–225, 2011 21804039

Cabaniss DL, Arbuckle MR, Moga DE: Using learning objectives for psychotherapy supervision. Am J Psychother 68(2):163–176, 2014 25122983

Doran GT: There's a S.M.A.R.T. way to write management's goals and objectives. Management Review 70(11):35–36, 1981

Goldberg DA: Structuring training goals for psychodynamic psychotherapy. J Psychother Pract Res 7(1):10–22, 1997 9407472

Rojas A, Arbuckle M, Cabaniss D: Don't leave teaching to chance: learning objectives for psychodynamic psychotherapy supervision. Acad Psychiatry 34(1):46–49, 2010 20071725

Shanfield SB, Matthews KL, Hetherly V: What do excellent psychotherapy supervisors do? Am J Psychiatry 150(7):1081–1084, 1993 8317580

Sokol L, Fox MG: Training CBT supervisors, in Teaching and Supervising Cognitive Behavioral Therapy. Edited by Sudak DM, Codd RT, Ludgate J, et al. Hoboken, NJ, Wiley, 2016, pp 227–242

9

Using Process Notes and Audio and Video Recordings in Psychotherapy Supervision

Katherine G. Kennedy, M.D.
Theunis O. de Boer, B.A.
Randon S. Welton, M.D.
Frank E. Yeomans, M.D., Ph.D.

KEY LEARNING GOALS

- Use process material from therapy sessions to improve the quality of the therapy and the supervision.

- Use process notes to capture the therapist's affective responses, associations, and thoughts to allow the supervisor and supervisee a window into the complex interaction between patient and therapist.

- Use process notes to enhance the supervisee's appreciation of the patient's internal world.

- Understand the role of recordings in providing reliable data about the interactions within treatment and identify omissions or distortions made by the therapist using recall alone.

MANY SUPERVISEES expect to bring to supervision a patient's presenting problem, history of present illness, past history, mental status, and diagnosis. They may not understand how an "I said, they said" summary of the session accelerates their acquisition of psychotherapy skills. This reporting may take the form of process notes or an audio or audiovisual recording. Each method conveys various benefits and creates different challenges, but the use of videotaped material in supervision is considered by many to be the "gold standard." Session recordings provide the complete dialogue of the session but raise issues of trust, consent, and confidentiality. Process notes, written postsession, may be less intrusive but less accurate. Supervisors will want to work with supervisees to arrive at a mutually agreeable plan for how to approach this summary of exchange of words, affects, and other relevant clinical material. Process material, no matter what form is used, allows the supervisory dyad to reflect on specific interactions and content within the therapy that may become the focus of efforts to improve the treatment and the therapist's skills. In this chapter we consider these different forms of summarizing the therapy session.

Process Notes

Historically, supervisors may have imposed their preferred styles for process notes on supervisees; today, deciding how to create and what to include in process notes is best approached as a collaborative venture between supervisors and supervisees. *Process notes* are more than attempts at verbatim transcriptions of conversations. They may be defined as attempts to encapsulate the key components of a therapy session, such as snippets of dialogue, additional summarizing texts, observations of the patient's various nonverbal behaviors (gestures, body language, and the "feeling" in the room) and the therapist's affective responses, associations, thoughts, and countertransference. Psychodynamic psychotherapy focuses on helping patients gain awareness of previously unknown aspects of their minds, and patient defenses against these aspects may take various forms. Process notes can help the trainee become aware of emotions, nonverbal behaviors, transference, and countertransference that have an impact on the therapy.

In reviewing process material, the supervisor and the supervisee must decide which material to highlight or gloss over, given that a review of the transcript from an entire therapy session would leave little time for discussion. One approach is to have supervisees present an overview at the beginning of the session and then select for discussion the sections of the session they found most relevant, challenging, or affect-laden. The mutually determined goals for supervision will help guide this discussion. For example, if a supervisory goal is for the therapist to be more attentive to the patient's transference, the process notes would include the patient's comments about the therapy, other relationships, and the therapist's responses and reactions (see Chapter 8, "Setting Goals for Psychotherapy Supervision"). Process notes typically include the following material:

- "Opening" and "closing" session statements by the patient.
- Expressions of affect, including nonverbal, by either the therapist or the patient.
- Unusual verbal expressions, including slang and idioms.
- Recurrent themes, stories, and narratives about relationships and conflicts.
- Nonverbal communication, such as silences, by both therapist and patient, including the material that precedes and follows.
- The patient's dreams and fantasies.
- The therapist's associations, daydreams, and reveries during and after the session.
- Boundary-pushing behaviors and other efforts by the patient to disrupt the frame of therapy.

Additionally, the supervisor will want to bring up for discussion the method for how the therapist will create the process notes. For example, should process notes be taken contemporaneously or written postsession? Some therapists and patients find taking process notes during the session to be distracting—mental energy must be given to decisions about what to write, and patients can notice and react to the therapist's writing. Notes written after the session avoid these problems but depend on therapists' recollections. This can be a benefit, however, if therapists are encouraged to also include their own thoughts and emotional reactions about the session. In addition, material presented in this way reflects some of the therapist's conscious and unconscious processing, which may help organize the session dynamics—that is, what the supervisee presents in supervision will have already been filtered and structured to some extent by the supervisee's personal dynamics and theoretical understanding of the case. This can be an advantage or a disadvantage: at best, it can show supervisees how their thoughts, feelings, and actions with respect to the patient and the supervision (e.g., forgetting to take or bring notes) can illuminate some aspect of the therapy. When process notes are written after the therapy session, the supervisor can suggest that the supervisee schedule a period of time, say 25 minutes, immediately following therapy to craft the process notes. If this is not possible, finding time before the end of that particular day will help facilitate session recall.

How process notes are presented in the supervision can vary, and decisions about preferred modes will need input from the supervisory dyad. Will the supervisor receive a copy of the process notes in advance of the supervisory session? Will the therapist read the notes to the supervisor? Should a full session be reported before considering commentary? How will supervisors or supervisees know when to interrupt a presentation to discuss material? What happens when supervisees arrive with pressing questions or concerns that preclude session reporting? How will the dyad handle situations in which the notes take up most of the session time? For example, some supervisees rigidly adhere to reading lengthy process notes, perhaps to forestall deeper discussion that would make them uneasy and/or to shield themselves from potential critique. We suggest that supervisors and supervisees agree that any urgent development in the patient's life or condition will take precedence over immediately entering into process material. In general, it is best that the supervisor take an overall flexible attitude that maximizes the educational experience for the supervisee.

Process notes require extra time and energy for therapists to create, and require supervisees to make themselves vulnerable, by exposing their associations and affective responses. Supervisors will want to regularly address how this additional burden affects the supervisee. While initially challenging, developing the ability to access one's own internal experience is at the heart of becoming a psychotherapist. At times, process notes may assume a particular meaning for the supervisee, perhaps as a way to act out feelings about the supervisory relationship, or as a manifestation of a parallel process within the therapeutic relationship. For these reasons, being supportive about occasional lapses in note-taking can be helpful, but if conflicts around process notes become the rule, the supervisor will want to gently explore why.

One drawback to process notes is that they cannot convey the full range of verbal and nonverbal communication between therapist and patient. A therapist may consciously or unconsciously edit process material for a variety of reasons. Session recordings can help bring these omissions and distortions to light.

Recordings

In contrast to the more subjective nature of process notes, recordings allow supervisors to directly observe trainees working with patients. These recordings may more clearly identify how the actual therapeutic interaction is going, and can be supplemented by supervisees' comments on their subjective responses throughout the session. Recordings may be helpful in several ways:

- Helping trainees to improve their clinical skills (e.g., listening, reframing, clarifying).
- Allowing supervisors to recognize verbal and nonverbal material that therapists may be omitting or distorting, either consciously or unconsciously.
- Helping supervisors and supervisees to understand why a particular therapy may be "stuck."

The most common method used by supervisors to observe trainees at work is through audio or audiovisual recordings. With many low-cost, high-definition video cameras readily available, audiovisual systems are practically as affordable as audio-only systems, and recording and storing of audiovisual files varies little from that of audio files. The capability of audiovisual recordings to capture nonverbal cues makes them the preferred choice. Supervisors should ensure that therapists and patients have properly consented to the use of video, depending on clinic guidelines and government regulations. Trainees will need to document patients' consent to having their therapy sessions recorded and also provide patients with information on the purpose of the recording (i.e., supervision), how the recordings will be stored, which individuals within the health care system will be able to access the recordings, and when the recordings will be deleted (Crocker and Sudak 2017).

Trainees and patients may initially raise objections to the use of video in supervision. Trainees may be concerned that they are "exploiting" their patients, or they may fear undue exposure and/or worry about making themselves vulnerable with the use of video. When watching videos with their supervisors, therapists may have to acknowledge "mistakes" they made—or witness embarrassing or painful unconscious defenses and enactments that occurred—during therapy sessions that might otherwise have remained hidden. Trainees' anxiety about using video may alter their conduct in therapy or exacerbate potential issues with authority. One way to minimize self-consciousness about recording for both therapists and patients is to record all sessions rather than only those sessions that are to be presented in supervision; the process of recording then recedes into the background. In addition, to minimize concerns about recording, supervisors will need to balance being supportive with challenging the trainee. They can initiate discussions of the power differential in supervision, concerns about the evaluative component, and the trainee's antici-pated feelings of inadequacy. They can remind the supervisee that self-assessment is critical to lifelong learning, and that watching the actual ther-apy is a unique opportunity to learn about themselves as therapists (Gold-berg 1983; Haggerty and Hilsenroth 2011; Topor et al. 2017).

Many patients have difficulty learning to trust that the video will be used responsibly and stored appropriately. Several techniques can help minimize this discomfort. The patient can be reminded of personal or clinic policies that control the storage, use, and ultimate destruction of therapy videos. The impact of videos can be discussed explicitly with pa-tients, and their concerns acknowledged and addressed. As trust develops over time, the fear of intentional misuse of the video often resolves. All parties can be reminded that videos are ultimately to help improve thera-pists' skill and the quality of the therapy they are providing (Alpert 1996; Goldberg 1983; Haggerty and Hilsenroth 2011; Topor et al. 2017).

Even with patients and therapists who express comfort with being re-corded, participants might have a tendency to alter their behavior because they are being monitored (i.e., the Hawthorne effect) (Haggerty and Hilsenroth 2011). Being on camera may hold various meanings for partic-ipants. For example, some patients may experience the videotaping in a paranoid way, as tantamount to a "taped confession," and withhold infor-mation; more narcissistically organized patients may view the videotaping as confirmation of how special they are. Exploration with patients about the meanings of the videotaping may help to increase comfort with the re-cording. A literature review of 27 studies examining factors that influenced consent to videotaping therapy sessions found that eventually almost all patients felt comfortable with the camera present (Ko and Goebert 2011).

Reviewing session video together allows supervisors and supervisees to observe verbal and nonverbal communications and provides objective data about trainees' clinical skills. Video exposes the alterations in recall that come with trainees' emotional distortions or countertransference (Alpert 1996; Goldberg 1983; Topor et al. 2017). Watching video enables the supervisor to observe and comment on firsthand data from the session rather than needing to rely only on the trainee's report. This increases the accuracy of the assessment and the impact of the feedback (Haggerty and Hilsenroth 2011).

> A resident presented a new case of a 28-year-old married mother of three children who sought therapy for help with a chronically depressed mood and difficulty applying herself at work, which had led to her being fired from a series of jobs. The situation was complicated by stress in her mar-

riage due to her loss of interest in sexual relations with her husband and his frustration that she was not contributing to the family finances.

In the first supervisory session, the resident discussed his initial two meetings with the patient and offered a diagnostic impression of dysthymic disorder with possible avoidant personality disorder. He presented written process material that suggested that the patient felt uncomfortable speaking freely about herself. She suffered from a conflict between a wish to connect with the other and anxiety based on the expectation of being judged and related difficulty in trusting. The supervisor helped the therapist see themes of an anxious attachment.

In the second supervision session, the resident brought a video recording. The supervisor and the therapist observed the video together and came to a very different understanding of the case. Although the patient's words communicated the same themes as had been discussed previously, the nonverbal communication and the "feel" of the session conveyed themes that were quite different.

> SUPERVISOR: Watching the tape, I've noticed that your patient looks very dressed up. Although she talks about the lack of joy and relationships in her life, in the session she is wearing makeup, her nails are polished, and she is dressed like she is going out to a party. She doesn't seem anxious—in fact, she seems subtly flirtatious and seductive.
>
> RESIDENT: You're right. Actually I look more anxious than she does. And maybe she isn't really as depressed as she says she is.
>
> SUPERVISOR: Well that may be, but what interests me more is whether she is dressing up for you.

The resident described his primary countertransference as feeling confused and unclear about what was going on. The supervisor suggested that this response might be due to the discrepancy between the patient's verbal communication and her nonverbal communication. As is the case with many early-career therapists, this resident focused more on listening to the patient's words than on "reading" the interaction. Aided by the video material, the supervisor helped the resident become more attuned to the latter. Going through this process led to a reformulation of the case, and rather than seeing the patient as an anxious woman fearful of the judgment of others, they saw narcissistic traits that involved attempts to win over (seduce) the newly encountered, and probably idealized, person in her life and then, as revealed by her marriage and job history, a devaluation of those persons with whom she had become close. This revised formulation had a major impact on the handling of the case.

Some consideration of the impact of video recordings on the supervisory dyad is warranted. Creating a supervisory alliance is fundamental to the work of supervision and requires multiple interactions over time. If the supervisory space is focused largely on watching videos, there may be less time to deepen the relationship. The video might also increase the tendency for a microanalysis of the session wherein the supervisor focuses on brief segments of the video rather than on learning about the entire session and understanding the segment within a larger therapeutic context. Prioritizing the supervisory alliance and allowing the trainee to relate the gist and highlights of the therapy session before watching the video can help address these concerns (Haggerty and Hilsenroth 2011).

Supervisors differ in their opinions about how videos should be used in supervision. Some supervisors may want to watch the entire video in supervision; this is not advised, because it eliminates the opportunity to discuss the session. Other supervisors may ask residents to review the video before supervision in order to discuss what they observed on tape and how it differed from what they remembered about the therapy session. Still other supervisors prefer to review the video of the therapy session before the supervision session or will ask to see specific parts of the recorded session (e.g., the beginning, the ending, the most confusing aspects). Trainees may select clips from segments in which they felt something went well or poorly, or they may display parts of the session in which they experienced uncertainty (Barnett 2011). Regardless of the approach adopted, supervisors and supervisees will need to address considerations regarding what to include, how much pre-supervision preparation time is realistically available, and how much time for discussion during supervision is desired.

SUPERVISOR: So what seemed to be the most confusing moment with your therapy patients this week?
TRAINEE: This week, that's easy. I was working with Mr. Y, and he suddenly became angry. I mean he was really pissed off. We worked through it, and he calmed down, but I hadn't seen that before. I had heard him talk about his temper, but he had never shown it.
SUPERVISOR: Do you remember what was going on just before he got so angry?
TRAINEE: At the time I was completely blindsided. I went back and watched the tape afterward though. I had made a comment about his interaction with his daughters, and I think he took it as a criticism or even an insult. I didn't mean it that way of course, but I think that's what he heard.
SUPERVISOR: Let's watch that part of the tape.

Table 9–1 summarizes the differences between process notes and audiovisual recordings of sessions.

Table 9–1.   Differences between process notes and audiovisual recordings of therapy sessions

Characteristics of reporting method	Process notes	Audiovisual recordings
Captures verbal communications (including dialogue, tone, and voice)	Clinical material is filtered through the supervisee's perspective	Supplements and/or challenges the therapist's memory of the therapy session
Captures nonverbal communications (including silences, gestures, and other physical aspects)	Clinical material is filtered through the supervisee's perspective	Supplements and/or challenges the therapist's memory of the therapy session
Intrusion into the therapeutic space	Less intrusive, especially if notes are written postsession	More intrusive—requires discussion and informed consent; patient may have additional concerns about confidentiality; "Hawthorne effect"[a] may occur
Reveals therapist's associations, fantasies, and affective responses	Yes, and such content is often also intercalated into the recollections of process material	No; such content must be solicited by the supervisor
Fosters a shared reality of clinical material	Effects are dependent on the supervisee's perspective and the supervisory relationship	Offers more objective data and more easily fosters a shared reality

[a] Hawthorne effect: Tendency of subjects in a study to alter their behavior when they are aware that they are being observed.

Conclusion

How process material is collected reflects the focus of the supervisory work. Written notes use the filter of the therapist to open a valuable window into the treatment and its dynamics, while direct recordings reveal actual therapist–patient interactions and provide more reliable data for direct feedback about specific techniques. Which modality is used will depend on discussions among the triad of individuals involved—supervisor, therapist, and patient—and the circumstances of the therapy and the supervision.

References

Alpert MC: Videotaping psychotherapy. J Psychother Pract Res 5(2):93–105, 1996 22700270

Barnett JE: Utilizing technological innovations to enhance psychotherapy supervision, training, and outcomes. Psychotherapy (Chic) 48(2):103–108, 2011 21639653

Crocker EM, Sudak DM: Making the most of psychotherapy supervision: a guide for psychiatry residents. Acad Psychiatry 41(1):35–39, 2017 27909977

Goldberg DA: Resistance to the use of video in individual psychotherapy training. Am J Psychiatry 140(9):1172–1176, 1983 6614223

Haggerty GH, Hilsenroth MJ: The use of video in psychotherapy supervision. British Journal of Psychotherapy 27(2):193–210, 2011

Ko K, Goebert D: Factors influencing consent to having videotaped mental health sessions. Acad Psychiatry 35(3):199–201, 2011 21602443

Topor DR, AhnAllen CG, Mulligan EA, et al: Using video recordings of psychotherapy sessions in supervision: strategies to reduce learner anxiety. Acad Psychiatry 41(1):40–43, 2017 27558629

10

When Psychotherapy Supervision Is Virtual

Seamus Bhatt-Mackin, M.D., C.G.P.
Aimee Murray, Psy.D., L.P.
Magdalena Romanowicz, M.D.
Anne E. Ruble, M.D., M.P.H.
David R. Topor, Ph.D., M.S.-H.P.Ed.

KEY LEARNING GOALS

- Understand the similarities and differences between in-person and videoconferencing psychotherapy supervision in regard to therapeutic presence, alliance, and boundaries.

- Use special strategies to build and maintain the supervisor–supervisee relationship in the virtual environment.

- Use practical strategies to help supervisees navigate clinical situations commonly encountered in virtual psychotherapy.

TRADITIONALLY, PSYCHOTHERAPY supervision occurred with the supervisor and the supervisee meeting in person. As communication technology has improved (Rousmaniere 2014), clinical innovators have noted many potential benefits of virtual psychotherapy supervision, including increased access to high-quality supervisors in underserved or rural locations (Gammon et al. 1998; Wood et al. 2005) and across national boundaries (Fishkin et al. 2011; Inman and Luu 2019), more flexibility in scheduling (Rousmaniere 2014), and novel methods of recording, reviewing, and live-viewing sessions (Nadan et al. 2020; Rousmaniere and Ellis 2013). Despite these advantages, many psychotherapists have remained skeptical of virtual formats, holding negative beliefs about what is possible in virtual psychotherapy (Sucala et al. 2013), which likely inform their views on virtual psychotherapy supervision. In 2020, the COVID-19 pandemic disrupted many traditions of our health care systems and necessitated the emergency development of remote psychotherapy, remote teaching, and remote forms of psychotherapy supervision.

> Dr. Adams enjoyed her weekly supervisory meetings with Dr. Smith. She liked his comfortable office and how she could grab a cup of coffee on her walk there. Then the COVID-19 pandemic started, and Dr. Adams's residency training program directed all residents and faculty to move their supervision to videoconferencing. Initially, supervision by videoconferencing felt impersonal. After a while, Dr. Adams noticed that she and Dr. Smith took turns more easily to avoid interrupting each other. She began to email brief summaries of her sessions and questions to Dr. Smith prior to their meetings, and this helped to structure the supervision. Because she called him from her home, Dr. Adams was able to make her own coffee, and this became her new pre-supervision ritual.

The term *virtual* refers to the fact that the supervision is not taking place in person. There are multiple possible formats for "virtual" psychotherapy supervision, including instant messaging, email, telephone, and videoconferencing. Based on a review of trends in the literature (Inman et al. 2019) and our own experience of providing supervision during the COVID-19 pandemic, this chapter focuses on providing psychotherapy supervision by internet-mediated videoconferencing, a technology that allows for face-to-face contact using synchronous audio and video connections. Our recommendations are based on case reports in the literature and our own experiences, as systematic research is not robust (Martin et al. 2018).

We organized our chapter around three core areas of practice important for in-person psychotherapy: presence, alliance, and boundaries. We begin with a brief review of each area as it is currently understood in videoconferencing for psychotherapy. We then discuss the impact of each area on the supervisory relationship. Finally, we describe commonly encountered dilemmas in psychotherapy conducted by internet-mediated videoconferencing and offer practical supervision strategies.

Core Areas of Practice Common to Both Virtual Psychotherapy and Virtual Psychotherapy Supervision

Telepresence

Telepresence refers to experiencing the online environment as if you were engaging with the patient in person. The word *telepresence* derives from "therapeutic presence," which involves therapists using their whole selves in a presence-centered relational stance to engage patients in therapy. Therapeutic presence correlates with a sense of safety, a deepened therapeutic relationship, and effective therapy (Geller and Porges 2014). Telehealth platforms change therapists' frameworks for using their "whole selves" by limiting their perceptual and contextual cues. Even with these limitations, exploratory research suggests that a higher level of telepresence in remote psychotherapy predicts a stronger therapeutic relationship and facilitates use of intersubjectivity (Haddouk et al. 2018). Emerging research is examining the necessary clinical training for cultivating telepresence in remote psychotherapy to maintain strong therapeutic relationships (Geller 2021). To increase engagement, the therapist needs to pay special attention to factors that can enhance or detract from telepresence.

Attending to the Alliance Virtually

The supervisory alliance corresponds to the patient–therapist alliance, which is an interpersonal process of mutual collaboration operationalized into three components: agreement on treatment goals, agreement on tasks involved in reaching those goals, and a positive bond (Horvath et al. 2011). Studies of the alliance in videoconferencing psychotherapy (VCP) have shown a correlation between the alliance and patient outcome (Flückiger et al. 2018; Norwood et al. 2021). In a meta-analysis comparing in-person psychotherapy with VCP, the alliance in VCP was found to be inferior in regard to the strength of the alliance but not in regard to patient outcomes (Norwood et al. 2018). Given the potential in VCP for technological problems and for missing nonverbal cues, it is recommended that psychotherapists prepare patients for the possibility of an alliance rupture, inquire regularly to rapidly identify ruptures, and actively work to repair any ruptures that occur (Dolev-Amit et al. 2021).

Managing Boundaries Online

Boundaries are sets of guidelines governing the relationship between therapist and patient. Boundaries are protective for both patient and therapist; they set expectations, help build a therapeutic alliance, and minimize harm (Drum and Littleton 2014). Boundary issues in office settings may relate to meeting place, length and frequency of sessions, payment, gifts, physical touch, language, clothing, self-disclosure, and sexual contact (Gutheil and Gabbard 1993). Supervisors can help trainees recognize aspects of boundaries that may require additional attention in the virtual space, such as adhering to structured time frames, conveying professionalism, and avoiding unintentional self-disclosure (Drum and Littleton 2014). It is important to maintain clear start and end times for sessions. This can help patients understand the length of time they will be expected to engage in challenging work. Wearing professional clothing can help differentiate teletherapy from friendship. It is recommended that therapists carefully review objects in the camera view to reduce the risk of involuntary personal disclosures. Another option for avoiding unintentional self-disclosures is to use a virtual background (Drum and Littleton 2014; Markowitz et al. 2021). These guidelines also apply to maintenance of boundaries within the supervisory relationship.

The Supervisor–Supervisee Relationship in the Virtual Environment

Maintaining Engagement

> A supervisee presents to remote psychotherapy with a dim background while patting down a cowlick he noticed on camera. The supervisor observes that the supervisee has poor eye contact, and she hears typing sounds. Assuming that the trainee is distracted, she moves closer to the camera to capture his attention, but the camera angle misses a lot of her body language. The supervisor is also preoccupied, because thoughts about an email she read from the head of her department just before the supervision session started keep creeping in. As supervision winds down, the supervisee is feeling rushed to cover his patients, and the supervisor is wondering whether she missed pertinent details. Both are feeling detached.

In an interview study of Australian psychologists that examined the experience of conducting supervision via videoconferencing, Miller and Gibson (2004) found that a notable number of supervisees and supervisors reported a sense of detachment in remote interactions. Many of the participants found the interaction impersonal and lacking in warmth. In the vignette above, increasing telepresence could decrease feelings of detachment (Miller and Gibson 2004). In this scenario, telepresence could be improved in a number of ways, including the following: 1) improve the supervisee's lighting; 2) discuss the differences in eye contact online; 3) have the supervisee explicitly share why he is typing (in this scenario, he is taking notes, and the supervisor does not know); 4) have the supervisor distance herself further from the screen to optimize the supervisee's ability to see as many nonverbal cues as possible, while optimizing distance for sound quality; and 5) have both participants turn off their self-view to reduce the distraction of seeing themselves (Markowitz et al. 2021).

In the vignette above, the supervisor had just read an email from the department head and could not get her mind fully back to supervision. Leroy (2009) described a phenomenon called *attention residue*, in which thoughts from a previous task persist into the next task. Individuals experiencing attention residue are likely to demonstrate poor performance on their next task, in this case clinical supervision. An expectation that both parties will silence their cell phones, close their email, and use the initial 2–3 minutes to mentally shift focus can increase engagement.

Martin et al. (2018) note that a pitfall of remote supervision is the tendency to reserve emotional issues for in-person meetings. The individuals in this scenario appear to be hesitant to discuss the issues that are occurring in the midst of supervision, which may also reduce the engagement that individuals experience in the online environment. Discussions with emotional content can increase telepresence and are an essential component to incorporate (Bouchard et al. 2011).

One of the key components of supervision is teaching; hence, findings from research in remote education may offer some insight into strategies for engagement in remote supervision (Miller and Gibson 2004). Online learner research shows higher levels of engagement when an instructor demonstrates a sense of caring (Arghode 2018). In this vignette, the supervisor could also take some time to check in with the supervisee, talk more explicitly about the supervisee's experiences online, and ask how she might improve the supervision experience.

Building a Supervisory Alliance

Dr. Shah, a volunteer faculty psychotherapy supervisor, is supervising via VCP for the first time. Although she is a bit intimidated by the technology and worried that Dr. Ruffin, the supervisee, will be more tech-savvy than she is, Dr. Shah is enthusiastic about saving travel time. At the first meeting, she provides no orientation to the medium, assuming that Dr. Ruffin is already familiar with it. She also does not invite discussion about using videoconferencing for supervision, despite the fact that Dr. Ruffin has a strong preference for in-person face-to-face supervision (which Dr. Shah would have learned, had she asked). Dr. Shah insists that they "keep to the new frame and restrict additional contact to only their supervision time, with no in-person meetings and no emailing in between." Both leave the first supervision session confused and discouraged; Dr. Shah's negative view of VCP is strengthened, and Dr. Ruffin is pessimistic about the benefits of supervision.

Recommendations for addressing the problems depicted in this vignette include the following: 1) use videoconferencing supervision only if its use is in the best interests of patients and supervisees, never solely for the convenience of the supervisor; 2) provide clear procedures and guidance in the technology; and 3) involve supervisees in the decision of whether to use telesupervision (Rousmaniere 2014). Some have recommended that the supervisory dyad initially meet in person and later transition to videoconferencing (Martin et al. 2018), while others have found that this is not necessary (Jordan and Shearer 2019; Tarlow et al. 2020). Communication outside the supervisory hour can be an asset; secure email can be used to assist with setting agendas, giving written feedback, and confirming the treatment plan (Yellowlees 2019). Given the newness for many in working this way, it is recommended that supervisors and supervisees regularly assess and discuss the effectiveness of their communication in the virtual space (Sørlie et al. 1999) and that they practice together how to communicate verbally that which is usually conveyed nonverbally. For example, the supervisor might adopt a formal, slower speaking style with short pauses to allow for interruption. In addition, the supervisor might ask the supervisee to convey the need to interrupt by using a hand signal.

Attending to Professional Boundaries

Dr. Chundalal, a supervisor, is meeting with Dr. Carl, a second-year psychiatry resident, for their first supervision session and notices that the supervisee logs in a few minutes late, against the backdrop of an apartment kitchen. Dr. Chundalal begins the session by orienting Dr. Carl to the importance of setting a therapeutic frame and maintaining boundaries via teletherapy. They talk together about starting and ending appointments at agreed-upon times and obtaining the patient's location in case of emergency. Dr. Chundalal directs Dr. Carl to seek supervision if a patient has difficulty with either of these issues, as there may be therapeutic implications. The two then role-play how Dr. Carl will explain to a "patient" (the supervisor) how to ensure a safe, private location and problem-solve challenging scenarios with regard to time and place boundaries, including an agreement to verbally alert the therapist if another person walks into the room during a session. At the close of the supervision session, Dr. Chundalal is surprised to see the resident's two roommates in the camera view, and the sounds of meal preparation are picked up by the microphone. Dr.

> Carl thanks Dr. Chundalal for guiding her through her first psychotherapy supervision of her residency and logs off before any further conversation can take place.

A vital part of the supervision process is ensuring that a resident understands the purpose, structure, and expectations of psychotherapy supervision (Crocker and Sudak 2016; Watkins 2020). In this vignette, the resident seems not to understand the private nature of supervision and also does not understand that the teaching provided on boundaries for psychotherapy sessions also applies to boundaries in psychotherapy supervision. Because Dr. Carl is a junior resident just beginning to see outpatients, she may assume that supervision is similar to a didactic experience and be unaware of the need for privacy to maintain patient confidentiality. Setting expectations in advance can help decrease difficulties in the supervisory relationship, and this applies to videoconferencing supervision as well. A supervision contract can address how to discuss dissatisfaction with the supervision directly (Ellis 2017) and encourages the supervisee to bring concerns to the attention of the supervisor, discouraging avoidance of conflict in the supervision relationship.

How Supervisors Can Help Supervisees Through Scenarios Common in Virtual Psychotherapy

Mitigating Disengagement With Patients

> During supervision, Dr. Calloway, a supervisee, reports to Dr. Anderson, the supervisor, that one of her patients spends much of the session "staring off into space." Dr. Calloway is frustrated because the therapy is taking place online. She exclaims, "If we were meeting in person, there is no way that he would be so disengaged."

The supervisee in this scenario is frustrated with the online format and likely sees this context as being the primary issue. She may feel upset that she cannot engage the patient, and displaces her discomfort onto the virtual format. The supervisor can validate the supervisee's frustration before moving on to a discussion of the patient, and can gently explore other possible explanations for the patient's behavior and steps that the supervisee could take. For example, the patient could be experiencing distracting symptoms, and the supervisee could be encouraged to check in with the patient or collateral informants. Attempting to engage the patient in exploring the behavior might lead to increased verbal participation by the patient. The patient's relative silence might also indicate that they are ready to terminate therapy but do not feel comfortable expressing this thought. Discussion about this range of possibilities may help the supervisee move past her focus on the immediate context.

> A supervisee reports on a therapy session in which she observed her patient using his cell phone during online psychotherapy. She notes that the patient tries to be discreet with his use and has his phone just off-screen. However, she expresses reluctance to confront the patient, because she does not want to replicate his experiences of his parents' controlling style.

The fact that this vignette takes place in a virtual environment is a significant piece of the picture. The supervisor should address the supervisee's discomfort, validate the supervisee's concerns by recognizing the importance of her conceptualization, and then consider ways that the patient could still be approached without duplicating a negative interaction pattern in the family.

Establishing a Working Alliance

> A supervisee reports that all of her patients struggle with the technology involved in VCP and that walking people through the steps of logging on to the platform, positioning the camera for visibility, attending to lighting, adjusting the audio sufficiently, and other standard practices requires time away from "really doing the therapy that I want to do."

When conducting psychotherapy in person, therapists do not usually need to provide patients with detailed instructions on all of the steps involved in "taking a seat" at the clinical office. However, VCP may require more guidance. This work may present an opportunity if it is considered to be part of the therapy endeavor itself rather than a necessary condition for the therapy to begin. The process of building a therapist–patient alliance is iterative and interactional in VCP (Norwood et al. 2021). How this initial goal—to be able to see and hear one other—is achieved may provide the foundation for the work that comes next.

> A supervisee reports that his therapy patient gives only one-word responses to the therapist's remarks and questions. This patient presents each week early to the VCP waiting room, appears attentive, stays the entire time, but seems to be in chronic emotional distress. Attempts at validation and clarification have illuminated nothing. After four sessions, the goals of treatment remain unclear. The supervisee is frustrated with this process and wants to end treatment to work with another patient.

This situation is not unique to VCP. The supervisor has little information to help guide this supervisee, apart from the trainee's obvious frustration. However, there is one strategy that might be useful. Remote live supervision is an approach in which the supervisor joins the videoconferencing platform muted with video off to silently observe the session (Rousmaniere and Ellis 2013). This method can be paired with instant messaging during the session to provide prompts to the novice therapist to help with this dilemma. Informed consent by the patient for this practice would be necessary prior to initiating remote live supervision.

> A psychiatry resident brings to supervision a technologically mediated microaggression that occurred when he met with a new psychotherapy patient via videoconferencing for the first time. At the beginning of the session, the audio was working but the video was not working. They decided to proceed to talk together about the patient's history, current difficulties, and goals for treatment. Near the end of the meeting, the video suddenly started working, and the psychiatry resident was initially relieved. However, the patient looked genuinely surprised at the appearance of the psychiatry resident and blurted out, "I thought that you were a white man. I guess this will be OK," and then looked embarrassed and quickly logged off. The psychiatry resident asked for advice in supervision about what to do next. The respective social identities of supervisor and supervisee—including racial identity—had not yet been discussed in supervision.

In this scenario, the suddenness of the appearance of visual cues may have prompted an unconscious patient reaction. This vignette highlights how racial and other aspects of social identity can emerge at any time. Indeed, residents have called for more attention to this issue in psychotherapy supervision (DeSouza et al. 2021). A best practice for supervisors is to broach the topic of cultural similarities and differences early in psychotherapy supervision with all supervisees (Jones et al. 2019). In this situation, the supervisor's first priority would be attending to the supervisee's request for help with next steps, while also acknowledging that this topic needs greater exploration within the supervision.

Maintaining Therapeutic Boundaries

> A supervisee has been seeing a patient weekly for several months. At their most recent session, the supervisee was startled to note that the patient was wearing only a loosely belted bathrobe. The supervisee was uncertain how to deal with the patient's unusual manner of dress. He was reluctant to upset or offend the patient, so he continued with the session as if she were fully clothed.

Professional role boundaries require focused attention and practice in VCP. For example, both the patient's and the supervisee's prior experiences with video modalities may have been primarily social (e.g., video chats with friends and family) (Drum and Littleton 2014). In the scenario depicted in this vignette, the supervisor can assist this supervisee in developing ways to help patients change their attire that are sensitive to the situation and to the patient's diagnosis. A patient with severe depression may need gentle encouragement and support, including validating that symptoms of depression can affect one's ability to engage in daily tasks and allowing the patient to attempt to get dressed or to reschedule for another time after a brief safety assessment. A patient with an eroticized transference may need orientation (or reorientation) to how a professional relationship is different from a friendship or romance. Maintaining role boundaries in dress allows the patient to stay safe and builds trust in the therapy. If the supervisee is unsure about what might be causing a patient's anomalous garb, a simple statement—such as "It seems that I have caught you at an inconvenient time. I will leave the session and come back in a few minutes to allow you some time to get dressed for the visit"—can convey a sensitive reminder to the patient that his or her apparel is inappropriate in the current setting.

> A supervisee reports to his supervisor that his patient was upset with him because he declined to conduct the therapy session while the patient was driving home from work in her car. Another supervisee divulges that one of her patients engages in household tasks during their sessions.

In the first situation, the supervisor can clearly instruct the supervisee that it is not safe to conduct therapy with a patient who is driving. The patient can park the car in a safe location and confirm the physical location of the car, or the patient can reschedule for another time when a private, safe location is available.

In the second situation, the therapist should consider both how long the patient has been receiving psychotherapy and the current working diagnosis. The patient may be unfamiliar with therapy and may not understand that performing other tasks is unhelpful to therapy sessions; a direct conversation about psychotherapy is indicated. The patient could also simply be nervous about engaging, so an empathic statement could be made about how it can be challenging to focus on the work of therapy with so many distractions in the home environment, followed by problem-solving together to create space for therapy in one's routine. Additionally, diagnoses such as anxiety, ADHD, and hypomania or mania may play a role in a patient's attentiveness during a session and should be discussed in supervision as possible factors in engagement.

Summary and Recommendations

Innovators in psychotherapy supervision have a history of adopting new technologies as soon as they become available (Wood et al. 2005). However, during the COVID-19 pandemic, nearly all psychotherapists and psychotherapy supervisors were forced to familiarize themselves with remote technologies through the internet. As we write this chapter, remote technologies such as videoconferencing are currently a standard part of clinical practice. However, systematic studies are limited, and more investigation is needed to inform practices and policy. For example, despite the fact that there are no head-to-head studies comparing telephone psychotherapy and VCP (Markowitz et al. 2021), the latter is assumed to be more effective and is currently the only format that is reimbursable.

Many therapists have taken techniques that are known to work well in person and have adapted these to working remotely (Fernández-Álvarez and Fernández-Álvarez 2021). In this chapter we followed a similar approach by focusing our review on the core features of clinical and supervisory encounters (presence, alliance, boundaries). However, conducting psychotherapy and psychotherapy supervision virtually may prompt new ways of thinking or facilitate a shift in focus. For example, Cataldo et al. (2021) consider the technology to be not just a vehicle of communication but also an "invisible third party" that is itself involved in the system of communication. Attending to the supervision in this way may prompt supervisees and supervisors to more often consider the environment of care and the systems in which we are all embedded.

In addition, there may be disorders and problems for which virtual psychotherapy is more effective than in-person psychotherapy (Kocsis and Yellowlees 2018), and there may be clinical supervision situations for which virtual supervision is preferred. As we move forward, it will be important for clinicians to be aware of our biases for (Yellowlees 2019) or against (Sucala et al. 2013) new technologies and to work to improve our knowledge and skills both through our experiences and through systematic study.

References

Arghode V: Engaging instructional design and instructor role in online learning environment. European Journal of Training and Development 42(7/8):366–380, 2018

Bouchard S, Dumoulin S, Michaud M, Gougeon V: Telepresence experienced in videoconference varies according to emotions involved in videoconference sessions. Stud Health Technol Inform 167:128–132, 2011 21685654

Cataldo F, Chang S, Mendoza A, Buchanan G: A perspective on client-psychologist relationships in videoconferencing psychotherapy: literature review. JMIR Ment Health 8(2):e19004, 2021 33605891

Crocker EM, Sudak DM: Making the most of psychotherapy supervision: a guide for psychiatry residents. Acad Psychiatry 41(1):35–39, 2016 27909977

DeSouza F, Mathis M, Lastra N, Isom J: Navigating race in the psychotherapeutic encounter: a call for supervision. Acad Psychiatry 45(1):132–133, 2021 33058047

Dolev-Amit T, Leibovich L, Zilcha-Mano S: Repairing alliance ruptures using supportive techniques in telepsychotherapy during the COVID-19 pandemic. Counselling Psychology Quarterly 34(3–4):485–498, 2021

Drum KB, Littleton HL: Therapeutic boundaries in telepsychology: unique issues and best practice recommendations. Prof Psychol Res Pr 45(5):309–315, 2014 25414540

Ellis MV: Clinical supervision contract and consent statement and supervisee rights and responsibilities. The Clinical Supervisor 36(1):145–159, 2017

Fernández-Álvarez J, Fernández-Álvarez H: Videoconferencing psychotherapy during the pandemic: exceptional times with enduring effects? Front Psychol 12:589–536, 2021 33679513

Fishkin R, Fishkin L, Leli U, et al: Psychodynamic treatment, training, and supervision using internet-based technologies. J Am Acad Psychoanal Dyn Psychiatry 39(1):155–168, 2011 21434749

Flückiger C, Del Re AC, Wampold BE, Horvath AO: The alliance in adult psychotherapy: a meta-analytic synthesis. Psychotherapy (Chic) 55(4):316–340, 2018 29792475

Gammon D, Sørlie T, Bergvik S, Høifødt TS: Psychotherapy supervision conducted by videoconferencing: a qualitative study of users' experiences. J Telemed Telecare 4 (suppl 1):33–35, 1998 9640727

Geller S: Cultivating online therapeutic presence: strengthening therapeutic relationships in teletherapy sessions. Counselling Psychology Quarterly 34(3–4):687–703, 2021

Geller SM, Porges SW: Therapeutic presence: neurophysiological mechanisms mediating feeling safe in therapeutic relationships. Journal of Psychotherapy Integration 24(3):178–192, 2014

Gutheil TG, Gabbard GO: The concept of boundaries in clinical practice: theoretical and risk-management dimensions. Am J Psychiatry 150(2):188–196, 1993 8422069

Haddouk L, Bouchard S, Brivio E, et al: Assessing presence in videoconference telepsychotherapies: a complementary qualitative study on breaks in telepresence and intersubjectivity co-construction processes. Annual Review of Cybertherapy and Telemedicine 16:118–123, 2018

Horvath AO, Del Re AC, Flückiger C, Symonds D: Alliance in individual psychotherapy. Psychotherapy (Chic) 48(1):9–16, 2011 21401269

Inman A, Bashian H, Pendse CD, Luu LP: Publication trends in telesupervision: a content analysis study. The Clinical Supervisor 38(1):97–115, 2019

Inman AP, Luu LP: Cultural competence in the context of telesupervision, in Cases in Multicultural Supervision: New Models, Lenses, and Applications. Edited by Burnes TR, Manese JE. San Diego, CA, Cognella Academic Publishing, 2019, pp 395–408

Jones CT, Welfare LE, Shekila M, et al: Broaching as a strategy for intercultural understanding in clinical supervision. The Clinical Supervisor 38(1):1–16, 2019

Jordan SE, Shearer EM: An exploration of supervision delivered via clinical video telehealth (CVT). Training and Education in Professional Psychology 13(4):323–330, 2019

Kocsis BJ, Yellowlees P: Telepsychotherapy and the therapeutic relationship: principles, advantages, and case examples. Telemed J E Health 24(5):329–334, 2018 28836902

Leroy S: Why is it so hard to do my work? The challenge of attention residue when switching between work tasks. Organizational Behavior and Human Decision Processes 109(2):168–181, 2009

Markowitz JC, Milrod B, Heckman TG, et al: Psychotherapy at a distance. Am J Psychiatry 178(3):240–246, 2021 32972202

Martin P, Lizarondo L, Kumar S: A systematic review of the factors that influence the quality and effectiveness of telesupervision for health professionals. J Telemed Telecare 24(4):271–281, 2018 28387603

Miller RJ, Gibson AM: Supervision by videoconference with rural probationary psychologists. International Journal of Innovation in Science and Mathematics Education 11(1):22–28, 2004

Nadan Y, Shachar R, Cramer D, et al: Behind the (virtual) mirror: online live supervision in couple and family therapy. Fam Process 59(3):997–1006, 2020 32594527

Norwood C, Moghaddam NG, Malins S, Sabin-Farrell R: Working alliance and outcome effectiveness in videoconferencing psychotherapy: a systematic review and noninferiority meta-analysis. Clin Psychol Psychother 25(6):797–808, 2018 30014606

Norwood C, Sabin-Farrell R, Malins S, Moghaddam NG: An explanatory sequential investigation of the working alliance as a change process in videoconferencing psychotherapy. J Clin Psychol 77(6):1330–1353, 2021 33482015

Rousmaniere TJ: Using technology to enhance clinical supervision and training, in The Wiley International Handbook of Clinical Supervision. Edited by Watkins CE Jr, Milne DL. Oxford, Wiley-Blackwell, 2014, pp 204–273

Rousmaniere TJ, Ellis MV: Internet-based one-way mirror supervision for advanced psychotherapy training. The Clinical Supervisor 32(1):40–55, 2013

Sørlie T, Gammon D, Bergvik S, Sexton H: Psychotherapy supervision face-to-face and by videoconferencing: a comparative study. British Journal of Psychotherapy 15(4):452–462, 1999

Sucala M, Schnur JB, Brackman EH, et al: Clinicians' attitudes toward therapeutic alliance in E-therapy. J Gen Psychol 140(4):282–293, 2013 24837821

Tarlow KR, McCord CE, Nelon JL, Berhard PA: Comparing in-person supervision and telesupervision: a baseline single-case study. Journal of Psychotherapy Integration 30(2):383–393, 2020

Watkins CE Jr: The psychotherapy supervisor as an agent of transformation: to anchor and educate, facilitate, and emancipate. Am J Psychother 73(2):57–62, 2020 31902226

Wood JAV, Hargrove DS, Miller TW: Clinical supervision in rural settings: a telehealth model. Professional Psychology: Research and Practice 36(2):173–179, 2005

Yellowlees P: Virtual or hybrid supervision, in Supervision in Psychiatric Practice: Practical Approaches Across Venues and Providers. Edited by DeGolia SG, Corcoran KM. Washington, DC, American Psychiatric Publishing, 2019, pp 45–53

11

Supervising Integrated Psychotherapy and Pharmacotherapy

David Mintz, M.D.
Marina Bayeva, M.D., Ph.D.

KEY LEARNING GOALS

- Attend to psychological pressures within the therapeutic milieu and the training environment that push toward an anti-integrative approach.

- Help trainees recognize when they may be using pharmacotherapy defensively against providing psychotherapy, and vice versa.

- Cultivate and model a capacity to deftly shift gears between levels of meaning and biology and to foster this capacity in one's trainees.

- Recognize the strains of learning an integrated approach to combined treatment.

Supervising psychotherapy, especially psychodynamic psychotherapy, is a complex task, requiring attention to the patient's therapeutic goals, their conflicts and resistances, and the transferences that fuel and complicate treatment. Simultaneously, the supervisor must consider the functioning of the therapeutic dyad, attend to the trainee therapist's technique, and monitor countertransferences that covertly pull against the therapeutic task. The task of supervising pharmacotherapy might seem straightforward until the multiple psychosocial factors that influence pharmacotherapy outcomes are recognized (Ankarberg and Falkenström 2008; Mintz 2005; Mintz and Flynn 2012) and addressed in supervision.

The task of supervising combination treatment with psychotherapy and pharmacotherapy is exponentially more complicated than supervising either form of treatment alone. Besides simultaneously supervising the psychotherapy and the pharmacotherapy, the supervisor is also attending to the complex dialectic between psychotherapy and medications, deftly shifting gears between biological and psychological frames of reference, while also addressing the complicated ways in which each frame may either augment or be used defensively against the other by patient and trainee alike.

Although the complex skill set of combination treatment with psychotherapy and pharmacotherapy is arguably the sine qua non of psychiatry (Belcher 2020), the teaching and supervising of combined treatments has received scant attention in the academic psychiatry literature. Beginning in 2001, the Psychiatry Residency Review Committee of the Accreditation Council for Graduate Medical Education briefly included combined psychotherapy with psychopharmacology as one of the five core psychotherapeutic competencies required of all U.S. psychiatric residents (Mellman and Beresin 2003). Unfortunately, the strains on training programs to teach five different psychotherapy modalities to the level of "competence" led to this requirement being dropped within 5 years, before significant research could be done to establish an evidence or practice base.

In 2001, the American Association of Directors of Psychiatric Residency Training (AADPRT) published a description of the core knowledge, skills, and attitudes that constitute competency in combining medications and psychotherapy (Sargent et al. 2001). This document addressed what should be learned in residency, but not how to teach it. A number of psychiatric educators have similarly addressed the benefits, techniques, and challenges of combining psychotherapy and pharmacotherapy (Cabaniss 2017; Gorman 2016; Kay 2009; Mintz 2023; White and Koehler 2021), but these writings focused on clinical issues and offered little guidance on how to foster this competency in trainees. On the other side, writings that addressed improvements in the pedagogy of pharmacotherapy neglected the topic of supervising its integration with psychotherapeutic treatment. One notable exception was Riba et al. (2018), who devoted a chapter of their book on combined treatment to the topic of supervision.

Establishing an Integrative Perspective

Trainees who are trying to learn (and supervisors who are trying to teach) combination treatment with psychotherapy and pharmacotherapy often find themselves within a system where anti-integrative pressures subtly undermine the trainee's capacity to master the integrative perspective. The split between the role of prescriber and the role of therapist is often built into the very structure of training, with different psychotherapy and psychopharmacology supervisors routinely assigned to the trainee for the same patient. This approach inadvertently divides the treatment and the training into "biological" and "psychological" parts and implicitly pushes the trainee to bring different aspects of the work to two separate supervisors, with limited opportunity for cross talk.

Coding procedures also unintentionally encourage trainees to think of clinical appointments as having discrete parts devoted either to psychotherapy or to psychopharmacology. Documentation templates that prompt clinicians to assign the exact number of minutes spent on medications and therapy create a strong sense of disconnect between the two. This, in turn, interferes with the trainee's ability to experience medication discussions as grist for the psychotherapy mill and to consider how psychotherapeutic exploration of issues related to pharmacotherapy enhances the patient's optimal use of medications.

Implicit anti-integrative pressures in the treatment and/or training can powerfully shape the trainee's view of combination treatment as a simple sum of its parts, rather than a unique clinical approach. This misassumption must be addressed directly in supervision. In addition, residency training directors and supervisors should be aware of the specific anti-integrative pressures within their individual systems and should explicitly address these during training. Despite the dearth of psychiatrists who specialize in the supervision of combined psychotherapy–psychopharmacology cases, all psychotherapy supervisors can directly acknowledge the systemic pressures that threaten integration and alert trainees to hidden aspects of the curriculum that inadvertently teach anti-integrative lessons.

Bringing an Integrative Perspective to Pharmacotherapy Supervision in Combination Treatment

Supervision of the pharmacological aspects of combined psychotherapy–pharmacotherapy should not simply focus on which medication to prescribe for a particular diagnosis or symptom; it should also address how to prescribe the medication (Mintz and Flynn 2012), taking into account a patient's defensive constellations, the special meanings that may be attached to illness and caretaking, and other psychological factors. In addition to having a command of the evidence base for psychotropic medications and their use in psychiatric disorders, the supervisor should also be knowledgeable about research related to effective prescribing processes and nonpharmacological aspects of medications (Mallo and Mintz 2013; Mallo et al. 2014; Mintz 2022; Mintz and Flynn 2012). Familiarizing the trainee with both sets of empirical evidence is an important aspect of the supervisory task for combined treatment.

Crucially, trainees should be alerted to the importance of the therapeutic alliance in pharmacotherapy, given that the alliance appears to be a more powerful predictor of treatment outcome than the actual medication prescribed (Krupnick et al. 1996). Elements such as warmth and empathy, support for patients' agency, and collaborative decision-making promote a more positive therapeutic alliance (Frank et al. 1995; Zuroff et al. 2007). Optimally, trainees should be helped to appreciate the distinction between a true alliance, in which there is room for negotiating difference and partnership, and a defensive compliance, in which agreeableness by either or both parties is used to avoid conflict. A deeper psychotherapeutic understanding of the patient permits the prescriber to consider the patient's multilayered and often conflicting goals and to incorporate these into the prescribing approach.

Given that patient ambivalence about medications is common and is known to affect outcomes (Piguet et al. 2007; Sirey et al. 2001), the supervisor's role includes helping trainees identify and explore the patient's resistances to a healthy use of pharmacotherapy. Trainees should be encouraged to explore the patient's conscious feelings regarding medications (e.g., fears of side effects, stigma of mental illness, anxieties about dependency) so that these can be directly addressed to support adherence. On a deeper level, uncovering the psychological meanings that patients attach to symptoms, such as an unconscious connection between being ill and receiving caring attention, can help therapists to address sources of treatment resistance (Plakun 2012; van Egmond and Kummeling 2002). Negative transferences (e.g., expecting harm or negligence from caregivers) may interfere with the effective use of pharmacotherapy and should be a focus of supervisory work.

In an integrative approach, the aim of pharmacotherapy extends beyond symptom management to encompass issues of functioning, including specifically the patient's ability to use psychotherapy. The supervisor of combination treatment may support the dual roles of psychotherapy and pharmacotherapy by helping the supervisee to consider how medications might facilitate the patient's growth through engagement in psychotherapy. For example, when a patient is unable to engage more deeply in therapy because they become easily overwhelmed by affect, the supervisee may be encouraged to recommend medications that are more likely to reduce emotional reactivity.

Conversely, supervisors can help trainees to identify situations in which medications are used countertherapeutically (Mintz 2019, 2022; Mintz and Belnap 2006). Beyond simple misuse of medications for pleasure rather than health promotion, patients may, for example, use the meaning of medications as a proof of the "biological" nature of an illness over which they would like to think they have no control. Making the observation that this reasoning allows patients to abdicate responsibility for destructive behaviors or impairs their agency to actively pursue recovery may be more helpful to patients than prescribing new medications. Similarly, patients may use pills to squelch distressing but important emotions, such as grief, anger, or loneliness. The supervisor's task is to illuminate for the supervisee the patient's anxious and defensive efforts to avoid facing and mastering painful emotions, thereby helping the trainee avoid overprescribing and instead find ways to better address the psychological conflicts that may be keeping the patient stuck.

Medications and Meaning

From the psychotherapeutic perspective, pharmacotherapy and the pharmacotherapeutic task are fraught with meaning. As with Einstein's recognition that the photon was both a particle and a wave, medications are both biologically and symbolically active (Plakun 2006). Indeed, medications may be so imbued with meaning that they serve as important object relationships (Tutter 2006), rivaling the importance of people in some patients' lives. Like the exploration of a dream, the exploration of the meaning of medications may illuminate important aspects of the patient's inner life (Powell 2001). Variously, medications may come to represent the illness, the diagnosis, the prescriber, or biomedicine in general; medications can also represent aspects of the patient's self. In combined treatment, medication discussions should be perceived through that lens. The supervisor can help bridge mind–body splits in the supervisee (and in the patient) by encouraging exploration of the patient's fantasies about and relationship with medications. Often, a patient's relationship with medications will mirror the patterns of other relationships in the patient's life (e.g., patients who are counterdependent[1] in personal relationships may also struggle to adhere to medication regimens).

Regarding positive meanings, the prescribing of medication may be experienced transferentially as an act of caring or concern, a recognition of suffering, an offer of support, or, in the oral metaphor, as a form of nurturance. Whether medications are experienced in this way is likely to be determined by factors such as the prescriber's actual feelings, the quality of the therapeutic alliance, and the patient's predominant object relations. In the latter instance, it is not uncommon for the prescribing of medication to enact for one or both parties a relationship between a caring and competent parent and a dependent and needful child. As prescribers, novice psychiatrists-psychotherapists may wish, consciously or unconsciously, to foster, exploit, and later ignore positive caregiving transferences, fearful that drawing attention to the placebogenic aspects of the relationship might lessen placebo responses. However, such an approach runs the risk of depriving patients of self-understanding, self-determination, and self-recognition of their own self-healing capacities. Supervisors can help supervisees to recognize medication-related idealizing (and also potentially disempowering) transferences, which are often overlooked or minimized, as well as the transitional object functions of pills and the role that the patient plays in positive pharmacotherapy outcomes.

On the other hand, prescriptions, and the diagnoses they may represent, can be experienced as concrete symbols of defect, or as signifiers of hopelessness or powerlessness. Transferentially, the therapist's act of prescribing may be experienced by the patient as a rejection, a giving up, an objectification, an effort at control, or even a sexual intrusion. Particularly when patients have experienced abuse or neglect at the hands of caregivers, such negative transferences will be easily mobilized, undercutting the alliance (both pharmacotherapeutic and psychotherapeutic) and the effectiveness of the overall treatment.

---

[1] *Counterdependency* is defined here as a refusal of attachment, denial of personal needs, and fear of dependency.

Supervising the Psychotherapy of Pharmacotherapy

In supervising treatment consisting of the combination of these two modalities, the supervisor can help the trainee learn to explore the meanings of medications in ways that contribute to the patient's self-understanding and reveal disguised aspects of the transference. However, as Freud (1912/1958) noted in "On Beginning Treatment," it may not be necessary to interpret transference until transference becomes a source of resistance.

When the meanings of medications threaten to undermine the working alliance, supervisors should help therapists address this critical issue. Supervisors may help supervisees listen to the patient's associations for manifestations of disguised negative transferences. They may facilitate the trainee's capacity to shift gears (Cabaniss 1998) by listening to the patient's reports of side effects as representing both a description of the concrete physical effects of medications and a communication of a disguised negative transference. When a patient attaches harmful meanings to pharmacotherapy, the supervisor may help the trainee to tactfully explore potential unconscious motivations for an attachment to treatment-interfering attitudes. For example, medications (or what they signify) may have been recruited by the patient to serve defensive functions. Trainees may be unaware of the subtle and indirect routes by which a patient's defenses may simultaneously hide, transform, and express (and then often punish) forbidden feelings, wishes, and impulses that become attached to pharmacotherapy.

Defensively, for example, patients may attach the meaning of "I'm incapable" or "It's not my fault" to pharmacotherapy. The prescription thus serves as an "inexact interpretation" (Glover 1931; Mintz 2019, 2022; Nevins 1990) that is used defensively by these patients to absolve themselves of responsibility for their situation, which is now interpreted as a manifestation of aberrant biology, with no real meaning. Moreover, an attempt to "medicate away" troublesome emotions deprives these patients of such emotions' developmentally important guidance, an outcome that fosters loss of self-efficacy and runs counter to the goals of therapy.

Medications may also be used unconsciously to communicate unacceptable feelings. For example, patients who require continual medication adjustments may use medications to express the feeling "I'm afraid that if I get better, you will abandon me." Other patients may report repeated harm by medications because they cannot directly express their anger about past harms by caregivers, and so instead tell their story through these complaints, using medication side effects as a story-telling vehicle. Only when these defensive maneuvers are put into words can these patients begin to find healthier and more direct ways to express their feelings.

Finally, pharmacotherapy may be recruited by patients or their physicians to serve defensive functions within the psychotherapeutic relationship. Supervisors can help trainees attend to the ways in which medication discussions may be used by either party to control or regulate the therapy. For example, supervisors may highlight how medications often become a focus of sessions when patients are feeling frustrated by their lack of progress. In this situation, a patient's raising the issue of medications may be used to sidestep uncomfortable aspects of the transference or as a way of expressing their lack of faith in psychotherapy. On the other side of the dyad, supervisors may help trainees identify situations in which they introduce the question of medications as a defense against painful feelings (e.g., hopelessness, helplessness, grief, anger) in themselves or in the patient. When trainees are helped to recognize how medical action may be used by therapists as a defense against a fuller encounter with the patient's affective life (Main 1977), this insight can clear the way for forging a deeper and more healing engagement with the patient. Through sustained attention to the meaning of medication discussions, trainees can learn to recognize such discussions as significant events in the psychotherapy.

The Challenge of Shifting Gears

Medication management discussions may occur at the beginning or end of the session, or throughout. The capacity to skillfully shift gears between medical and psychotherapeutic functions is thus one of the more significant achievements in learning to provide combination treatment (Cabaniss 1998). This skill requires a capacity for mental integration (e.g., thinking of medications as both medical and psychological) as well as a sense for when and how to shift gears clinically. The supervisor may facilitate trainees' acquisition of this skill by elucidating the strengths and weaknesses of different strategies for shifting between roles. Rather than teaching the "right" way to integrate the two functions, the supervisor can shed light on the complexity of the combination treatment approach and help trainees pay closer attention to the interface between therapy and medication work within each session.

Clinicians may, on the one hand, start the session with the pharmacological agenda. This provides ample time to explore all medication-related questions and psychological ramifications. Moreover, by introducing medications directly, the clinician signals attentiveness to the pharmacological aspects of treatment, which could otherwise be eclipsed by the intensity of the psychotherapeutic work. However, by opening with medication-related questions, the therapist disrupts the usual psychotherapeutic frame (wherein the patient's thoughts and feelings are prioritized), potentially foreclosing a topic that the patient may have wished to explore. The power imbalance that is introduced when the therapist sets an agenda can be partially mitigated by initially asking the patient whether there is something more pressing to discuss than medications.

Another approach is to leave medication discussions for the end, mitigating the risk of having the psychiatrist's agenda shape the session or signal that pharmacological issues take priority over therapy. The clinician may even defer pharmacological discussions to the following session if the patient is sharing something important and medication issues are nonurgent. This approach, however, carries the risk of allotting insufficient time for medication-related issues. For example, a simple inquiry about side effects may uncover a major problem that, if immediately addressed, would extend the session beyond its time boundary. Moreover, time constraints may not permit exploration of relevant psychological issues related to prescribing.

Regardless of whether pharmacotherapy is allotted space at the beginning or at the end of a session, either approach risks fostering a mind–body split in the patient's self-experience, with a divide in the session implying a divide in the patient. Educating patients about mind–body interactions in pharmacotherapy and continuously modeling the integration of these perspectives may ameliorate the divide, yet a discrete distinction between the two modalities remains entrenched in both approaches. Another concern is that both methods alter the usual flow of the therapy session, and, as with any impingement on the frame, patients will react in line with their own expectations and transference predispositions.

A third approach to the integration of psychopharmacology into psychotherapy is to address medication issues as they emerge organically during the session. In this approach, patients are explicitly empowered to communicate their questions or concerns about medications rather than being expected to wait to be asked. Treaters must listen to the patient's associations for veiled references to medications and be prepared to explore medication issues in response. Artfully applied, this method allows for optimal integration, as the clinician shifts seamlessly between the two modalities, going from medication issues to their meanings (defenses, conflicts, or ambivalence related to medications), and vice versa. However, this approach potentially sets the stage for important enactments. Clinicians and patients who are uncomfortable in a charged transference–countertransference field can switch into a "medical mode" to avoid discomfort. Intense emotions, such as anger, grief, or dependent longing, can be defensively treated as symptoms to be medicated rather than as feelings to be understood. For this reason, medication discussions could serve to distract from, rather than to facilitate, psychotherapy. Similarly, patients may unconsciously (or deliberately) bring up medication questions or report side effects during the last few minutes in an attempt to extend the session or to challenge the time boundary. With this approach, supervisors should be particularly alert to nonmedical uses of medication discussions and should encourage trainees to explore such patterns with the patient. At the other extreme, relying on patients to introduce medication concerns runs the risk of neglecting pharmacological issues, especially when therapy is compelling. A reluctance to interrupt free associations may inhibit appropriate questioning related to pharmacological treatment. Attending to symptoms primarily for their communicative value may also lead to undertreatment of such symptoms.

Beyond setting an integrative frame, there are psychological challenges to the trainee's ability to shift from a biomedical to a psychological perspective. In prescribing, the psychotherapist-pharmacotherapist is actively intervening in the patient's life in a concrete way, and thus relinquishes a position of abstinence and neutrality, a role alteration that poses special dilemmas for psychotherapy and its supervision. By becoming less of a neutral screen, the therapist-prescriber has effectively taken sides in the patient's struggle. In this sense, the line between the transference and the real relationship has become blurred—which, in turn, can make it more difficult to perceive and illuminate for the trainee the ways in which the patient may be experiencing the therapist through the lens of the transference. It may be difficult, too, for the prescribing therapist to differentiate countertransference from reality. For example, a patient complains of the harmfulness or the impotence of medications. Because the supervisee has actively provided something concrete that the patient experiences negatively, the supervisee's feelings of guilt or inadequacy may be experienced more concretely, whereas a unimodal psychotherapist might more easily experience such feelings as projective identifications, providing information about the patient's inner life. Supervisors should be aware of and attentive to the ways that the dual relationship may render supervisees more vulnerable to accepting painful projective identifications in an unquestioned way and may make it harder for them to sort out what is real and what is fantasy.

The dialectic between meaning and medication is so potent and complex that when patients report improvement after starting a new medication, it is typically not possible to know how much improvement stems from the medication and how much emanates from placebogenic factors associated with the prescription. This honest and humble recognition may pose a challenge to the emerging sense of competence of the psychiatric trainee. Part of the task of the supervisor of combination pharmacotherapy–psychotherapy is to support the trainee's capacity to recognize and bear the ambiguity inherent in combined treatment. This may require supervisors to attend to the defensive and narcissistic needs of their trainees (Brightman 1984–1985) as they come to recognize and accept their limitations in knowledge and potency and learn to find a useful place for negative feelings.

Like their patients, trainees struggle with ambiguity, ambivalence, and inner conflict. The capacities that trainees develop to manage their own conflicts go a long way toward creating a safe space for patients to successfully grapple with theirs. These capacities, in turn, may be shaped, in a parallel process, by witnessing and experiencing the capacities of supervisors and other role models to tolerate the ambiguity and complexity of combination treatment. Having successfully navigated this challenge, trainees are in a better position to nondefensively shift gears (Cabaniss 1998) between biomedical and psychological frames of reference and to be curious about and interested in areas of conflict, rather than moving toward defensive certainty.

Conclusion

As acknowledged in the original five psychiatric core psychotherapy competencies mandated by the Psychiatry Residency Review Committee, the integration of psychotherapy and pharmacotherapy is a unique skill set that is distinct from either psychotherapy or pharmacotherapy. Regrettably, not only are the unique skills of combined treatment often given short shrift in residency education, but psychotherapy and pharmacotherapy are often taught in a way that fosters disintegration, as if the two skills do not interact with and shape one another in profound ways. Supervisors, too, may not be sufficiently trained in integrating these dual functions.

These deficiencies become especially important when one considers the likely practice patterns of today's graduating residents. Among residents who will be conducting psychotherapy after graduation, the vast majority will be providing combined treatment rather than psychotherapy alone. Ideally, given that residency should prepare residents for their future practice, psychiatric training should focus more on teaching combined psychotherapy–pharmacotherapy than on teaching psychotherapy alone. At a bare minimum, psychiatric residents should have at least one psychiatrist supervisor who supervises both pharmacotherapy and psychotherapy in an integrated manner. Even if a single supervisor is not sufficient to bring trainees to the level of "competence," having a supervisor who is experienced in integrating pharmacotherapy into psychotherapy treatment will orient trainees to the inherent complexities of combination treatment and provide an initial understanding that allows trainees to apprehend future learning needs. Without such supervisory experiences, trainees might not recognize a need to develop a practice that considers an integrative approach.

Common sense suggests that patients who receive combination treatment in which pharmacotherapy and psychotherapy are poorly integrated will likely experience no advantage over patients who receive split treatment. The true benefits of combined treatment emerge when the psychiatrist is fully attuned to the ways in which medications and therapy can be facilitating and/or conflicting and has the skills needed to provide truly integrated care. Supervision of combined treatment should prepare trainees to thoughtfully use medications in ways that enhance the therapeutic alliance and support the patient's capacity to engage in psychotherapy. At the same time, the training of the pharmacotherapist-psychotherapist should foster an awareness of the myriad ways in which irrational processes (in both patient and psychiatrist) can set the goals for psychotherapy and pharmacotherapy unconsciously at odds, undermining the growth and effectiveness of one or both treatments. This risk is particularly salient in regard to patients with treatment-refractory and difficult-to-treat mental illness, who increasingly constitute the caseloads of psychiatrists, and who have complicated relationships with medications, care, or health itself. Practicing at the true "top of [one's] psychiatric license" (Mintz 2018; Welton 2019) rests in the ability to integrate psychopharmacological knowledge with psychotherapeutic skills in ways that support the optimal use of both functions, leading to enhanced outcomes. Skilled supervision of combined treatment is crucial to providing psychiatric trainees with the skills needed to address the needs and dilemmas posed by our most complicated and challenging patients.

References

Ankarberg P, Falkenström F: Treatment of depression with antidepressants is primarily a psychological treatment. Psychotherapy (Chic) 45(3):329–339, 2008 22122494

Belcher R: Psychotherapy and the professional identity of psychiatry in the age of neuroscience. Acad Psychiatry 44(2):227–230, 2020 31734936

Brightman BK: Narcissistic issues in the training experience of the psychotherapist. Int J Psychoanal Psychother 10:293–317, 1984–1985 6511192

Cabaniss DL: Shifting gears: the challenge to teach students to think psychodynamically and psychopharmacologically at the same time. Psychoanalytic Inquiry 18(5):639–656, 1998

Cabaniss DL (with Cherry S, Douglas CJ, Schwartz A): Psychodynamic Psychotherapy: A Clinical Manual, 2nd Edition. New York, Wiley, 2017

Frank E, Kupfer DJ, Siegel LR: Alliance not compliance: a philosophy of outpatient care. J Clin Psychiatry 56 (suppl 1):11–16, discussion 16–17, 1995 7836346

Freud S: On beginning the treatment (further recommendations on the technique of psycho-analysis I) (1912), in The Standard Edition of the Complete Psychological Works of Sigmund Freud, Vol 12. Translated and edited by Strachey J. London, Hogarth Press, 1958, pp 121–144

Glover E: The therapeutic effect of inexact interpretation: a contribution to the theory of suggestion. The International Journal of Psychoanalysis 12:397–411, 1931

Gorman JM: Combining psychodynamic psychotherapy and pharmacotherapy. Psychodyn Psychiatry 44(2):183–209, 2016 27200462

Kay J: Combining psychodynamic psychotherapy with medication, in Textbook of Psychotherapeutic Treatments. Edited by Gabbard GO. Washington, DC, American Psychiatric Publishing, 2009, pp 133–161

Krupnick JL, Sotsky SM, Simmens S, et al: The role of the therapeutic alliance in psychotherapy and pharmacotherapy outcome: findings in the National Institute of Mental Health Treatment of Depression Collaborative Research Program. J Consult Clin Psychol 64(3):532–539, 1996 8698947

Main TF: Traditional psychiatric defences against close encounter with patients. Can Psychiatr Assoc J 22(8):457–466, 1977 597809

Mallo CJ, Mintz DL: Teaching all the evidence bases: reintegrating psychodynamic aspects of prescribing into psychopharmacology training. Psychodyn Psychiatry 41(1):13–37, 2013 23480158

Mallo CJ, Mintz DL, Lewis KC: Integrating psychosocial concepts into psychopharmacology training: a survey study of program directors and chief residents. Psychodyn Psychiatry 42(2):243–254, 2014 24828593

Mellman LA, Beresin E: Psychotherapy competencies: development and implementation. Acad Psychiatry 27(3):149–153, 2003 12969837

Mintz DL: Teaching the prescriber's role: the psychology of psychopharmacology. Acad Psychiatry 29(2):187–194, 2005 15937266

Mintz D: Practicing at the top of your license. May 25, 2018. Available at: https://austenriggs.org/blog-post/practicing-top-your-license. Accessed May 23, 2021.

Mintz D: Recovery from childhood psychiatric treatment: addressing the meaning of medications. Psychodyn Psychiatry 47(3):235–256, 2019 31448987

Mintz D: Psychodynamic Psychopharmacology: Caring for the Treatment-Resistant Patient. Washington, DC, American Psychiatric Association Publishing, 2022

Mintz D: Combining medications and psychotherapy, in Gabbard's Textbook of Psychotherapeutic Treatments, 2nd Edition. Edited by Crisp H, Gabbard GO. Washington, DC, American Psychiatric Association Publishing, 2023, pp 743–760

Mintz D, Belnap B: A view from Riggs: treatment resistance and patient authority–III. What is psychodynamic psychopharmacology? An approach to pharmacologic treatment resistance. J Am Acad Psychoanal Dyn Psychiatry 34(4):581–601, 2006 17274730

Mintz DL, Flynn DF: How (not what) to prescribe: nonpharmacologic aspects of psychopharmacology. Psychiatr Clin North Am 35(1):143–163, 2012 22370496

Nevins DB: Psychoanalytic perspectives on the use of medication for mental illness. Bull Menninger Clin 54(3):323–339, 1990 2207466

Piguet V, Cedraschi C, Dumont P, et al: Patients' representations of antidepressants: a clue to nonadherence? Clin J Pain 23(8):669–675, 2007 17885345

Plakun EM: A view from Riggs: treatment resistance and patient authority, III: what is psychodynamic psychopharmacology? An approach to pharmacologic treatment resistance. J Am Acad Psychoanal Dyn Psychiatry 34(4):579–580, 2006 17274729

Plakun E: Treatment resistance and psychodynamic psychiatry: concepts psychiatry needs from psychoanalysis. Psychodyn Psychiatry 40(2):183–209, 2012 23006116

Powell AD: The medication life. J Psychother Pract Res 10(4):217–222, 2001 11696647

Riba MB, Balon R, Roberts LW: Competency in Combining Pharmacotherapy and Psychotherapy: Integrated and Split Treatment. Core Competencies in Psychotherapy. Gabbard GO, Editor. Washington, DC, American Psychiatric Association Publishing, 2018

Sargent J, Mohl P, Beitman B, et al: AADPRT Psychotherapy Combined With Psychopharmacology Competencies. Revised November 21, 2001. Available at: https://portal.aadprt.org/public/vto/categories/Virtual%20Classroom/Psychotherapy%20Competency%20Tools/57fc01d1a2f73_Psychotherapy%20Combined%20with%20Psychopharmacology%20Competencies.pdf. Accessed May 23, 2021.

Sirey JA, Bruce ML, Alexopoulos GS, et al: Stigma as a barrier to recovery: perceived stigma and patient-rated severity of illness as predictors of antidepressant drug adherence. Psychiatr Serv 52(12):1615–1620, 2001 11726752

Tutter A: Medication as object. J Am Psychoanal Assoc 54(3):781–804, 2006 17009655

van Egmond J, Kummeling I: A blind spot for secondary gain affecting therapy outcomes. Eur Psychiatry 17(1):46–54, 2002 11918993

Welton RS: How can psychiatrists practice to the "top of their license"? Psychiatric News 54(17):14–15, 2019. Accessed at: https://psychnews.psychiatryonline.org/doi/10.1176/appi.pn.2019.9a29. Accessed May 25, 2021.

White M, Koehler H: Integrating medication and therapy, in Psychotherapy: A Practical Introduction. Edited by Brenner AM, Howe-Martin LS. Philadelphia, PA, Wolters Kluwer, 2021, pp 363–390

Zuroff DC, Koestner R, Moskowitz DS, et al: Autonomous motivation for therapy: a new common factor in brief treatments for depression. Psychotherapy Research 17(2):137–147, 2007

12

Termination of Psychotherapy Supervision

Rebecca Nejat, M.D.
Natasha Chriss, M.D.

KEY LEARNING GOALS

- Recognize common reasons for terminating psychotherapy supervision and understand why avoiding an explicit discussion about termination may have potential negative consequences.

- Explain the four crucial steps in planned supervisory terminations: set a date, express feelings, give and receive feedback, and say goodbye.

- Describe how the termination of supervision can serve as an experiential teaching tool to facilitate clinical terminations.

- Understand the importance of using supervisory termination as an opportunity to assess and evaluate the educational goals that have been set during supervision.

Dr. Cortes, an early-career psychiatrist, establishes private outpatient psychotherapy supervision with Dr. Benton, a supervisor she enjoyed working with during training. At the beginning of private supervision, Dr. Cortes and Dr. Benton discuss a frame for supervision that includes frequency and payment. Dr. Benton encourages Dr. Cortes to voice her concerns and preferences, including thoughts about wanting to end supervision, if they arise in the future. After 2 years of supervision, Dr. Cortes starts feeling more confident in her clinical work. Although she continues to enjoy the supervisory relationship, she feels less need for supervision and finds herself exploring new ways of thinking and working that differ from the approaches of her supervisor. At the same time, she feels unsure about what she might do without supervision when clinical difficulties arise. Uncertain about how to bring up these concerns, Dr. Cortes continues supervision.

Dr. Benton starts noticing that Dr. Cortes's enthusiasm for supervision seems diminished, and that she now spends much of their time together looking for approval of already formulated hypotheses and clinical choices. Dr. Benton takes this opportunity to ask Dr. Cortes about her experience in supervision and whether it has changed over time. Dr. Cortes acknowledges that she feels that her need for supervision has decreased, but she feels anxious about working completely independently. Dr. Benton asks Dr. Cortes to say more about what she imagines she might lose and gain from ending supervision. Dr. Benton is then able to normalize Dr. Cortes's feelings and respond with warmth and encouragement. She reflects on Dr. Cortes's professional development and competency. Together they collaborate in thinking through ways for Dr. Cortes to continue to develop professionally after supervision ends. They also identify managing uncertainty in clinical work as an educational goal to focus on in the ending phase of supervision. They set an end date 3 months in advance and continue the supervision up until this date.

In this final phase, Dr. Cortes and Dr. Benton continue to reflect on the experience of working together, acknowledge the loss around ending supervision, and focus on the remaining learning goals. In addition, by speaking openly about terminating supervision and receiving feedback from Dr. Benton about her growth and development, Dr. Cortes feels emboldened to share some of her new ideas that challenge those of her supervisor. She feels gratified when Dr. Benton welcomes them and considers them seriously. Dr. Cortes looks forward to potentially working with Dr. Benton as a colleague in the future. As supervision ends, Dr. Cortes is excited about taking the knowledge acquired in supervision and building on it to further develop her own evolving clinical perspective.

Termination describes the process of ending a working relationship. The main goal of terminating psychotherapy supervision is to bring the supervision to a deliberate, meaningful, and reflective end. As with all important relationships, endings can bring up a wide variety of emotions for both supervisor and supervisee. When the relationship has been mutually rewarding and successful, positive feelings of accomplishment, gratitude, and connection may be particularly strong, alongside more painful feelings such as loss and anxiety. When the relationship has been more conflictual, feelings of guilt, frustration, anger, and relief may also be present.

Due to the intensity of feelings and the fear of conflict, the topic of terminating supervision may be avoided by both parties. When this happens, both the supervisor and the supervisee miss opportunities for growth. Supervisors cannot receive feedback or model a thoughtful ending phase. Supervisees are unable to collaboratively reflect on their feelings and professional development. Terminating psychotherapy supervision is a valuable opportunity to deepen the work, further the goals of supervision for both participants, and model for the supervisee how to terminate a therapeutic relationship.

Terminations occur in many different settings and for a variety of reasons. In this chapter we first review a suggested model for managing the termination of supervision, which has been illustrated in the opening clinical vignette. We then review common problems that may arise in the termination of supervision. Because of the diverse circumstances in which terminations occur, a planned ending, while preferable, is not always achievable. Even when termination is not brought up in advance, this model can still be used to encourage explicit discussion of and reflection on terminating supervision. Such discussion and reflection can allow a more meaningful ending to occur and can consolidate the experience of supervision for both supervisor and supervisee.

Assessing Readiness for Terminating Supervision

Throughout supervision, the supervisor should be thinking about the growth of the supervisee and listening for the possibility that the supervisee may be signaling readiness to end. Whether in private supervision where the termination date is open-ended or in a training program where a termination date has been predetermined, attending to and verbally noting signs of the supervisee's progress is crucial, and will ultimately facilitate a conversation about termination that is natural and productive. Supervisors should be aware of how supervisees make use of the supervision and how this may change over the course of working together. This involves paying attention to potential ways that supervisees may indicate that they have started thinking more autonomously. What types of advice are they seeking from the supervisor? How urgently are they grasping for help with clinical management? Can they construct a case formulation with increasing levels of nuance?

Readiness to end supervision can manifest differently in different supervisees. For some supervisees, such readiness takes the form of asking more questions as their understanding of theoretical complexity advances. For others, readiness can manifest as asking fewer questions as clinical knowledge is consolidated and trusted. Problems can arise both in ending supervision precipitously and in prolonging supervision with a supervisee who may benefit from more independent practice. We strongly recommend that supervisors help supervisees end the supervision according to their own personal preferences, even if this means that supervisees end supervision before supervisors believe that they are fully ready to do so. By preserving supervisee autonomy, the supervisor leaves open the possibility of future work, which the supervisee may need.

Steps in Terminating Supervision

Once a supervisor and a supervisee have agreed to terminate, and when a planned termination is possible, there are four critical steps for the supervisor to take when ending a supervision, as illustrated in Table 12–1: 1) setting a date for the final session, 2) reflecting on the feelings that come up around ending supervision, 3) giving and receiving feedback on the educational experience, and 4) saying goodbye. Managing psychotherapy termination in this way strengthens the clinical and educational objectives that supervision can achieve.

Discussing Termination and Setting a Date

Ideally, at the start of a supervision, supervisors should invite supervisees to bring up the topic of termination when it is on their mind. This opens the door to straightforward communication and gives the supervisee permission to bring up this difficult topic. When termination has not been discussed in the framing of supervision, supervisors can bring it up at any point if they believe it would be helpful. Most important is to be open, warm, and respectful in discussing termination whenever the topic arises.

Once termination has been agreed to, the first step is collaboratively choosing an end date with the supervisee. Choosing a specific date helps both parties recognize the finite time they have remaining to work together. The pair can then intentionally choose how to spend this time and what goals a supervisee may wish to focus on in the time remaining. Without setting an end date, this final working period goes unidentified, leaving the ending abrupt, unobserved, and lacking in educational focus.

As with clinical work, the length of the termination phase of supervision should be proportional to the length of the supervision. We suggest allocating approximately 20% of the full supervision length for the termination phase. However, as few as one to three supervisory sessions may also be adequate. Occasionally, the process of discussing termination may change this timeline; thus, maintaining flexibility and being attuned to the supervisee's needs and desires is most important. For example, discussing what clinical skills have been developed and what is left to work on may

Table 12–1.   Steps in terminating supervision

1. **Set a date.**
   - Discuss termination explicitly.
   - Set a date for the final supervision session.

2. **Acknowledge feelings.**
   - Reflect on what emotions come up for supervisees around terminating supervision.
   - Discuss the importance of self-awareness of these feelings, particularly in how they may ultimately relate to clinical terminations.

3. **Give and receive feedback.**
   - Reflect on what educational goals have been accomplished.
   - Identify what educational goals remain for future learning.
   - Solicit feedback from supervisees about your own supervisory skills.

4. **Say goodbye.**
   - Discuss a plan for future contact.
   - Acknowledge the change in the nature of the professional relationship (from mentor/teacher to colleague).
   - Consider marking the occasion (e.g., lunch, a small gift).
   - End the supervision.

lead supervisees to choose to spend a bit longer in supervision than they had initially envisioned when they brought up termination. In other circumstances, discussing difficulties with time and money or deeper conflicts in supervision may help highlight a supervisee's wish to terminate more quickly. Regardless of the specific circumstances, it is important to lean toward the supervisee's opinion of when to stop and to facilitate ending the supervision on the supervisee's terms.

Acknowledging Feelings That Arise in Response to Terminating Supervision

Dr. Steele is a fourth-year psychiatry resident approaching graduation. During supervision, he tells his supervisor, Dr. Kim, about his frustration with one of his psychodynamic psychotherapy patients, with whom he will soon have to terminate. Dr. Steele describes feeling guilty for "leaving" his patient after she has become attached to him, knowing how painful it was for the patient when her last therapist graduated. He wonders whether the patient is having strong feelings about this upcoming termination but isn't acknowledging them. Dr. Kim hears him expressing aggravation about managing this clinical termination and notices that he is attributing potential feelings of loss only to his patient. She also notices that Dr. Steele has not mentioned his own feelings of loss related to the clinical treatment or to the supervision. Dr. Kim herself feels quite sad that their productive working relationship is nearing an end, and she realizes that they have not discussed the upcoming end of their supervision.

Dr. Kim asks Dr. Steele if he is feeling a sense of sadness about the forced clinical termination with his patient. After Dr. Steele acknowledges some sadness, Dr. Kim notes that it is not just his clinical relationship that is ending, but because he is graduating, their supervisory relationship is also ending. Noticing a shift in emotion for a moment, Dr. Kim decides to share a personal experience about feeling quite overwhelmed with sadness during her own supervision as a trainee when she had both a clinical case and a supervision co-terminating at the end of training. She discloses that acknowledging her own sense of sadness helped her to be more emotionally available to her patient during the clinical termination process. After hearing this, Dr. Steele admits to feeling quite emotional himself. He realizes how meaningful this patient has become to him and how appreciative he feels for his time in supervision, which is coming to an end. After more reflection, Dr. Steele notices that he feels surrounded by loss and sadness about his upcoming graduation because it requires him to end many important clinical and professional relationships. He had felt he could not acknowledge these feelings, because they didn't fit with his idea of what he was "supposed" to feel as a doctor.

Dr. Kim invites him to share his thoughts about endings in supervision, related either to clinical or to supervisory termination. They discuss how to make use of the remaining time in supervision, including educational goals and a plan for future contact. The two decide to leave open the option of working together in private supervision after Dr. Steele's graduation if he desires. Most importantly, Dr. Kim continues to normalize and acknowledge Dr. Steele's feelings of loss when they are voiced. As a result of acknowledging the depth of his feeling of loss, the meaningfulness of his patient, and his connection with his supervisor, Dr. Steele stops feeling frustrated with his patient and instead starts asking more direct questions about what ending is like for her, as Dr. Kim had with him. Where at first he feared and avoided thinking about his patient's experience of termination, he now feels ready and able to receive the patient's communicated experience.

Once a date has been set for the final supervision, feelings about the termination will arise in both supervisor and supervisee. Supervisors can consider mentioning and normalizing common feelings that tend to arise during terminations, including both positive feelings (e.g., gratitude, connection, support) and painful feelings (e.g., loss, sadness, anxiety), among others. Supervisors should encourage supervisees to be aware of and reflect on the feelings that may arise around ending during this final phase of supervision. Supervisors also can suggest that supervisees use the experience of ending supervision to think more broadly about how endings generally affect them (Schlesinger 2005). Such thinking fosters self-awareness in the supervisee that can be utilized in clinical work, particularly around understanding countertransference reactions during clinical terminations.

Although using an upcoming termination to stimulate affective awareness in supervisees can be fruitful, it is important to keep in mind that supervisors' relationships with their supervisees are not clinical relationships. Therefore, personal and professional boundaries in exploring feelings should be maintained. Supervisors can encourage supervisees to think about these personal feelings and to feel free to share them in supervision if they feel comfortable doing so, or to simply reflect on them privately.

When supervisory termination coincides with clinical termination, the feelings that arise may be particularly intense, as in the vignette with Dr. Steele. Helping supervisees work through these feelings will help them navigate both supervisory and clinical terminations more effectively. The wider the range and depth of feelings therapists can identify, feel, and manage, the more their patients will be able to identify, feel, and manage. Additionally, feeling seen and understood by a supervisor during the termination phase of supervision can be deeply supportive.

In the vignette above, Dr. Steele was unable to experience his patient's feelings about termination because he himself was unaware of and trying to avoid his own grief about the multiple endings he was facing. One way his supervisor helped highlight Dr. Steele's feelings of loss was to notice that she herself felt sad about the supervision ending but had not explicitly initiated a discussion about supervision ending. This is an example of parallel process, wherein a supervisor's affect reflects and mimics an affect occurring in the clinical relationship between therapist and patient (Zetzer et al. 2020). During these periods of more intense affect, the countertransference of the supervisor and of the supervisee can be essential clinical tools in clarifying and deepening a treatment.

Graduation from training is a common setting for terminating supervision. This represents a type of forced termination in which a date for ending supervision is set in advance by a third party. It is important to recognize that any forced termination can cause supervisors or clinicians to unwittingly avoid feelings and discussions around the termination of supervision or psychotherapy, because the date is preset. Graduation is unique among forced terminations because trainees are experiencing both supervisory and clinical termination along with many other changes, including collegial, social, institutional, and potentially geographic (Bostic et al. 1996). This may make feelings about termination more intense, which may further contribute to a desire to avoid discussions around termination.

Giving and Receiving Feedback

Giving and receiving feedback is an essential task in terminating psychotherapy supervision. Having a supervisor who speaks candidly about their progress helps supervisees to develop a more accurate self-appraisal of their strengths and weaknesses. Having their supervisor provide positive feedback about what supervisees have excelled at can be exciting for them and can foster greater self-confidence in independent work. Feedback is often more difficult for both parties when discussing continued areas for growth. Providing such feedback in a tactful and encouraging manner is essential. Similarly, assessing the need for more supervision, either together or with another supervisor, can be helpful.

Ideally, educational goals have been discussed early on in supervision. During termination, the pair can then discuss what specific progress has been made and consolidate the knowledge acquired. They can also identify what goals remain that the supervisee may wish to focus on in the future. Based on this collaboration, the pair can more intentionally decide how to use their limited time together most effectively. Even when educational goals have not been previously discussed, explicitly asking about such goals in the final phase of supervision can be highly beneficial. The supervisor can use setting a termination date as an opportunity to ask about the supervisee's educational goals for the remainder of the supervision. This discussion can help realign the supervisory relationship so that the end of supervision continues to be as educationally rich as the rest of the supervision.

It is helpful to acknowledge in this phase of supervision that the work of personal and professional development is never fully complete, even after ending a productive supervision. Such an acknowledgment by supervisors can help supervisees who may struggle with accepting the fact that uncertainty, confusion, and conflict will always be a part of clinical work, no matter how far they advance. Supervisors have an opportunity to model for supervisees that the work of professional growth is always ongoing. This invites supervisees to continue to develop and add to the work of supervision, even after the supervision has terminated.

Feedback should also be bidirectional, allowing supervisors to receive information about their own supervisory skills and to identify areas for improvement in the future (Jacobs et al. 1995). Supervisors should ask explicit questions about areas for their own development. While hearing about one's own potential shortcomings can be deflating, demonstrating an open and receptive stance to negative feedback is an invaluable skill to model for supervisees.

Saying Goodbye

Finally, the last supervision meeting will arrive, and it will be time to say goodbye. The supervisory relationship often remains an important professional connection for the supervisee. It is important to discuss with supervisees how to stay in touch after supervision ends, particularly if they are graduating and beginning a practice. At the end of a supervision, it can be helpful to acknowledge the potential transition in the relationship from a mentoring relationship to a more collegial professional relationship. It can be meaningful to mark this transition with a joint experience (e.g., coffee or lunch), a small gift (e.g., a book), or a formal acknowledgment of the supervisee as a junior colleague (e.g., acknowledging a graduation). When there has been a good working relationship that has been mutually meaningful, and both parties agree, the two may decide to leave open the option of future contact in the form of mentoring or professional collaboration.

Managing Conflicts in Supervisory Termination

The following vignette demonstrates some difficulties supervisees may face in bringing up termination, especially in the context of having some negative feelings toward the supervisor.

> Dr. Joyce is an outpatient psychiatrist who would like to learn more about managing patients with substance use disorders. He reaches out to a more senior professional colleague, Dr. Hackett, and begins a private once-weekly supervision. After 9 months, Dr. Joyce feels that the supervision has been very helpful. He feels more confident in treating patients with substance use and, although the supervision has been highly productive, he now wishes to have more free time for clinical practice and wants to be more financially conservative. However, termination has never been discussed, and Dr. Joyce is highly apprehensive about expressing his desire to end supervision, fearing that he will offend Dr. Hackett. He also begins to feel frustrated by Dr. Hackett's nonacknowledgment of the progress he has made in managing substance use cases over the course of the supervision.
>
> Dr. Joyce decides to avoid these discussions and instead tries to decrease the cost of supervision by intermittently canceling supervisory sessions and "spacing them out." As time passes, he becomes increasingly resentful about supervision, despite considering that it was a highly valuable experience overall. He feels guilty about wanting to stop and worries he will hurt Dr. Hackett's feelings by communicating this desire. Eventually, Christmas is approaching, and Dr. Joyce tells Dr. Hackett that scheduling has become difficult, so they should hold off on scheduling "for a while," but that he will be back in touch. The two do not meet again and do not discuss termination further. Their relationship ends, and Dr. Joyce worries about encountering Dr. Hackett again in professional contexts.

If a supervisor has any concerns that a supervisee is bringing up the topic of termination because of a problem in the working relationship, it is the supervisor's responsibility to empathically ask about the potential issue and to be open to feedback for improvement. It is important to consider this possibility, even when a supervisee frames the desire to terminate as being due to external stressors. For example, in the vignette above, Dr. Joyce cites an external stressor, time, as the reason he desires to end supervision in order to avoid a more uncomfortable confronting of the fact that he is ready to practice more independently and feels frustrated that Dr. Hackett has not acknowledged his progress. When this occurs, we suggest that supervisors first ask explicitly about the external stressor the supervisee has brought up (often time or money). After being sensitive to and acknowledging the real contribution of the external stressor, the supervisor can explore collaboratively with the supervisee whether there is anything else that may be making the supervision unsatisfactory. It is crucial for the supervisor to be aware of and sensitive to the power dynamic between the supervisor and the supervisee that may stifle the supervisee's expression of frustration or readiness to stop.

In this vignette, even though the supervision has been a very positive experience for Dr. Joyce, his supervisor's lack of attention to his progress and his signs of readiness for termination led to a conflict within the relationship and a missed opportunity for a productive and meaningful termination. Often, when no external date has been set in advance for the termination of supervision, the burden of terminating supervision inappropriately falls on the supervisee, as in the case with Dr. Joyce. It is the supervisor's responsibility to share this burden and to ensure that the issue of termination is not left for the supervisee to manage alone. Most importantly, supervisors must maintain awareness about whether they themselves are avoiding discussing ending supervision for personal reasons, such as financial benefit or to maintain self-esteem.

Discussion of potential difficulties in the supervision may lead to important feedback for supervisors, which is essential for improving supervisory skills. It may be difficult to listen to such feedback, and supervisors may, at times, feel a sense of narcissistic injury (Jacobs 2001). It is important for supervisors to recognize this possibility and process it self-reflectively, rather than transmit their feelings of devaluation to supervisees. Discussing difficulties in the relationship may or may not lead to resolution of the issue. If an issue cannot be fully addressed and resolved, supervisors should be open to referring a supervisee to another supervisor. Furthermore, if after considering and discussing a supervisee's reasons for wanting to terminate, the supervisor and the supervisee still do not agree on what is truly causing the conflict, it is important for supervisors to let supervisees leave for their own stated reasons. A supervisee's explanation should be respected, even if the supervisor senses that other factors may be contributing. This will leave open the option for future work, either together or with another supervisor, if the supervisee desires to do so in the future.

Issues of Identity and Bias Leading to Termination

In the following vignette, a supervisor alienates the therapist who had engaged him for private supervision by asserting a patient formulation that exposes his own biases.

> Dr. Lowe is an early-career psychiatrist who sought supervision for assistance with a new 35-year-old patient now in twice-weekly psychodynamic psychotherapy. At her first meeting with Dr. Thorp, her new supervisor, Dr. Lowe presents her patient's history and her chief complaint about depressed feelings in the setting of a recent romantic breakup. After listening to the case presentation, Dr. Thorp states that he thinks that her patient is a "therapy emergency." Dr. Lowe feels immediately confused, since there are no clinical safety concerns, and she asks for clarification. Dr. Thorp responds by forcefully asserting that a 35-year-old single woman who wants children is a "therapy emergency," alluding to the fact that he is concerned that if the patient doesn't engage in therapy and work out her relationship issues, she will never be able to have children. Dr. Lowe is both offended and frustrated by this formulation. Dr. Thorp is judging her patient in exactly the same rigid way that the patient is judging herself, heightening her shame around the recent breakup and its implications for her future. Dr. Lowe feels overwhelmed and demoralized, now worrying that she won't be able to get a more nuanced understanding of the case, and also feeling unsure about whether she can fully trust Dr. Thorp's clinical acumen. As a result, Dr. Lowe starts to think about ending this private supervision.

It is critical to recognize that issues of racism, sexism, implicit bias, and other forms of identity discrimination may play a role in the supervisory relationship and may be an unspoken reason that a supervisee wants to end a supervision. It is the supervisor's job to be aware that these biases can and do affect supervisory relationships. The supervisor should be open to noticing the overt and more subtle ways that these biases impact the supervisory relationship. These biases may influence how the supervisor thinks about the supervisee and/or the supervisee's patient. If a supervisee brings up concerns about potential implicit or explicit issues of racism, sexism, ableism, or other areas of potential discrimination, it is imperative that the supervisor be sensitive and receptive to these concerns. The supervisor must listen to feedback and preferences carefully and be open to discussing and respecting any such concerns. A nondefensive and self-reflective tone can be extremely helpful. Although they can be difficult to acknowledge, such conflicts do frequently come up in supervision.

One contributory factor is that there are often generational differences in the supervisory relationship, as younger supervisees seek clinical help from more experienced and more senior colleagues of an older generation, who may be unaware of their own cultural and social biases. Supervisors should be open to learning about these issues and should work to be more self-aware and to invite thoughtful correction by their supervisees around all issues, especially ones related to implicit and explicit bias.

Terminations Initiated by the Supervisor

Just as a supervisee's needs and desires may evolve over the course of a supervision, the supervisor's needs may also change over the course of working with a particular supervisee. These changes may include changes in the supervisor's personal life, such as availability, health, finances, and the desire to continue supervising. These changes may also manifest in the supervisor's professional life, such as changes in jobs, institutions, or geographical location. When a supervisor becomes aware of a change and would like to initiate a termination, it is important to bring this change up as early and as transparently as possible. There may be circumstances in which advance notice is not possible, such as sudden illness, and termination may be unexpected or premature. In these situations, acknowledging the circumstances and their difficulty to whatever extent possible can be helpful.

Once the supervision has terminated, it can be useful for supervisors to reflect on their supervisory experience. What feedback was received? Just as was suggested for supervisees, supervisors should reflect on their own work to identify opportunities for further development, including thinking about how to support further personal growth—for example, through additional didactic education or peer supervision.

Conclusion

Setting a frame for ending supervision can be a highly enriching experience for both supervisor and supervisee. However, discussing and planning for termination can be difficult and complicated, causing the topic to be avoided by both supervisor and supervisee. In this chapter we have provided vignettes addressing different potential scenarios to help supervisors understand a variety of supervisee experiences that might make discussion of terminating supervision challenging. We have also outlined a model approach for supervisors to help supervisees address the feelings, thoughts, and didactic questions that may arise around ending supervision.

Additional Resources

Bostic JQ, Shadid LG, Blotcky MJ: Our time is up: forced terminations during psychotherapy training. Am J Psychotherapy 50(3):347–359, 1996

Jacobs D, David P, Meyer DJ: The Supervisory Encounter. New Haven, CT, Yale University Press, 1995

References

Bostic JQ, Shadid LG, Blotcky MJ: Our time is up: forced terminations during psychotherapy training. Am J Psychother 50(3):347–359, 1996 8886234

Jacobs D: Narcissism, eroticism, and envy in the supervisory relationship. J Am Psychoanal Assoc 49(3):813–830, 2001 11678239

Jacobs D, David P, Meyer DJ: The Supervisory Encounter. New Haven, CT, Yale University Press, 1995

Schlesinger HJ: Endings and Beginnings: On Terminating Psychotherapy and Psychoanalysis. New York, Routledge Taylor & Francis Group, 2005

Zetzer HA, Hill CE, Hopsicker RJ, et al: Parallel process in psychodynamic supervision: the supervisor's perspective. Psychotherapy (Chic) 57(2):252–262, 2020 31944805

PART III

Factors That Affect Psychotherapy Supervision

13

Race, Culture, and Ethnicity in Psychotherapy Supervision

Dionne R. Powell, M.D.

KEY LEARNING GOALS

- Recognize that as psychiatric practitioners, we engage with our patients in the most significant complexities surrounding hate, aggression, envy, sex, paranoia, anxiety, trauma, and sexuality without hesitation; however, race, ethnicity, and culture continue to remain outside of our clinical and supervisory purview, potentially limiting the therapeutic potential for patients of color, the relevance of psychotherapy training for trainees of color, and the educational application of psychotherapeutic ideas for an increasingly multiracial, multiethnic society for all trainees.

- Promote deeper levels of engagement and understanding in each space by increasing curiosity and reflection about race, culture, and ethnicity in both the supervisory and the therapeutic dyads.

- Open up the pedagogical space to discuss race and culture with supervisees. Breaking silence about race and culture is the supervisor's responsibility regardless of the trainee's or their patient's race and/or ethnicity. This dynamic aspect of self is a critical subject of exploration if approached with cultural humility, integrity, and openness.

- Confront hierarchies of power within the supervisory relationship that can silence discussions about race and ethnicity, and work toward better self-awareness of unconscious biases and prejudices about race, ethnicity, and culture, especially those that become manifest with racially different supervisees.

IT IS REASONABLE to state as fact that America is a multicultural, multiethnic, and multiracial society (U.S. Census Bureau 2021). However, this reality has not been fully integrated into psychiatry and psychology training centers, especially when addressing dynamic psychotherapy training and supervision. There is a history of psychodynamic training that consciously and unconsciously excludes issues surrounding race, ethnicity, and culture from three vantage points. First, until the end of the twentieth century, America was considered to be a melting pot—a place where individuals could assimilate into a culture that was not defined by one's historical immigrant roots, but rather by one's ability to integrate (i.e., adopt) current sociocultural norms. These norms were exclusively Eurocentric, Western, and focused on the individual more than the family or the community—in short, heterosexual, patriarchal, and white.[1] Thus, the way a person ate, spoke (English only), dressed, and greeted others; the privileging of the nuclear family over the extended family; and the favoring of independence over interdependence were all part of an unconscious but dominant set of aspirations, with subtle and overt influences, that continue to resonate within psychotherapy training centers as educational aspirations and in some instances as educational standards (Sue and Sue 1999).

The second factor contributing to the silence surrounding issues related to race, ethnicity, and culture within psychodynamic training centers is how the psyche was privileged as being both universal and individual, thus moving away from consideration of cultural and ethnic contributions in

---

[1] In this chapter I designate upper case for Black, speaking to the collective experience and shared cultural identity of African peoples in the Americas and larger Diaspora, while attempting to dismantle white, such as the *New York Times* has done, as a monolithic nondescriptor, as brown refers to "a wide range of cultures…and white doesn't represent a shared culture and history in the way Black does" (Coleman 2020) (see also Baquet and Corbett 2020).

the development of concepts of the mind (Stoute 2017). Cultural, ethnic, and racial factors thus became the purview of sociologists, not of psychiatrists or clinical psychologists (Bobo 2001, 2004; Bonilla-Silva 2015).

And finally, the history of American independence and nation building is intertwined and directly linked with the history of racism and the enslavement of African people concurrent with the destruction of the land's original indigenous inhabitants. This double helix of democracy and slavery, and the aftermath of slavery—its legacy, including Jim Crow laws; forced labor; inequities in housing, employment, education, and health; the appropriation of Black-owned farms; the forced relocation of urban communities of color; the destruction of Black communities (Greenwood-Tulsa, OK; Rosewood, FL; Wilmington, NC); and the forced use of Black bodies without anesthesia to perfect surgical techniques, along with other experiments, including Tuskegee and Henrietta Lacks—have traumatized the Black community for more than 400 years (Alexander 2010; Anderson 2016; Briggs and Krakauer 2020; DeGruy 2005; Grier and Cobbs 1968; Guthrie 1976; Hannah-Jones 2019; Hoffman et al. 2016; Luhrmann 2010; Skloot 2010; Staples 2020; Washington 2006; Vaughans 2015; Wilkerson 2020). Individuals who are Black, indigenous, and people of color (BIPOC) are increasingly speaking of these racial traumas within their own psychotherapy, a change mirroring that taking place in the larger society (Davidson 1987; Gay 2016; Holmes 2006, 2016, 2019, 2021; Pierce 1974; Powell 2012; Stoute 2021; Tummala-Narra 2007, 2009, 2013; Tummala-Narra et al. 2017).

This change is also captured in the new edition of *Gabbard's Textbook of Psychotherapeutic Treatments* (Crisp and Gabbard 2023). As section editor for Part VII, on racial and ethnic diversities in psychotherapy, I brought together eight authors writing about the African American (Hart, Powell), Asian American (Ueng-McHale, Chin), South Asian American (Tummala-Narra, Kanwal), and Latinx (Gaztambide) experience in psychotherapy, and also about the development of racial concepts in children (Stoute). These chapters expose the challenges and opportunities of working clinically with diverse populations, as well as the training experiences of psychotherapists of color (Gaztambide 2023; Powell and Hart 2023; Stoute 2023; Tummala-Narra and Kanwal 2023; Ueng-McHale and Chin 2023).

This chapter is intended to highlight for readers the paucity of attention given to race, culture, and ethnicity within the supervisory relationship, which—in addition to trainees' individual psychotherapy (increasingly voluntary)—is the quintessential setting for experiential learning to occur. Goals of this chapter include 1) opening up this aspect of supervision to facilitate a deepening appreciation of the influences of race, ethnicity, and culture on the dual relationships of trainee–patient and supervisor–supervisee and 2) highlighting frequently experienced racial assumptions (transferences) held by supervisors, supervisees, and the supervisory dyad that contribute to avoidance of topics related to cultural, racial, and ethnic components of the psychic self. Unaddressed racial silence within the supervisory relationship can limit the trainee's learning experience, adversely affect the therapeutic relationship with patients, and discourage trainees of color from pursuing psychotherapy practice as a career option (Powell 2018). Vignettes illustrating supervisory principles will be presented to highlight these points, along with suggestions on integrating issues relating to race, culture, and ethnicity into the supervisor's pedagogic armamentarium.

Race, Culture, and Ethnicity in Psychotherapy and Supervision

I begin with a very brief history of the absence of the racial/ethnic or cultural self within the supervisory relationship. There are sufficient data and collective experience to confirm that race is a complex and challenging phenomenon within the therapeutic and supervisory dyad, particularly when it is not addressed. From Freud to Winnicott, there have been active attempts to bring the "cultural experience" into the psychodynamic as foundational. We are aware, from Freud in 1915 writing about the implosion of civilized man during war (WWI), that "we are mistaken in regarding our intelligence as an independent force and in over looking its dependence on emotional life. Our intellect…can function reliably only when it is removed from the influences of strong emotional impulses; otherwise it behaves merely as an instrument of the will and delivers the inference which the will requires" (Freud 1915/1957, p. 287).

Racism and privilege in American society, in how one views "the other," is the "strong emotional influence" that shapes us all, results in us automatically moving away from rationality, and makes race and the effects of racism, prejudice, and privilege unique and important, whether in our personal lives, in the consulting room, or within supervision. In the United States, where racist sociopolitical systems subjugate large numbers of the population, race serves as a unique flash point in society and within our training centers (Powell 2020). The sheer concept of race is a sociopolitical construction that requires constant vigilance to mitigate its deleterious effects (Hammonds and Herzig 2008; Roberts 2011).

Winnicott described the in-between state of inner psychic reality and external reality as an area of potential space to play, to bring together, within the dyad, whether supervisor–supervisee or clinician–patient (Winnicott 1967, 1968). It is within this contextual dynamic framework that I approach race in the clinical and supervisory situation. And with acceptance of the intersubjective components of the dyad, whether supervisory or therapeutic, we appear to be at a moment of consolidation of how the intrapsychic and race can be integrated in mind. What both Winnicott and Freud were also advocating goes beyond the intellectual didactic experience and speaks to the necessity for an experiential exchange for transformative learning to occur, that interplays with the instinctual, the uncanny, and the biopsychosocial. The pedagogical space most aligned to the potentialities of the development of a trainee's experiential knowledge as pertains to race and culture is within the supervisory relationship. As Tummala-Narra (2004, p. 300) noted, "integration of racial and cultural diversity related issues in clinical supervision is an essential component of the clinical and teaching competence, which has important implications for the provision of services to ethnic minorities and, more broadly, to better addressing the full realm of clients' intrapsychic and interpersonal worlds."

Differences in race tend to confound these motivations of connection due to the long-held silence surrounding race, and the racial imbalance and white hierarchy of training centers. Examples of the absence of diversity within training centers abound, with the lack or minimal training of BIPOC trainees, BIPOC patients, and BIPOC faculty. Their collective experiences are beginning to emerge (Cooke 2017; Dunlap et al. 2020; Harpe 2021; Hart 2020; Milloy and Lawson 2020; Shim 2020; Tummala-Narra 2004; White-Davis et al. 2016).[2]

Psychiatry residency and psychology graduate training are experienced as one of the last bastions of white exclusivity. One may easily surmise when encountering the mental health care training situation (psychiatry residency or clinical psychology graduate school) that one has entered an exclusive white club. What makes this particularly jarring for trainees of color is that most training centers are located in major urban centers at the heart of communities of color, with access to professional and academic BIPOC communities that should provide a steady engagement for potential faculty, trainees, and patients. Worsening the situation is the ab-

---

[2] Association of American Medical Colleges data from 2020 indicate that the percentages of U.S. medical school graduates who are African American (7%), Latinx/Hispanic (6%), and American Indian/Alaska Native (0.2%) remain strikingly low for the population and will continue to contribute to health disparities (Association of American Medical Colleges 2021).

sence of racial trauma in the *Diagnostic and Statistical Manual of Mental Disorders* as a causative agent in posttraumatic stress disorder. Failure to represent this at the training and treatment level continues to highlight the magnitude of racial inequities in terms of access to mental health care services and providers of care. The dual events of the 2020 pandemic of COVID-19 and the pandemic of racism affecting brown and Black people, culminating in the May 25, 2020, murder of George Floyd, have brought these disparities to full public and academic awareness (Egede and Walker 2020). The cumulative effects of these disparities on Black, brown, and Asian communities have shattered the myth of the United States as a colorblind society with equal access to and opportunities for health care, employment, housing, and long life expectancies. Recent data from the *Washington Post* database "Policing in America" (www.washington-post.com/police-america/), which in 2015 began to log every fatal shooting by an on-duty police officer, showed that the number of police shootings are still at the same level as they were at the time of George Floyd's murder, despite protests and vigorous advocacy for police reform. People of color are pursuing mental health care services at increasingly high rates (Bahrampour 2013; Milloy and Lawson 2020) but are unable to access health care when searching for mental health care providers of color, who often have full private practices or no available appointments within clinic settings. These needs will increase the demand that supervisors become experienced in treating a diverse patient population and supervising all trainees as multicultural, multiethnic, and multiracial populations become the norm and not the exception (Hart 2019b).

For trainees of color, there are more pronounced racial hurdles that must be faced during training, including microaggressions, discriminatory gestures, prejudices, and biases that follow them from medical school into psychiatry residency (Hart 2019a; Pierce 1974; Thomas and Sillen 1972). Studies indicate that underrepresented minority medical students are less likely to speak up and give presentations on rounds, a circumstance that can negatively affect their ultimate evaluations, especially in clerkships (Teherani et al. 2018), as well as their competitiveness for residency positions. Medical students of color have described answering questions on clinical rounds and being ignored, while later, a white student provides the same answer and receives praise and recognition from attending physician. Repeated experiences with this form of microaggression and disavowal can silence trainees of color, leading the medical or graduate student to turn away from psychiatry or clinical psychology as a career or conditioning the psychiatry resident of color to remain silent (Rojek et al. 2019).

The following personal example illustrates what I have frequently heard from mental health care trainees of color, a form of erasure that can be potentially damaging to a young trainee:

> I am the only psychiatrist of color in a peer supervision group of six psychiatrists who had been meeting bimonthly for 8 years at the time of this incident. One colleague wanted to discuss a difficult clinical dilemma. I was the only one who responded, and my response opened up a different understanding of the enactment that had unfolded with the colleague's patient that they found helpful. After some moments of silent reflection, the colleague who began the inquiry turned to another colleague and thanked them for making *my* comment. My colleague, and friend, was convinced that in this small setting I could not be the person who made the comment that deepened their understanding, even with the others confirming what had just transpired. Unfortunately, as documented by trainees of color who have shared their experiences in medical school, graduate school, residency, or analytic training, receiving acknowledgment for their clinical or academic contributions is rare; instead, credit for their contribution is often given to a non–person of color, thus confusing the trainee of color and discouraging them from voicing their thoughts in the future. One can imagine how negative stereotypes can be attributed to a quiet trainee of color, with whites not exploring their complicity in this silencing, minimizing, or ignoring of the contributions of trainees of color.

Another perspective on the problem of mental health care and the failure to match patients with clinicians of color or those with racial and cultural sensitivity is demonstrated by the following data: More than 50% of persons of color (POC) drop out after their first psychotherapy session (Sue and Sue 1999). These attrition rates speak to the failure of engagement by clinicians working with racially and ethnically diverse patients. If these patients feel unrecognized or misunderstood, they will turn away from treatment. Thus, it is imperative that the clinician quickly correct any potential early misattunements that jeopardize the beginning treatment for BIPOC patients. The burden of and responsibility for creating a receptive environment for all patients must rest on the clinician.

Recent investigations reveal that more than 90% of whites have "whites only" friendship groups (Chang 2018), a finding that suggests that for most white trainees, their first in-depth engagement with people of color may occur within the intimate professional confines of the therapeutic relationship. With multiculturalism increasing among younger cohorts, psychiatrists and psychologists in training may potentially be more familiar and engaged with multicultural milieus than are their supervisors (Constantine and Sue 2007). This may lead to uncomfortable silences as therapists stay quiet, waiting for the patient of color or the white supervisor to open up the conversation on racial matters. If the patient follows the lead of the therapist, stemming from what has been modeled or silenced in supervision, race will be ignored—potentially to the patient's detriment. If supervisors do not emphasize the importance of race/culture and ethnicity within the therapeutic encounter, supervisees will never bring these issues into their clinical understanding, thus leaving them outside the therapeutic relationship. As an African American psychiatrist and psychoanalyst, I often have to explicitly bring race and culture into the supervisory experience, regardless of the race of the trainee or of their patient. It is essential for supervisors to open up the pedagogical space to discuss race and culture with their supervisees. In my over 30 years of supervisory experience, supervisees in training rarely will.

In their 2018 article (Schen and Greenlee 2018), Dr. Cathy Schen, a white supervisor, and Dr. Alecia Greenlee, an African American psychiatry resident, thoughtfully considered their interactions and how they brought race into their supervisory experience. For Schen, Greenlee was the first African American resident to be assigned to her for supervision in her 20-year experience teaching in a major urban area, signifying the absence of trainees of color and the possible tensions when race is not integrated into the teaching and supervisory model. For Greenlee, the inherent tension of medical school and psychiatry residency, laced with microaggressions (Pierce 1974), along with a desire to learn, and not wanting by default to be *the voice* of African Americans and other underrepresented minorities, combined to bring potential dynamic tension into the supervisory space. Schen and Greenlee's article provides a granular exploration of the conscious and unspoken assumptions that each was able to explore and articulate with increasing mutual vulnerability, thus promoting a deeper learning and supervisory experience.

Effects of Stereotypes, Biases, and Prejudice on the Supervisory Relationship

Increasing our awareness of the unconscious influences that are embedded in stereotyping is essential to maximize our supervisory potential. As I stated in my 2020 paper, "Racial differences are signified in childhood often as traumatizing or confusing moments of development. Inevitable intergenerational racial and ethnic stereotyping occurs. Who we fear and why we fear are imprinted through our caregivers and typically not from a negative experience with the other" (Powell 2020, p. 424). As clinicians and supervisors, we are reluctant, afraid, embarrassed, and ashamed in not knowing what to do when race enters the clinical or supervisory situation. It is this very unknowing that requires conscious reflection and acknowledgment within the supervisor and within the supervisor–supervisee dyad. Or as stated by Powell and Hart (2023): "A prejudiced orientation, held either consciously (in the form of attitudes and beliefs), unconsciously (in the form of biases), or both, represents a person's curtailment of their own original curiosity—a curiosity that, at the beginning of life, orients itself toward everything and everyone new and unknown. One can begin to understand how built-up prejudices and biases can limit the capabilities of human interactions and therefore curtail the imaginative capacities of mind" (p. 476). The challenge of getting in touch with one's "inner racist" (Davids 2011) or one's "racist states of mind" (Keval 2016) takes us away from the pejoratives that infect any considerations or conversations about race, allowing us to be open, curious, and exploratory about the underlying sources of racial stereotypes, biases, and prejudices that are within us all. By this perspective, racial prejudice, which is frequently and reflexively polarized toward the binary of whether someone is good or bad, becomes a universal feature of humanity and therefore worthy of acknowledgment and discussion instead of silence and shame.

> As a personal example of how race can present itself in treatment, in this instance as a defensive retreat from more painful affects: I accused my analyst of "talking like a white woman," with overt claims that she couldn't understand me due to her whiteness (Powell 2020). She responded with: "Well, I *am* a white woman, but is that what's between us?" I came to appreciate that my accusation in the mid-phase of my analysis was easier to tolerate than to confront and work through my rage and destructiveness, with its historical familial roots, and ultimately my fears and anxieties, or my dependence on and need of my analyst. We eventually reached these deeper levels, but my emphasis here is on my use of a prejudicial remark to distance myself from my analyst. My increasing curiosity about our engagement and my analyst's ability to lean into this moment with me rather than retreating in silence, with mutual attempts to pursue this further, led to deeper levels of engagement and understanding. This example and others solidified that race—its explication and exploration—is a significant factor in the clinical and supervisory experience.

While one's own prejudices, anchored in memories and fears, can best be explored in personal analysis and/or in supervision, the ability to explore issues related to race is dependent on the clinician's or supervisor's self-reflective capacities, as the above vignette illustrates.

We are acutely aware of the enigma of the other and the human tendency to seek out points of connectivity in every encounter. This is similarly true within the supervisory relationship, in which direct collaboration supports trainees' ability to view and engage with their patients from multiple perspectives (developmental, conflictual or ego psychological, various self states, attachment theory, relational theory, and object relations theory, to name a few) by providing a method of learning essential skills, with subjective and objective elements. There are assumptions that are automatic in any dyadic encounter, typically relating to characteristics that are most noticeable: race, culture, religion, gender, presence of an accent, style of dress, education, and so forth. In addition, we all seek points of confluence to make connections, and we all have assumptions about the other, whether confirmed or not. Within the supervisory pair and/or the treating pair, if there are racial, ethnic, or cultural differences, supervisors should assist trainees to be open and curious, while demonstrating cultural humility and creating a space for racial and cultural meanings and experiences to have free expression (Hart 2017; Watkins and Hook 2016). Davidson (1987), writing about the supervisory relationship, encouraged trainees to ask about their patients' culture and to admit ignorance when necessary. At the 110th Annual Meeting of the American Psychoanalytic Association in 2021, Otto Kernberg (2021) spoke of his early experiences at the Menninger Clinic in Topeka, Kansas. He described lengthy history taking, with inquiries about the patient's developmental history, including community and the cultural/ethnic influences, that provided an in-depth perspective of the patient presenting for treatment. The supervisory experience should provide a model for and promote an engagement with supervisees to be equally curious and in conversation with all elements of the therapeutic dyad, including the racial and ethnic; nothing should be left to conjecture.

According to Watkins and Hook (2016), development of "cultural humility" involves "a *willingness and openness to reflect on one's self as an embedded cultural being,* an awareness of one's personal limitations in understanding the cultural other and in guarding against culturally unfounded, automatic assumptions; interpersonally, cultural humility involves being *open to hearing and striving to understand aspects of the other's cultural background and identity*" (p. 490). Although we have accepted the need to acknowledge the existence of the racial or ethnic other, we continue to ignore or disavow the need to acknowledge its presence at the training level. We all carry stereotypes. As stated by Powell and Hart (2023, p. 478):

> Stereotyping, like all forms of prejudice, protects people from the unsettling feelings associated with encountering situations and interactions that are unfamiliar; it provides the illusion that the world, and other people in it (including those who are different from us, and thus "other") are already known. However, although stereotyping provides an immediate

sense of security (”I know what they are like,” “I know what is going on,” “I know what to expect”), it invariably has a long-term cost due to its reliance on oversimplification and distortion of the existing complexities of reality.

Prior to the supervisory encounter, supervisors should be in touch with their own forms of stereotyping and educate themselves about this, including their racist states of mind (Keval 2016; Kovel 1970) or being in touch with their inner racist (Davids 2011).

Part of the challenge for supervisors is to confront the hierarchies of power within the supervisory relationship that can potentially silence discussions about race and ethnicity (e.g., if the supervisor does not show, model, or suggest the importance of race within both the therapeutic and the supervisory encounter). Supervisors should recognize their power to control what is considered to be important in psychotherapy. They can use their influence either to encourage and model discussion of racial, cultural, and ethnic issues or to tacitly silence these vital discussions, to the detriment of both clinical and supervisory experiences.

There are a set of assumptions, professionally referred to as transferences, that draw our attention when there are manifest differences between the therapist and the patient or among the supervisor–patient–supervisee triad. Attempts must be made to explicate these assumptions, which frequently present unconsciously, requiring a type of self-exploration that is essential for supervisors. Below are a few examples of racial assumptions or stereotypes that require vigilance and exploration:

1. *The angry or aggressive African American supervisee or patient of color.* The history of the African in America is one of resilience in the face of racial trauma. From cradle (higher infant and maternal mortality in POCs) to grave (children with poorer educational experiences, mass incarceration), increased mortality for BIPOC, racial bias in pain assessment, the cumulative effects of unrecognized racial trauma, and the physical and mental health consequences for POC can manifest in anger (Alexander 2010; Goldstein and Parlapiano 2021; Hoffman et al. 2016; Metzl 2010; Pagán et al. 2020; Schaeffer et al. 2021). This is contextually related to frustration regarding the unaddressed, underlying racial issues at play. Having worked with patients of color from across the economic spectrum, I have not had an experience in which issues of racial trauma were not an aspect of my patients' clinical experiences. In my work underneath anger is the fear of not being acknowledged for the pain of racial trauma, and not being taken seriously for the complaints being voiced (Stoute 2021).

2. *Providing a course on "cultural competence" as being sufficient to bring race and culture into the training experience.* There is a false assumption that the racial other can be "taught" in a seminar on diversity. This stereotype not only minimizes the complexities of race, ethnicity, and culture that privilege whiteness as the foundational educational standard of training but also leaves diversity at the margins. Until ethnic and racial diversity is integrated into the curriculum and supervision, trainees will not experience and incorporate these aspects into their psychodynamic thinking.[3]

3. *BIPOC people have too many realistic social problems to benefit from dynamic psychotherapy.* This assumption reflects socioeconomic class biases when working with trainees of color. With prominent artists and athletes (e.g., Naomi Osaka, Simone Biles) speaking out about their mental health challenges, including dealing with racial trauma, this assumption is being actively confronted. As illustrated by my colleagues of color's experiences, the demand for mental health care services has never been greater and is expanding, primarily from the BIPOC community (Bahrampour 2013; Milloy and Lawson 2020).

Supervisors' Blind and Bright Spots

As stated earlier, supervisors have unconscious biases and prejudices about race, ethnicity, and culture that become manifest with racially different supervisees. These racial "blind spots" or impediments to the supervisory work must be worked through in the supervisor's mind; it is not the trainee's responsibility to explain such issues to the supervisor as if the trainee were an expert on race, culture, and ethnicity. Mitigating the assumptions and biases held by supervisors that can impede and inflict damage on trainees of color requires self-study and/or study groups (Baldwin 1962; Crenshaw 2016; Eng and Han 2018; Fanon 1952; Gay 2016; Gherovici and Christian 2019; Grier and Cobbs 1968; Jones-Marlin 2020; Noah 2020; Peele 2017; Pogue White 2002; Sharpe 2016; Stevenson 2014; Wilkerson 2010).[4] Supervisors must be willing to reveal their

---

[3] A personal example: I was the only African American throughout my 4 years of psychiatric residency training. At one point, a minority fellowship grant became available, and I proposed applying to support my having an African American supervisor for one of my long-term psychodynamic therapy patients. At the time, there was no African American faculty in my residency. My proposal was declined; instead, I was told that if I were to obtain the fellowship, I could create a seminar on race and cultural competence for my fellow residents. I refused to apply.

own lack of familiarity and expertise when certain racial and ethnic issues arise. It can be challenging for supervisors to put themselves in this awkward position of "unknowingness" when it comes to issues surrounding race, culture, and ethnicity.

Biases in a different direction can come to light when the supervisor and the supervisee appear to have similar backgrounds; in this situation, there can be an equally unexamined assumption of familiarity when none actually exists. These "bright spots" can lead white trainees to dispense with certain curiosities about race, culture, and ethnicity in an attempt to model themselves toward their supervisor's approach, abandoning their nascent curiosities (Goldberger 1993). What is included and essential, and what is peripheral and irrelevant within supervision is entirely shaped by the supervisor. This influence has career-long consequences for supervisees and highlights the importance of supervisors' self-study, both intrapsychically to mitigate prejudice, bias, and racist overtones and interpersonally to familiarize themselves with the ethnic, cultural, and racial experiences of the patient and the supervisee. Such efforts promote a mutual learning experience for both supervisor and supervisee.

One of the challenges of supervision is to refrain from moving into a clinical psychotherapy role with supervisees. If racial differences between the supervisory or treatment pairs are never explored, there is a greater tendency for supervisees to remain aloof and distant within the supervisory encounter. This nonengagement can lead to dissatisfaction on both sides, including a form of scapegoating in which the supervisor's discomfort with the racial tension and the lack of exploration of what is occurring within the supervisory space is blamed on the supervisee (White-Davis et al. 2016). In a paper by White-Davis et al. (2016, p. 353), the following areas were highlighted in supervisees' statements about what they were seeking from their supervisory encounters:

1. "Issues related to how my interpretations of the lives of my Black and Hispanic patients are assessed mostly by middle class white supervisors." (Asian/Pacific Islander supervisee)
2. "I wanted to discuss how certain observations to me seemed culturally normal instead of pathological." (Latinx supervisee)
3. "[I would like to] Address a subtext that is often at work in the supervisory relationship…learn how to better address it with colleagues;

---

[4] My intentional inclusion of outside reading and visual sources in this chapter is provided for those readers who are attempting to further their self-study, which is essential for an ongoing contemporary supervisory experience.

become more aware of my implicit bias and my impact on colleagues and patients as a white trainee." (white supervisee)

In Chapter 3 of this book, a psychiatry resident of color describes their experience in supervision: "I resolved to be the good trainee. I channeled enthusiasm, professionalism, and collegiality. I trained myself to be exquisitely attuned to my supervisors' anxieties, knowing when a shift in their gaze or a change in their tone meant I would need to maneuver myself back into their good graces." One can imagine the limiting experience of a supervisee who, instead of conveying what they have learned from the patient interaction, has to focus their attention and curiosity to pleasing or accommodating someone in power, in this instance their supervisor (Eng and Han 2018). Enactments within the supervision can occur when issues of race within the treatment setting are not brought up by supervisors with their supervisees, a situation exemplified in the following vignette:

A Latinx psychiatry resident, in working with her white patient, notices that the patient is late to appointments, misses sessions without notice, and expects the therapist to make up for these changes by finding additional times for them to meet or extending the time of their sessions. The therapist's attempts to accommodate this patient lead to disruption of her schedule and increasing frustration, as well as critical responses from colleagues and faculty about her tardiness that hold racial undertones (i.e., microaggressions). One day the patient describes, for the first time, her beloved childhood Latinx nanny, who was present and available when her parents frequently were not. The supervisee begins to feel like the mistreated nanny, sacrificing her time and changing her schedule to accommodate the patient.

None of this is questioned by the resident's white supervisor, and the supervisee continues to feel intruded upon by the patient. Eventually the supervisee unintentionally misses two consecutive supervisory sessions, an event that finally causes the supervisor to wonder what is going on. However, the parallel process is not taken up in supervision; the supervisor never connects the resident's absences to the clinical material, while the resident, although sensing that her missing of supervision sessions may be connected to her patient, remains silent. This extended enactment could have been avoided if there had been more open questioning by the supervisor about the patient's relationships, both past and present, including the power dynamic along racial lines of the patient with her nanny. The enactment—the two consecutively missed supervisions—served as the clue that something more transferential was occurring, but by then, the treatment was close to ending, and this content was never addressed, with both the clinical and the supervisory experience being lost for further exploration.

This vignette illustrates the need to bring issues relating to race, culture, and ethnicity into the psychodynamic lexicon that shapes the mind, development, and nature of object relations; no longer seeing these areas as being outside the purview of the intrapsychic or the psychodynamic.

Although both supervisor and supervisee can potentially learn from these encounters, it is important that supervisors acknowledge when they do not know about or understand a cultural concept that may be a part of the ethnic experience of the patient or the communicative style of the supervisee. Encouraging supervisees to discuss their impressions of their patients' material, including their transferences and countertransferences, supports trainees' dynamic curiosity as being paramount to an engaging supervisory experience.

Getting to know supervisees at the inception of supervision mitigates stereotyping and prejudice. In most of my supervisory encounters, I emphasize that "my job is to help you learn and become a more effective clinician."[5] I will frequently ask about supervisees' residency or graduate school experience, the challenges and opportunities, and discuss the goals of supervision. This is optimally achieved when supervisors share aspects of their professional development and make clear that they are there to support their trainees' clinical skills in the face of exposure to often complicated and confusing clinical presentations. During these initial meetings, a spirit of open curiosity regarding patients being presented and supervisees' thoughts and feelings about what they are experiencing should be promoted. If supervisees become silent, this is a prime opportunity for supervisors to share their impressions or to highlight an aspect of the material—particularly if racial, cultural, or ethnic in origin—to demonstrate that the supervisory space can be utilized in this fashion as well. Parallel to the clinical experience, the ideal supervisory experience should over time become more nuanced and immersive within a framework of experiential learning. Race, culture, and ethnicity should be of interest to supervisees, similar to how other aspects of patients are important. Often these areas can be included when listening for the developmental history and the history of the patient's object relationships, with supervisors demonstrating their curiosity. Supervisors should not make tacit assumptions about the race of a patient and of her/his/their objects.

---

[5] While not scripted, in initial meetings with supervisees, my intention is to convey the following about my role: Within this process, we are going to typically discuss uncomfortable material, with the goal of deepening the understanding of your patient and increasing your comfort in speaking to your patient, that is in part discussing some of your feelings toward the patient and their material with me. Within this, nothing is left out of the discussion, including race, culture, community, fantasies, sex, religion, aggression, depression, fears, wishes, and anxieties, to name a small few.

If race is not stated, the supervisor should inquire, in the service of addressing and mitigating the default to whiteness (wherein race is mentioned only if a patient is not white).

"As American as Chinese Food"…"As American as the Taco": The White Supervisor–White Supervisee Pair

What currently represents what is *American*? It depends on your audience, but I would argue that if Americans were to speak through their stomachs, it would not be apple pie in the twenty-first century, but rather the taco or Chinese food that would more aptly capture America's culinary desires. However, our intrapsychic landscape has not fully reconciled with external reality when it comes to racial diversity. If race is rarely mentioned with biracial participants, whether supervisor, supervisee, or patient, what transpires when all participants are white? I believe that there is a total absence of speaking to and about race, even if it is within the clinical material (White-Davis et al. 2016). An understanding of whiteness is essential to understanding the tenacity of assumptions, prejudices, biases, and stereotypes that compromise the potential to train and treat an increasingly diverse society (Altman 2006).

Whiteness is a nondynamic, defensive cover that obscures the individual and their ethnicity/ethnicities or cultural roots. When European immigrants came to the United States in the twentieth century, they were often initially met with great opposition and discrimination by the current citizenry; however, the relative ease with which these white European immigrants were able to enfold themselves into whiteness has played a role in maintaining systems of institutional racism (Desmond 2019; Meacham 2020b; Wilkerson 2020). Psychosocial norms are molded and shaped by this monolithic pseudoculture that dismantles the immigrant's cultural and familial roots, with their rich complexities—which are lost or reduced once they identify as white, along with the accompanying uniqueness of a multicultural, multiethnic, multiracial society. Society is beginning to experience the fault lines of whiteness as a concept (Diangelo 2018; Irving 2014; Kovel 1970; Metzl 2019; Moss 2006, 2021; Rao 2021). These factors—the unconscious guilt and shame in acknowledging our complicity in racial hatred, and the hierarchical structure of training, where power and position can make or break a training experience—deserve thoughtful consideration in every supervisory encounter, but especially in racially mixed supervisory pairs, or when the patient is a POC.

Final Remarks: The Perils and Benefits of Including Race, Culture, and Ethnicity Within the Supervisory Experience

The author Ta-Nehisi Coates (2015) noted that society needs to lean into the discomfort of race for its reparative value. As psychiatric practitioners within the clinical setting, we are accustomed to engaging with our patients in discussing significant complexities and intimacies surrounding hate, aggression, envy, sex, paranoia, anxiety, trauma, and sexuality, often without hesitation or pause. However, the fact that issues related to race, ethnicity, and culture continue to be considered as external to our clinical and supervisory purview requires our thoughtful engagement as we begin to dismantle systemic forms of institutional and intrapsychic racism.

Addressing issues of race, ethnicity, and culture within the supervisory encounter requires active engagement to bring these vital aspects of self into the therapeutic and educational discourse. This is not an easy task. It is unfortunate, but many a supervisee has revealed to me privately that their initial supervisory encounter began with the question "What are you?" This form of Othering does not promote a positive supervisory experience, and actually creates its opposite.

Instead of remaining silent when issues of race, culture, and ethnicity emerge, supervisors can explore their own internal biases, privileges, and racist states of mind, while practicing cultural humility and openness with integrity, thereby demonstrating and encouraging the emergence of these vital aspects of the self in the learning experience of their trainees. This more-encompassing approach with our supervisees and their patients can facilitate a transformational shift in how we think about and approach all patients and trainees in this multicultural, multiethnic, and multiracial society, and conceptually can promote an anti-racist attitude (Kendi 2019; Meacham 2020a).

References

Alexander M: The New Jim Crow: Mass Incarceration in the Age of Colorblindness. New York, The New Press, 2010

Altman N: Whiteness. Psychoanal Q 75(1):45–72, 2006 16482960

Anderson C: White Rage: The Unspoken Truth of Our Racial Divide. New York, Bloomsbury, 2016

Association of American Medical Colleges: Total U.S. MD-Granting Medical School Graduates by Race/Ethnicity and Sex, 2016–2017 through 2020–2021. 2021. Available at: https://www.amc.org/systems/files/2021...12/2021_Facts_Table_B-4. Accessed July 2021.

Bahrampour T: Therapists say African Americans are increasingly seeking help for mental illness. The Washington Post, July 9, 2013

Baldwin J: The Fire Next Time. New York, Vintage Books/Random House, 1962

Baquet D, Corbett P: Uppercasing "Black" (memo). New York Times Company, June 30, 2020. Available at: www.nytco.com/press/uppercasing-black. Accessed January 31, 2022.

Bobo LD: Racial attitudes and relations at the close of the twentieth century, in America Becoming: Racial Trends and Their Consequences. Edited by Smelser N, Wilson WJ, Mitchell F. Washington, DC, National Academy Press, 2001, pp 262–299

Bobo LD: Inequalities that endure? Racial ideology, American politics, and the peculiar role of the social sciences, in The Changing Terrain of Race and Ethnicity. Edited by Krysan M, Lewis AE. New York, Russell Sage Foundation, 2004, pp 13–42

Bonilla-Silva E: The structure of racism in color-blind, "post-racial" America. American Behavioral Scientist 59(11):1358–1376, 2015

Briggs W, Krakauer J: The massacre that emboldened white supremacists. The New York Times, August 28, 2020

Chang A: White America is quietly self segregating. Vox, August 31, 2018

Coates T-N: Between the World and Me. New York, Penguin Random House, 2015

Coleman N: Why we're capitalizing Black. The New York Times, July 5, 2020, p. A2

Constantine MG, Sue DW: Perceptions of racial microaggressions among black supervisees in cross-racial dyads. Journal of Counseling Psychology 54(2):142–153, 2007

Cooke M: Implicit bias in academic medicine: #WhatADoctorLooksLike. JAMA Intern Med 177(5):657–658, 2017 28264084

Crenshaw K: The urgency of intersectionality. TED Talk. 2016. Available at: www.ted.com/talks/kimberle_crenshaw_the_urgency_of_intersectionality?referrer=playlist-10_great_talks_to_celebrate_bl. Accessed January 31, 2022.

Crisp H, Gabbard GO (eds): Gabbard's Textbook of Psychotherapeutic Treatments, 2nd Edition. Washington, DC, American Psychiatric Association Publishing, 2023

Davids MF: Internal Racism: A Psychoanalytic Approach to Race and Difference. London, Springer Nature Limited, 2011

Davidson L: The cross-cultural therapeutic dyad. Contemporary Psychoanalysis 23(4):659–675, 1987

DeGruy J: Post Traumatic Slave Syndrome: America's Legacy of Enduring Injury and Healing. Milwaukie, OR, Uptone Press, 2005

Desmond M: In order to understand the brutality of American capitalism, you have to start on the plantation. The New York Times. August 14, 2019

Diangelo R: White Fragility: Why It's So Hard for White People to Talk About Racism. Boston, MA, Beacon Press, 2018

Dunlap CE, Dennis E, Desouza F, et al: Management of race in psychotherapy and supervision. Psychcast: Official podcast feed of MDedge Psychiatry, part of the Medscape Professional Network. June 22, 2020. Available at: https://_www.mdedge.com/psychiatry/article/224275/ptsd/management-race-psychotherapy-and-supervision/page/0/4. Accessed May 5, 2022.

Egede LE, Walker RJ: Structural racism, social risk factors, and Covid-19: a dangerous convergence for Black Americans. N Engl J Med 383(12):e77, 2020 32706952

Eng DL, Han S: Racial Melancholia, Racial Dissociation: On the Social and Psychic Lives of Asian Americans. Durham, NC, Duke University Press, 2018

Fanon F: Black Skin, White Masks. Translated by Philcox R. New York, Grove Press, 1952

Freud S: Thoughts for the times on war and death (1915), in The Standard Edition of the Complete Psychological Works of Sigmund Freud, Vol 9. Translated and edited by Strachey J. London, Hogarth Press, 1957, pp 275–301

Gay V: On the Pleasures of Owning Persons: The Hidden Face of American Slavery. New York, International Psychoanalytic Books, 2016

Gaztambide D: There is no such thing as Latinx: race, intersectionality, and immigration in clinical work and supervision with Latin American communities, in Gabbard's Textbook of Psychotherapeutic Treatments, 2nd Edition. Edited by Crisp H, Gabbard GO. Washington, DC, American Psychiatric Association Publishing, 2023, pp 553–574

Gherovici P, Christian C: Psychoanalysis in the Barrios: Race, Class, and the Unconscious. New York, Routledge, 2019

Goldberger M: "Bright spot," a variant of "blind spot." Psychoanal Q 62(2):270–273, 1993 8502731

Goldstein D, Parlapiano A: The Kindergarten Exodus. The New York Times, August 7, 2021

Grier WH, Cobbs PM: Black Rage. New York, Basic Books, 1968

Guthrie RV: Even the Rat Was White: A Historical View of Psychology. London, Pearson, 1976

Hammonds EM, Herzig RM: The Nature of Difference: Sciences of Race in the United States From Jefferson to Genomics. Cambridge, MA, The MIT Press, 2008

Hannah-Jones N: The 1619 Project. The New York Times Magazine, August 2019

Harpe JM: Why I will not be attending my medical residency graduation. Medium.com, 2021

Hart A: From multicultural competence to radical openness: a psychoanalytic engagement of otherness. The American Psychoanalyst 51(1):12–27, 2017

Hart AH: The discriminatory gesture: a psychoanalytic consideration of posttraumatic reactions to incidents of racial discrimination. Psychoanalytic Social Work 24(April):2–20, 2019a

Hart AH: Why diversities? The American Psychoanalyst 53(3):8–10, 2019b

Hart AH: Principles for teaching diversity and otherness from a psychoanalytic perspective. Contemporary Psychoanalysis 56(2–3):404–417, 2020

Hoffman KM, Trawalter S, Axt JR, Oliver MN: Racial bias in pain assessment and treatment recommendations, and false beliefs about biological differences between blacks and whites. Proc Natl Acad Sci USA 113(16):4296–4301, 2016 27044069

Holmes DE: The wrecking effects of race and social class on self and success. Psychoanal Q 75(1):215–235, 2006 16482966

Holmes DE: Culturally imposed trauma: the sleeping dog has awakened. Will psychoanalysis take heed? Psychoanalytic Dialogues 26(6):641–654, 2016

Holmes DE: Our country 'tis of we and them: psychoanalytic perspectives on our fractured American identity. American Imago 76(3):359–379, 2019

Holmes DE: "I do not have a racist bone in my body": psychoanalytic perspectives on what is lost and not mourned in our culture's persistent racism. J Am Psychoanal Assoc 69(2):237–258, 2021 34039064

Irving D: Waking Up White and Finding Myself in the Story of Race. Cambridge, MA, Elephant Room Press, 2014

Jones-Marlin B: Breakthrough: The Trauma Tracer. YouTube Video, 2020. Available at: www.youtube.com/watch?v=pBkVx12yc2M. Accessed May 5 2022.

Kendi IX: How to Be an Antiracist. New York, Random House, 2019

Kernberg O: Perspectives From Seven Decades of Psychoanalytic Research (Science Department, Session 2). Presentation at the APsaA 2021 National Meeting (Virtual), Weekend 3, Saturday, 2–4 pm, February 27, 2021

Keval N: Racist States of Mind: Understanding the Perversion of Curiosity and Concern. London, Karnac, 2016

Kovel J: White Racism: A Psychohistory. New York, Columbia University Press, 1970

Luhrmann TM: Book Forum: The Protest Psychosis: How Schizophrenia Became a Black Disease (Metzl 2010). Am J Psychiatry 167(4):479–480, 2010. Available at: https://ajp.psychiatryonline.org/doi/10.1176/appi.ajp.2009.09101398. Accessed August 12, 2022.

Meacham J: His Truth Is Marching On: John Lewis and the Power of Hope. New York, Random House, 2020a

Meacham J: The South's fight for white supremacy. The New York Times, August 23, 2020b

Metzl JM: The Protest Psychosis: How Schizophrenia Became a Black Disease. Boston, Beacon Press, 2010

Metzl JM: Dying of Whiteness: How the Politics of Racial Resentment Is Killing America's Heartland. New York, Basic Books, 2019

Milloy C, Lawson W: Black psychiatrists are few. They've never been more needed. The Washington Post, August 11, 2020. Available at: https://www.washingtonpost.com/local/black-psychiatrists-are-few-theyve-never-been-more-needed/2020/08/11/7df9eeea-dbeb-11ea-8051-d5f887d73381_story.html. Accessed August 12, 2022.

Moss DB: Mapping racism. Psychoanal Q 75(1):271–294, 2006 16482968

Moss D: On having whiteness. J Am Psychoanal Assoc 69(2):355–371, 2021 34039063

Noah T: Trevor Noah Explains How Society Has Broken Its Social Contract on Black America. YouTube video, 2020. Available at: www.youtube.com/watch?v=QSyPy9vdA_s. Accessed May 5, 2022.

Pagán AM, Quintana V, Spotnitz J: Mitigating Black maternal mortality. Berkeley Public Policy Journal, Spring 2020

Peele J: Get Out [American horror film]. Written and directed by Jordan Peele. Produced by Jordan Peele, Jason Blum, Edward Hamm Jr., Sean McKittrick. Production Cos: Blumhouse Productions, Monkey Paw Productions, QC Entertainment, 2017

Pierce C: Psychiatric problems of the black minority, in American Handbook of Psychiatry. Edited by Arieta S. New York, Basic Books, 1974, pp 512–523

Pogue White K: Surviving hating and being hated: some personal thoughts about racism from a psychoanalytic perspective. Contemporary Psychoanalysis 38(3):401–402, 2002

Powell D: Psychoanalysis and African Americans: past, present, and future, in The African American Experience: Psychoanalytic Perspectives. Edited by Akhtar S. New York, Rowman & Littlefield, 2012, pp 59–84

Powell D: Race, African Americans, and psychoanalysis: collective silence in the therapeutic situation. Journal of the American Psychoanalytic Association 66(6):1021–1049, 2018

Powell D: From the sunken place to the shitty place: the film Get Out, psychic emancipation and modern race relations from a psychodynamic clinical perspective. The Psychoanalytic Quarterly 89(3):415–445, 2020

Powell DR: Introduction to Part 7: Racial and Ethnic Diversities in Psychotherapy, in Gabbard's Textbook of Psychotherapeutic Treatments, 2nd Edition. Edited by Crisp H, Gabbard GO. Washington, DC, American Psychiatric Association Publishing, 2023, pp 459–465

Powell DR, Hart A: African Americans and psychotherapeutic treatment: challenges and opportunities, in Gabbard's Textbook of Psychotherapeutic Treatments, 2nd Edition. Edited by Crisp H, Gabbard GO. Washington, DC, American Psychiatric Association Publishing, 2023, pp 467–493

Rao JM: Observations on the use of the N-word in psychoanalytic conferences. J Am Psychoanal Assoc 69(2):315–341, 2021 34039066

Roberts D: Fatal Invention: How Science, Politics, and Big Business Re-create Race in the Twenty-First Century. New York, The New Press, 2011

Rojek AE, Khanna R, Yim JWL, et al: Differences in narrative language in evaluations of medical students by gender and under-represented minority status. J Gen Intern Med 34(5):684–691, 2019 30993609

Schaeffer MW, Rozek CS, Maloney EA, et al: Elementary school teachers' math anxiety and students' math learning: a large-scale replication. Dev Sci 24(4):e13080, 2021 33382186

Schen CR, Greenlee A: Race in supervision: let's talk about it. Psychodyn Psychiatry 46(1):1–21, 2018 29480781

Sharpe C: In the Wake: On Blackness and Being. Durham, NC, Duke University Press, 2016

Shim RS: Structural racism is why I'm leaving organized psychiatry. STAT, July 1, 2020. Available at: www.statnews.com/2020/07/01/structural-racism-is-why-im-leaving-organized-psychiatry. Accessed January 31, 2022.

Skloot R: The Immortal Life of Henrietta Lacks. New York, Crown Publishers, 2010

Staples B: The burning of Black Wall Street revisited, The New York Times, June 19, 2020

Stevenson B: Just Mercy: A Story of Justice and Redemption. New York, Spiegel & Grau, 2014

Stoute BJ: Race and racism in psychoanalytic thought: the ghosts in our nursery. The American Psychoanalyst 51(1):10–29, 2017

Stoute BJ: Black rage: the psychic adaptation to the trauma of oppression. J Am Psychoanal Assoc 69(2):259–290, 2021 34039068

Stoute BJ: How our mind becomes racialized: implications for the therapeutic encounter, in Gabbard's Textbook of Psychotherapeutic Treatments, 2nd Edition. Edited by Crisp H, Gabbard GO. Washington, DC, American Psychiatric Association Publishing, 2023, pp 575–605

Sue DW, Sue D: Counseling the Culturally Different: Theory and Practice, 3rd Edition. New York, Wiley, 1999

Teherani A, Hauer KE, Fernandez A, et al: How small differences in assessed clinical performance amplify to large differences in grades and awards: a cascade with serious consequences for students underrepresented in medicine. Acad Med 93(9):1286–1292, 2018 29923892

Thomas A, Sillen S: Racism and Psychiatry. Secaucus, NJ, Citadel Press, 1972

Tummala-Narra P: Dynamics of race and culture in the supervisory encounter. Psychoanalytic Psychology 21(2):300–311, 2004

Tummala-Narra P: Skin color and the therapeutic relationship. Psychoanalytic Psychology 24(2):255–270, 2007

Tummala-Narra P: Teaching on diversity: the mutual influence of students and instructors. Psychoanalytic Psychology 26(3):322–334, 2009

Tummala-Narra P: Psychoanalytic applications in a diverse society. Psychoanalytic Psychology 30(3):471–487, 2013

Tummala-Narra P, Kanwal G: South Asian Americans, in Gabbard's Textbook of Psychotherapeutic Treatments, 2nd Edition. Edited by Crisp H, Gabbard GO. Washington, DC, American Psychiatric Association Publishing, 2023, pp 525–552

Tummala-Narra P, Claudius M, Letendre PJ, et al: Psychoanalytic psychologists' conceptualizations of cultural competence in psychotherapy. Psychoanalytic Psychology 35(1):46–59, 2017

Ueng-McHale J, Chin C: Contextualizing psychodynamic psychotherapy with Asian Americans: integration of transnational and intergenerational histories and Asian American racialization, in Gabbard's Textbook of Psychotherapeutic Treatments, 2nd Edition. Edited by Crisp H, Gabbard GO. Washington, DC, American Psychiatric Association Publishing, 2023, pp 495–523

U.S. Census Bureau: 2020 census results. October 28, 2021. Available at: www.census.gov/programs-surveys/decennial-census/decade/2020/2020-census-results.html. Accessed January 31, 2022.

Vaughans K: To unchain haunting blood memories: intergenerational trauma among African Americans, in Fragments of Trauma and the Social Production of Suffering. Edited by O'Loughlin M, Charles M. London, Rowman & Littlefield, 2015, pp 277–290

Washington HA: Medical Apartheid: The Dark History of Medical Experimentation on Black Americans From Colonial Times to the Present. New York, Anchor Books, 2006

Watkins CE Jr, Hook JN: On a culturally humble psychoanalytic supervision perspective: creating the cultural third. Psychoanalytic Psychology 33(3):487–517, 2016

White-Davis T, Stein E, Karasz A: The elephant in the room: dialogues about race within cross-cultural supervisory relationships. Int J Psychiatry Med 51(4):347–356, 2016 27497455

Wilkerson I: The Warmth of Other Suns: The Epic Story of America's Great Migration. New York, Random House, 2010

Wilkerson I: Caste: The Origins of Our Discontents. New York, Random House, 2020

Winnicott DW: The location of cultural experience. Int J Psychoanal 48(3):368–372, 1967 6053299

Winnicott DW: Playing: its theoretical status in the clinical situation. Int J Psychoanal 49(4):591–599, 1968 4180041

14

Gender Influences in Psychotherapy Supervision

Rosemary H. Balsam, FRCPsych (Lond),
MRCP (Edinburgh)

KEY LEARNING GOALS

- Help supervisees understand the history of gender and gendered attitudes in psychoanalysis to help inform their practice of psychodynamic psychotherapy.

- Recognize that there is no place for biological essentialism in the contemporary psychological assessment of people: "masculine" and feminine" are attitudinal qualities that belong to self- and social estimates.

- Foster supervisees' learning and growth and help supervisees recognize common theoretical psychodynamic concepts within the patient-therapist material.

IT SEEMS OBVIOUS that a person's sex and gender, partner status, and race will influence both a psychotherapy and a supervisory dyad. A new supervisee may think that this should go without saying. It may be enlightening, then, in the course of teaching, to provide trainees with a brief overview of the history of these psychodynamic ideas that have heightened personal awareness in the therapy encounter. The history of how therapists and patients view themselves, interact with each other, and listen and hear each other, and of how patients and therapists think about their emotional problems is subtly interwoven into the history of gender and sexuality (in the West), in our field.

Surprisingly, acute personal and cultural awareness in the therapy encounter is a relatively recent focus in conducting psychodynamic therapies. In college settings, it is now common for a therapist to say during introductions, "I'm so-and-so: my pronouns are [for example] he, him, his; or they, them, theirs—what are yours?" A therapist may wish to choose the moment for introducing pronouns, or wait to see where such an issue lies with the individual, especially if the client is older. But this is an example of the current changing social climate, and a newly acceptable question on meeting someone. Some say that it should become automatic, especially for cisgender individuals, so that queer-gender people need not feel uncomfortable, negatively "special," or "outed." There are also other factors that can influence the therapeutic dyad, such as age, ethnicity, and the mental health care discipline in which one was trained—medicine, psychology, social work, divinity school, and so forth. The demographics are less important as "facts" than as meanings that accrue with a particular supervisee, from the first meeting. For example, varying nervous expectations of the power differential that is inevitably inbuilt in a teacher–student dyad will affect how the individuals expect this interaction to proceed. These days we look on these differences as exploratory opportunities, rather than becoming stuck on the barriers they can present for a patient's treatment. Inevitably such issues will be reflected in the supervisory dyad as well.

Selected History Relevant to Gender Interaction in Psychotherapy and Supervision

Since Breuer and Freud began their in-depth psychological investigations in the late nineteenth century, members of a therapy or consultant dyad have always been aware of each other's similarities and differences at some level. Here, for example, are a descriptive few lines about the first analytic patient, Anna O., written in 1893 by Breuer, Freud's colleague: "This girl, who was bubbling over with intellectual vitality, led an extremely monotonous existence in her puritanically-minded family" (Breuer 1893/1955, p. 22). This was a more animated text than much analytic writing that came later! By the 1950s, say, the therapeutic intentions were to aim for cool "objectivity" and a lack of emotional involvement on the part of the therapist, in the belief that this attitude was "scientific" and in the best service of the study of the patient/subject's human mind. Even Breuer did not linger in that early text on his admiration for Anna O., for example, or on a possibly zealous fantasy of saving her from her strict family, as might be inferred from his lively description. In the first half of the twentieth century, psychodynamic psychotherapists and psychoanalysts saw themselves as being idealistically engaged in a positivistic scientific enterprise, where differences were sharpened, for example, between "the objective" and "the subjective;" "reality" and "fantasy." Importantly for this discussion, "masculine" behaviors were initially declared "active," versus "feminine" behaviors that were supposedly "passive," and there were aspirations to declare definitively what is "normal" gender versus the "perverse" or "deviant." Roughly around the mid-twentieth century, the philosophy of science became more complicated. Therapists were increasingly aware of being "participant-observers," as described in anthropology, and not just detached observers. Scientific authority concerning others' lifestyles was questioned. The sex and gender, and varying gendered attitudes, of therapists themselves were acknowledged openly to matter to a patient, and to affect the outcome of treatment (Kantrowitz 2019; Kantrowitz et al. 1989).

The atmospherics in treatment are thus far from "neutral." And the more awareness that therapists allow about their own participation, the more tolerable it will be to hear the patient's reactions and associations to these personal features. Both parties can learn a great deal—therapists mostly by being receptive to hearing while processing privately their reactions, and patients mostly by being responsive in their telling and not holding back.

The Time Factor in Evolving Transferences and Countertransferences

Hearing a patient's story unfolding over time in one's presence allows thinking space for the therapist and the supervisor together, to observe and appreciate paradoxes that are not rapidly explicable. Freud tried to elaborate a lack of clarity in "genders" he encountered in patients' descriptions, by noting mixed-gender sensibilities and theorizing an imagined sense of underlying physical "bisexuality." Over time, he realized *psychologically* that no one can actually be purely either "masculine" or "feminine." But Freud still believed that "masculine" was "active," and that the father was the all-important figure to both girls' and boys' gender portraiture. Modern therapists appreciate that *both* the mother (or other adult women) and the father (or other adult men) in the child's environment will become individually internalized psychologically and give a cast to how patients themselves then come across in the therapy space. I believe, based on my experiences, that the crucial adult/child pairings that become vital building blocks for mentalization are especially along same-body lines. If an adult patient, for example, has a consistent hatred and rejection for the same-sex parent (often for traumatic reasons), this will likely provide a special challenge to the patient's formation of a reliable and enjoyable gender portrait and aspirations in living. These kinds of internal clashes can be part of patients' problems that they bring to treatment. It is important that supervisees be helped to see how these problems arise, and to develop an empathic approach to this inner complexity. A beginner might think it helpful, say, to advise patients to be more forgiving of parents, or even to suggest that patients cut ties to "solve" their problem. In those cases, the supervisor—after exploring how such an intervention was thought to be helpful—might help direct a beginning therapist to wonder whether they pitied the patient's poor mother—perhaps overidentifying, as if it were their own mother who was being hurt. Over time, a student therapist can begin to perceive more of a patient's past as being integral to the present inner life that is enfolding the drama in the room.

The *style* of thinking in psychoanalysis and psychodynamic theory has changed in the last 40 or so years. Importantly, for example, being self-identified as queer, gay, or lesbian, or as transgender, is not seen as "arrested development" and deviant from some ideal "normal" development. These gender variants are instead perceived as alternative paths in development, where the commonness of heterosexuality and being cisgender is just one path, and not *the* singular path to maturity. Supervisees, regardless of age, have had a past too, and many people simply grow up with less tolerance in their original environments that may demand or even dictate clear-cut gender polarity as "mental health"—perhaps because it is simpler, if inaccurate, exclusionary, and merely biased.

Transference and Countertransference

It can be interesting for supervisees to learn that Freud first noticed his own interactional discomforts in a way that helped him think further about and theorize the experience, with the famous patient Dora, in 1905. She fled treatment after only a few months. Among other issues, it dawned on Freud, in retrospect, that his cigar smoke had been provocative to her, and that this sensory experience was likely connected in her memory with her conflicted fury and distaste of her noxious, sexually harassing family friend, Herr K. In retrospect, Freud made the crucial observation of "transference"—that is, the personal connections from experiences in the conflicted past that affected a present-tense therapy relationship. We of course encounter this constantly in conducting therapy. A supervisee can be comforted to know how easy it is to overlook such an impact—even Freud was blind. The good news is that it is never the last chance to understand such issues more fully, because transferences are repetitive.

Relevant as background to our topic, Freud followed this by recognizing "countertransference" in 1910: "We have become aware of the 'counter-transference,' which arises in [the analyst] as a result of the patient's influence on his unconscious feelings, and we are almost inclined to insist that he shall recognize this countertransference in himself and overcome it" (Freud 1910/1957, pp. 144–145). One can see instantly an injunction to try "to rid oneself" of this phenomenon, as a fixed barrier to "the therapy." The modern shift toward understanding the implications of countertransference for the treatment, rather than judging it negatively, touches on how we teach today. Changes in theory and technique allow for feelings concerning gender to be acceptable topics to air in supervision, rather than to ignore. In an older day, any negativity or "too much" sexual or gender attraction would be totally sequestered with the therapist's analyst. Personal privacy for a supervisee is still appropriate, but it is recognized as a part of the therapy supervision as well, with an opportunity to learn tolerance through identification with the senior therapist, and how to defer action in conducting psychotherapy. A supervisee who is learning well may say, "I'm not proud of this but…" and follow with a story of being afraid of being seduced by a good-looking queer client salivating about the great sex of the night before. Or, for example, a young male therapist being tempted to confess companionably to an older male patient who looks like his own father—but who has talked intensely of the sexual possessiveness he felt about his teenage daughter—a guilty tale of being aroused by his own toddler girl while giving her a bath. In either case, the supervisor might help the therapist explore how and why these elements may have been stimulated. The growth of interest in the mechanism of "projective identification" is also an aid to discussion, as it is a defense mechanism that is a "call and response" mechanism that unconsciously involves both patient and therapist. A trainee may like to know that this concept first emerged from Kleinian theory, due to Klein's focus on early interactions between baby and mother.

For many nowadays, mental health is increasingly associated with the idea of an expansive mind and ego functioning that is flexible enough to accommodate resonances of one's memories and past without fear and is able to recognize one's own patterns of response with a sense of choice of restraint. The aim of treatment is not to "resolve" trauma by dramatic ca-tharsis or "free" the mind radically (as in Alfred Hitchcock's movies). Su-pervisees may be relieved that their job need not entail banishing all of their patients' problems! Rather, the job may sometimes lie in helping pa-tients to tolerate and integrate more moderate and livable expectations that are different from ideals connected to their past.

Countertransferences are sought out in conducting and supervising psychotherapy, as we try to find out about what these responses tell us about the interaction with the patient. It is not so blameworthy as it once seemed, but rather is part of a working surface in the supervision and ther-apy. "Enactment" is another interactional concept that has gained traction since Jacobs (1986) first introduced it. It functions as a way of making dis-cussable aspects of the intercommunication and actions unfolding in the room, or outside it, that are unintentional and unusual for the therapist. Enactments may seem unremarkable at the time, signaling a form of blindness until they emerge more clearly as contributing (for example) to an impasse in conducting treatment. Supervision can help bring phenom-ena into view. Formerly, "acting out" was something undesirable that pri-marily needed to be stopped. Gendered aspects of the therapist–patient interaction are frequently involved in enactments (as illustrated in the clinical example in the section "Therapy Changes That Follow From In-vestigating Gender Portraiture" below). Supervisors may help trainees to detect examples of a theory being learned in the classroom, as well as as-sist them in consolidating and differentiating current and past psychody-namic knowledge and psychotherapy process knowledge for use during clinical work.

Masculinity and Femininity

Because of this cultural shift in outlook, it seems to have become clear that gender-binary distinctions between what is the purview of "masculinity" and "femininity" are variably interpretable by individuals rather than fixed phenomena. This is a change from the original sense of how gender is constructed in a linear form with girls becoming "feminine" in a prepat-terned way—say, to be modest and self-effacing or playing dumb at sci-ence, or of boys becoming "masculine" by being physically aggressive and boastful and good at science. The strict binary forms of gender are now seen as social constructions for group purposes. One sociopsychological purpose served by these constructions—inadvertent and unconscious, but often identified—is support for male hegemony and phallocentric atti-tudes, where women are dependent and subjugated (e.g., Balsam 2022). Feminism of both the second and third waves (represented by academic and psychoanalytic feminist writing in the United States) has played a role in enlightenment. I believe it is crucial to allow the validity of a binary distinction for "male" and "female" only in natal morphological differentiation that occurs at birth, but to realize that "masculine" and "feminine" are entirely attitudinal qualities that belong to self- and social estimates. Variety will therefore rule. There is no reliable place for biological essentialism in the contemporary psychological assessment of people—e.g., just because a woman gives birth, it would be mistaken to think (as formerly) that there is a "maternal instinct" that dictates automatically that she will love her child; or because a boy is aggressive, loving football would not automatically be a test of how "masculine" he is.

Therapy Changes That Follow From Investigating Gender Portraiture

In the case vignettes below, I illustrate some of the implications of gender flexibilities for the therapist–patient interaction in various therapies.

Case Vignette 1: A Gendered Enactment

Ms. T, a 21-year-old female undergraduate from a European country, was beginning therapy with Dr. Q, a young male psychiatrist, who discovered, from her accent on the phone, that she was from his favorite European vacation city. Dr. Q was openly delighted at the prospect of seeing this patient, and told me, his supervisor, that he looked forward very much to the prospect of getting a few tips for his next vacation—Ha-ha! There were beautiful girls in that city (indicating to me a slight boastfulness about his heterosexual proclivity). As we were new to each other too, Dr. Q added that of course he knew better then to act on such things! (This indicated to me his concern that I might judge him harshly for his sexual interests, or that he was concerned he'd act flirtatiously with this patient and look inexperienced in my eyes.) I agreed that he "knew better," ha-ha!

Ms. T came in, forlorn, weeping, and darkly gorgeous, petite, slender, gracefully limbed and showing her legs to advantage in Gucci high heels (which I noted as her showing off her genuine body assets of erotic attractiveness: thus signaling that, although she was miserable, she had retained some contact with a possible enjoyment in her identity that she'd like also to communicate). She described herself to Dr. Q as depressed and feeling very low ever since she had returned to school this semester. Dr. Q rapidly (and not inappropriately) arranged medications for her. I noted to myself that he barely listened to her story and seemed in a hurry to get her better. I elected not to say anything, as such speed often happens in a busy, pressured student health facility. They agreed to meet weekly during the semester. At the next visit, Ms. T reported feeling a little brighter, cried much less, and was talkative (indicating that arranging to see Dr. Q supported some hopefulness for her). Her father was mega-wealthy, and she had grown up in a luxurious large apartment overlooking the famous river that flowed through the city. She had hated growing up there, and started to tell of the violence of her father. Dr. Q listened also to her fear of the professors and her shame about underperformance.

Dr. Q then missed two consecutive supervision sessions with me. He left legitimate excuses. When he returned, he seemed interested in my assuring him that he had done nothing "wrong"—as if he were guilty in front of me. I reassured him, but asked why he was so worried, and privately wondered what more could be going on. To cut it short, there had been an enactment that touched on gender issues. Dr. Q had crossed paths with Ms. T two Saturday nights previously in a bar. He told me, stammering and blushing, that he had made a mistake; he had briefly introduced his male roommate to her, knowing he was crossing a confidentiality boundary. "I just described her as a friend. I said nothing about her being a patient. He doesn't know." OK, but my supervisee was on a slippery slope. The good news for me as supervisor was that Dr. Q was so conscious of his actions. The boundary crossing was not good, but in itself was not an *unconscious* "enactment." The more we talked, the more it became clear that he had had sexual fantasies about Ms. T—about their vacationing romantically in her family's villa in Europe (he referred to a "Roman Holiday"). Dr. Q was quite elaborately imaginative (an asset for a therapist). The part that became more pressured and less under his control was that his excitement had *almost* led him, he said, to push his roommate toward her, sparing himself, he thought, the boundary crossing of his fantasy. He would be innocent. "What stopped you?" I asked. "Well… that was it…after saying 'Hi' to me, she went over to her friends and gave a woman she was with…(he stammered)…a…a kiss." He almost spat out the last words. "They were all over each other the rest of the evening." He sighed. I could see his deep disappointment, and I thought it likely that he had fantasized about enjoying a relationship with Ms. T by proxy—he could be a voyeur through his roommate. (This, I thought, *may* be the unacceptable thinking that Dr. Q felt guilty about, and feared would emerge; thus, he had needed to keep away from me.) It emerged that in the following therapy session (i.e., the one that he would also have reported on freshly to me, had he kept that appointment), Ms. T talked about her lesbian relationship. In fact, her original upsettedness concerned a threat of loss of this important relationship.

Because of the original enactment of Dr. Q's missing the sessions with me, we could address his fear of revealing himself to me, an equally white grandmother-type, through his process work with Ms. T. He found himself angry at this young woman and unconsciously was afraid of inadvertently revealing in supervision his initial excitement, with its inevitable disappointed fairytale quality, in which Ms. T would play Audrey Hepburn to his Gregory Peck, and I would be the envious admiring bystander. Because Dr. Q was playfully imaginative, he began to wonder if—by almost pushing his roommate toward Ms. T, heterosexually, to play Gregory Peck for him—he had placed himself in the role of excluded admirer as well. I reminded him, as an actor in this triangle, that in the bar, he and Ms. T had seemed to engage in a scene where she had her lover's interest while he had, apparently, found himself in the voyeuristic stance, wishing that he could take the place of her female lover. Dr. Q then told me his sister was lesbian, too, and he had struggled with a deep sense of rejection that young women who were lesbian…he said hesitatingly…were offended at his manhood. And it hurt him. I used this feature as a teaching point, on how this view was not at all a *universal* feature of lesbian women. It used to be assumed, I said, from a strictly male (phallocentric) viewpoint, that this was the case, and in fact this supposition sometimes drew male rage and retaliation. We discussed this modern gender point intellectually. (I assumed that Dr. Q's anger and rejection had played a role in his not wanting to approach this topic previously in supervision, but I left that as a private guess.) The most important issue was that we were now able to discuss the enactment. Dr. Q took these fantasies and feelings at this point to his own private treatment, as they likely involved a conflicted family matter beyond our purview.

In using the enactment that had developed, I asked Dr. Q what imaginative sense he might make of it. What if Ms. T, knowing where he was sitting in the bar, had preconsciously or even consciously created a triangle composed of herself, her lover, and him as a watcher? I said I presumed there would be feelings she'd be interested in arousing in him. Dr. Q entered into the idea. He was an excellent and responsive therapist, as the reader sees here. He said that when he was joking around with me in the beginning, it was as if he wanted me to know he was capable of flirting with a beautiful woman who would be interested in him. I joked back, "Granma should encourage her boy!" He laughed, "Yeah…actually my grandmother was very strict with us about good behavior," he mused. And we went on to wonder whether Ms. T might be toying with the same tensions. What if—even though Dr. Q was thinking of himself as her brother—what if she thought of him as a dad who had been trying to push a "nice young man" on her romantically—and what if she longed for her father's admiration instead for her *own* choice of a "nice young woman"…as she was showing him their loving behaviors so vividly?

We agreed together that neither of us knew what was going on inside Ms. T's head in the bar as she reacted to his introduction of his roommate, and subsequently to the knowledge or fantasy that he was watching her with her friends afterwards. A capacity to hold uncertainty was a vital point of our therapist/supervisory agreement about this treatment. What we had co-created together was simply one tableau that could make emotional sense of this enactment. I can think of several others, too, but I was teaching Dr. Q how one can make great use of one's own "mistakes" to further the patient's knowledge of herself and discover more about, in this instance, Ms. T's feelings about her sexual partner choice and orientation and view of her own gender features. Dr. Q would begin this exploration by finding a tactful way to ask Ms. T what her further thoughts were about the encounter in the bar. We had talked together about his infatuation with her, in case Ms. T brought up with him that the encounter had been awkward for her. Dr. Q's facing his own emotional truth privately could allow Ms. T full expression of the reality of her awkward feelings.

Case Vignette 2: A Case of Pronouns

My supervisee, June, was a white heterosexual cisgender psychologist just starting to build her own private practice, and was eager to come across as pleasant to her new patient, Alex, a 26-year-old graduate student. She sensed, in the patient's hesitancies during the initial phone contact, a potential for a fragile therapeutic alliance. Alex was a tall person with a crew cut. In the office, sitting with thin legs tightly crossed, the patient had rounded hips, faint breast shapes, and was wearing a smart shirt and college-stripe tie. Alex forcefully announced: "People need to call me 'they.' That pronoun accurately addresses my gender status. 'He' or 'she' is ill-matched to me, and it is far too limiting." June repeated, "You'd like me to call you 'they.'" June later told me that she was feeling on edge, and was worried that she might become confused in the spontaneous back-and-forth of conversation and might inadvertently call Alex "she." She was afraid of "doing something wrong" with this patient. She was sophisticated about gender and sexuality scholarship, but here she felt she was being tested for her ability to encompass "otherness." The patient had already sacked four therapists, finding them wanting. After June cautiously repeated back the pronoun request, Alex snapped testily, "No—there won't be any need for *you* to use that pronoun in here, will there now?"

On reflection in supervision, we could see that this statement was of course accurate. One needs no other pronoun than "you" to address one's patient directly face-to-face. The therapist and the supervisor shared their confusions here, as shown in this extra effort to try to sort out the conditions of the right usage of the pronoun. The threat of being offensive (from the patient's point of view) was ripe within the tension of these uses of familiar versus unfamiliar everyday language—a concern in contemporary times, sometimes unfortunately trivialized as an effort motivated by "mere political correctness." "They" (Alex) were thus struggling to correct the terminology of everyday life. The older or the more conservative the therapist, the more befuddled the inner response to these pronouns, I believe. In supervision, this young therapist easily thereafter referred to Alex as "they," which I got used to also. For me there was a kind of "we" sense surrounding Alex, as if there were two or more entities rolled into one. Theoretically, of course, I could readily think of Nancy Chodorow's (1994) "Heterosexualities" as plural. Intellectually I am extremely intrigued and interested in gender plurality. Yet I believe I am not alone, even including some of the young therapists, in being capable of confusion in the immediacy of the moment. I hope my confusion does not represent a phobic response, but if it does, then it is better to be able to consider the uncertainty. I daydreamed in this case while I listened to the process notes and my supervisee speaking about Alex's troubles with their mother—I imagined that there must be a comfort in this plural identity, given the maternal barrages that any single identity would be even more demolished by! I imagined this natal-born girl expanding herself—as twins maybe, who could make themselves heard better, or protest more effectively than one alone. A boy and a girl together could flourish better. The "they" sense is much more expansive and encompassing than some conflictually internal "he versus she" sense that might form the substance of another person's gender issues. Each entity in a "they" internal sense can almost be fully accommodated, but perhaps not fully inhabited…or I wonder if I am off on a bourgeois path of assumption that singular means just that, and plural means just more than one. My supervisee and I needed to retranslate Alex's plurality of gender in their own world and in their own terms.

As this therapy went on, Alex and June became bonded. The gender portrait presented may not actually have conformed to any set prepattern that I am aware of—transgender was too narrow. The patient was polyamatory, which was consistent with the polyamorous responsiveness of their body also. I did not view any of these revelations as being conflictual as presented to June, and I saw the sexual choices as forms of mental health, and as appropriate young adult experimentation for this person. Alex was still youthful when they terminated. More of their life is there to be developed. The therapist mostly helped Alex with feelings—their detail and their meanings in the context of Alex's relationships. I believed that Alex still had much work to do in the matter of trust and finding comfort in intimacy—in the aftermath of their traumatic childhood. But Alex did very well academically. They had a buoyant zest for living as they ventured forth—brave, adventurous, and still a proud solo spirit that contained multiple internal identities, forging their own path into their future.

Conclusion

As with the powerful benefits gained from actually conducting psychotherapies, the accumulation of their own clinical examples, both difficult and gratifying, can demonstrate to trainees more than any academic teaching the necessity of often allowing oneself "not to know." One can then try to learn more from an actual live patient that one is encountering. It is essential, however, also to recognize, as a therapist, that simultaneously one *does* have a theory in mind garnered from one's living and psychological education up to that point. It is thus important to ask what one's assumptions are as one listens. This is a freeing move, so that one can then realize the aspects less applicable to that individual in the room. Working with gender issues in mind, it is important not to confuse "neutral" with "nonexistent." These pointers open the way to being able to try to keep thinking and absorbing what patterns may unfold with surprise. Theory legitimately keeps shifting; the interior of patients' lives shift; the social world excitingly keeps changing.

References

Balsam RH: Liberating "female" from "femininity": Helene Deutsch and the past to Dianne Elise and the present, in Psychoanalytic Explorations of What Women Want Today: Femininity, Desire and Agency. Edited by Cereijido M, Ellman PL, Goodman NR. London, Routledge, 2022

Breuer J: Fräulein Anna O, case histories from studies on hysteria, (1893), in The Standard Edition of the Complete Psychological Works of Sigmund Freud, Vol 2. Translated and edited by Strachey J. London, Hogarth Press, 1955, pp 19–47

Chodorow N: Femininities, Masculinities, Sexualities: Freud and Beyond. Lexington, University Press of Kentucky, 1994

Freud S: The future prospects of psychoanalytic theory (1910), in The Standard Edition of the Complete Psychological Works of Sigmund Freud, Vol 11. Translated and edited by Strachey J. London, Hogarth Press, 1957, pp 139–151

Jacobs TJ: On countertransference enactments. J Am Psychoanal Assoc 34(2):289–307, 1986 3722698

Kantrowitz J: The Patient's Impact on the Analyst. London, Routledge, 2019

Kantrowitz JL, Katz AL, Greenman DA, et al: The patient-analyst match and the outcome of psychoanalysis: a pilot study. J Am Psychoanal Assoc 37(4):893–919, 1989 2632628

15

Supervision of Psychotherapy With Lesbian, Gay, Bisexual, and Transgender Patients

Stewart Adelson, M.D.
Jack R. Keefe, Ph.D.
Frank E. Yeomans, M.D., Ph.D.

KEY LEARNING GOALS

- Identify unique developmental experiences of lesbian, gay, bisexual, and transgender (LGBT) patients in domains of sexual orientation, gender identity, and gender expression (e.g., nonconforming childhood gender expression, impact of stigma, being "in the closet" versus "coming out").

- Describe basic ways in which psychotherapy might require adaptation for LGBT patients in light of these unique experiences (e.g., for patients with identity concealment, rejection anticipation, family nonacceptance).

- Describe basic ways in which unique experiences of LGBT patients, supervisees, and/or supervisors might affect the supervision of psychotherapy (e.g., anticipation of gaps in understanding, shame, disclosure conflicts).

- Identify ways in which these unique experiences could influence transference, countertransference, and parallel processing among patient, supervisee, and supervisor (e.g., identifications, therapist/supervisor values, normative models).

THE AIM OF THIS chapter is to discuss areas of psychotherapy supervision that are specific to lesbian, gay, bisexual, and transgender (LGBT) people and to examine how these areas relate to general principles of psychotherapy supervision. LGBT people exhibit the same range of personality styles, have the same range of mental health needs, and may seek psychotherapy for the same range of problems, issues, and concerns as all people. In this sense, the principles of psychotherapy supervision for LGBT populations are the same as those for anyone else. However, LGBT people may have additional unique mental health needs related to their sexual orientation, gender experience, or both. These needs—whether they are a prime focus of treatment or affect other issues that motivated therapy— may benefit from consideration in psychotherapy.

In comparison with the general population, people who are LGBT are at increased statistical risk for certain psychiatric conditions. These include depression, suicidality, anxiety disorders, PTSD, substance use disorders, and possibly disordered eating (Institute of Medicine 2011). These mental health disparities in the LGBT population are frequently associated with exposure to various kinds of stigma. The minority stress hypothesis, a risk paradigm with much empirical evidence (Meyer and Frost 2013), holds that exposure to stigma causes increased risk for mental and physical illnesses.

Clinically and culturally competent psychotherapy with LGBT patients requires certain skills in psychotherapists and their supervisors (Drescher et al. 2003; Friedman and Downey 2002). These include the ability of clinicians to monitor not only their own knowledge base but also their own biases (whether explicit or implicit), personal values that might interfere with objective mental health care treatment, and reactions such as negative identification or overidentification with patients or within the supervisor–supervisee dyad that could affect treatment.

Supervisors must also be able to monitor their supervisees' explicit or implicit biases in reaction to a patient's nonconformity with sexual or gender norms. In addition, clinicians conducting psychodynamic psychotherapy must monitor transference and countertransference reactions to such biases. Supervisors must be able to assess supervisees' ability to amend any biases they may hold and to monitor their own countertransference. If they determine that supervisees do not have that ability, supervisors can consider transition to care with a therapist who does.

To assist supervisors of LGBT psychotherapy, this chapter builds on other chapters in this volume, adding detailed information about clinical competence with LGBT patients. The discussion of clinical competence is presented in two sections: one on Basic Information and the other on Basic Skills required for the supervision and psychotherapy with people who are LGBT.

Clinical Competence: Basic Information for Supervisors of Psychotherapy With LGBT Patients

Over the last 50 years there has been a dramatic shift in mental health care professionals' understanding of the mental health needs of LGBT individuals. Historically, LGBT sexual orientations and gender identities were viewed by the mainstream mental health care professions as being inherently pathological. For example, until 1973, the American Psychiatric Association's *Diagnostic and Statistical Manual of Mental Disorders* (DSM) defined homosexuality as a mental illness. However, such conceptualizations were not supported by empirical evidence and have accordingly undergone successive revisions.

Contemporaneously with a shift to empirical nomenclature beginning with DSM-III (American Psychiatric Association 1980), appropriately designed research showed that most gay and lesbian individuals are mentally healthy. Homosexual orientations were accordingly depathologized in subsequent editions of the DSM and the World Health Organization's *International Classification of Diseases* (ICD) (Bayer 1981). Empirical research examining historical efforts to use psychotherapy to change sexual orientation—so-called conversion therapies—has never provided any evidence that such "treatment" can achieve lasting change in an enduring pattern of nonheterosexual attraction (although patients experiencing conflict over their sexual orientation due to self-stigmatization can disavow a gay or bisexual identity and suppress same-sex behavior) (Drescher et al. 2016). Similarly, family dynamics that were hypothesized to cause homosexuality were found to be neither necessary nor sufficient to cause a nonheterosexual orientation. Based on the absence of any evidence of efficacy and the potential risks to mental health of reinforcing self-stigma and undermining protective factors such as self-acceptance, family connectedness, and identity pride, conversion therapies have been renounced in the official guidelines of mainstream mental health care bodies. Additionally, such treatments are increasingly legally proscribed by regulatory bodies, and the United Nations has called for a worldwide end to conversion therapies as a human rights issue (United Nations Human Rights Council 2020).

Diagnoses related to transgender identities have also been revised and are undergoing further research and revision. For example, the DSM-IV (American Psychiatric Association 1994) diagnosis of *gender identity disorder* was replaced with *gender dysphoria* in DSM-5 (American Psychiatric Association 2013). With this shift, transgender identities were recognized as variants rather than inherently pathological conditions. In contrast to gender identity disorder, gender dysphoria has as its core feature *distress* related to an incongruence between an individual's gender identity and their somatic sex or assigned gender. In ICD-11 (World Health Organization 2019), gender dysphoria was replaced with *gender incongruence,* from which the distress criterion had been removed. In keeping with this change, the diagnosis was reclassified outside the mental health chapter, further emphasizing the non-psychopathologizing conceptualization of transgender identities.

The rationale for providing a separate chapter on psychotherapy supervision with LGBT people relates to the unique psychotherapeutic needs of this population. These generally involve two areas. The first involves developmental experiences that are unique to the life course of LGBT people, such as having a sexual orientation, gender expression, and/or gender identity that differs from that expected by family, peers, and community. Although they may initially conceal these identities from others, these individuals may subsequently face the difficult dilemma of whether to reveal them, or "come out." The second area of unique psychotherapeutic needs relates to this population's increased risk for certain psychiatric conditions due to factors such as exposure to anti-LGBT stigma. Appropriate psychotherapeutic care for LGBT people often requires an understanding of the influences of unique life course experiences, developmental challenges, and stigma on mental health. Supervisors of psychotherapy with LGBT patients should be familiar with these issues, know how to teach them in didactic and clinical formats, and monitor for related transference/countertransference reactions in psychotherapy supervision involving LGBT patients, clinicians, and/or supervisors.

Psychotherapy treatments used with the general population sometimes require adaptation when used with LGBT people (Pachankis et al. 2015). The degree to which the empirical evidence base for psychotherapies can be generalized to LGBT patients is an important question that requires careful evaluation and clinical judgment in relation to specific elements of these patients' mental health needs. Although a full discussion of the appropriate adaptation of psychotherapeutic modalities to LGBT populations is beyond the scope of this chapter, supervisors should be aware that such adaptations have been published and should keep up to date with developments in the field. A number of practice guidelines, review articles, and other sources of information on these adaptations are available (Cabaj n.d.; Pachankis et al. 2019).

It is also important to note that significant gaps remain in the knowledge base of LGBT mental health and require further research. For example, knowledge about the basic epidemiology and developmental trajectories of transgender development within population samples is lacking. However, much evidence from clinical and convenience samples suggests that transgender people, like lesbian, gay, and bisexual people, may be at increased risk for depression and other conditions warranting care. Psychotherapy supervisors should keep abreast of developments in the field and communicate relevant information about treatment adaptations to those whom they supervise.

Unique Developmental Experiences Among LGBT People

In order to understand and supervise the psychotherapeutic treatment of LGBT people, supervisors should be familiar with three domains of gender and sexual development especially pertinent to this population. These domains are distinct but can overlap.

1. *Sexual orientation* refers to the sex of those to whom an individual is attracted. It comprises distinct *domains* of sexual *feelings*, *behavior*, and *identity* (both private and public, which can differ). These domains can be aligned or not. Behavior, and to some degree identity, can be chosen; feelings cannot. Identity or behavior may change over time; feelings vary over time more commonly in females then in males.
2. *Gender expression* refers to a person's behaviors that are culturally recognized as being masculine or feminine in areas such as clothing, grooming, and mannerisms. In children, gender expression may involve toy preferences, a predilection for or an aversion to rough-and-tumble play, and peer selection.
3. *Gender identity* refers to an individual's experienced gender as male, female, or sometimes another gender (e.g., between genders, nonbinary, agender). A person's gender identity might differ from their somatic sex or gender assigned at birth. A transgender, nonbinary, or other noncisgender identity can emerge at different points in the life course, including prepubertally, in adolescence/young adulthood, or later in life. Different ages of clinical presentation appear to be correlated with different developmental trajectories.

With increasing social awareness of transgender and nonbinary gender identities, terms such as *genderqueer* (having a gender that is not binarily male or female), *agender* (not identifying as having a gender per se), and *pansexual* (attraction to more than one gender identity, possibly including nonbinary ones) are increasingly being discussed in the mental health literature. Sometimes more expansive acronyms such as LGBTQ are used to denote these experiences. In this chapter we use the LGBT acronym to refer to the evidence base regarding what is currently known about the needs in these groups (including disparities in risk for mental health conditions). However, psychotherapy supervisors should know that other sexual and gender identities, including nonbinary ones, may be clinically salient.

Numerous studies of gender specialty clinic cohorts have found that developmental trajectories of individuals with gender dysphoria differ depending on the age at which the individual first seeks care for gender dysphoria. A stable transgender identity has been more frequently reported among individuals in whom the transgender identity presented in adolescence or adulthood, whereas a prepubertal transgender identity may be replaced by a reported cisgender identity in adolescence or young adulthood, most frequently associated with a nonheterosexual orientation. However, such studies usually have relatively brief follow-up periods. It is unknown how frequently a change from a prepubertal transgender identity to an adolescent cisgender identity reflects identity concealment and to what extent the developmental trajectories in specialty clinic cohorts are representative of the general transgender population.

Although these domains of sexual orientation and gender experience are distinct, they can overlap and be developmentally related. For example, prehomosexual males report having felt averse to rough-and-tumble play significantly more frequently than do heterosexual males (Bailey and Zucker 1995). A meta-analysis of 15 studies found a developmental association between gender-nonconforming behavior in childhood and nonheterosexual orientation in adulthood. Although its mechanism is unknown, this association is especially strong in males. Gender expression generally emerges by ages 2–4 years (Bailey and Zucker 1995). Gender-nonconforming behavior during childhood and adolescence may affect a youth's experiences of peer acceptance and self-esteem, because these can be strongly influenced by nonconformity to gender-typical patterns. Childhood gender nonconformity may thus be associated with feeling different and with being at risk for peer nonacceptance, family nonacceptance, or other experiences that affect long-term self-esteem. Among vulnerable individuals, such experiences may constitute a risk factor for the emergence of depression, anxiety, or other psychiatric conditions.

Mechanisms of Difference: Object Choice/Orientation Paradigms

Factors influencing sexual orientation, gender expression, and gender identity are complex and multifactorial. Biological, psychological, and social factors appear to interact to influence gender and sexual development. A number of biological influences have been found to affect sexual orientation and childhood gender expression, including genetic and prenatal neurohormonal factors (Adelson and American Academy of Child and Adolescent Psychiatry Committee on Quality Issues 2012). These factors operate differently in males than they do in females. Fraternal sibling birth order predicts sexual orientation in males. However, none of these biological influences entirely determine a person's sexual orientation or gender expression.

Factors influencing gender identity—whether transgender or cisgender—are even less well understood. Research examining brain gender has identified more than 2,000 sexually dimorphic CNS systems at various levels that can be masculinized or feminized. These include genetic, epigenetic, cellular, and anatomic gender differences, in addition to neuroendocrine, neurocognitive, stress-related, emotional, and other functional ones (Hines 2004; McEwen et al. 2015). Gender *mosaicism* refers to the fact that gender-dimorphic CNS systems can be masculinized, feminized, or both independently, in myriad ways in any given individual, creating a CNS gender mosaic. Ultimately, an individual could be "high" or "low" in overall feminization, masculinization, both, or neither.

On another level, sexuality and gender are also socially organized according to *sexual scripts* and *gender roles* that inflect the meaning of sexuality and gender in a cultural context. The interplay of biological and social influence takes on personal psychological meaning for an individual in the context of their temperament, attachment style, character, and developmental experiences to influence patients' mental health needs. For this reason, a comprehensive biopsychosocial understanding of the patient is a fundamental requirement for any psychotherapeutic treatment plan.

Stigma, Minority Stress, and Other Mental Health Risk Paradigms

Stigma describes a psychosocial phenomenon by which certain groups are labeled as different and/or devalued and are placed at risk for acts of discrimination. Stigmatization can occur at a number of levels, including interpersonal levels such as family nonacceptance or peer bullying for gender nonconformity or nonheterosexual orientation. Stigma can also be experienced individually as intrapsychic stigma, including identity concealment and rejection anticipation (Meyer and Frost 2013). The minority stress theory posits that exposure to stigmatization causes increased risk for poor mental health. This causal theory suggests that addressing stigma—including eliminating it when possible and, if not, supporting resiliency and coping—may be an important focus of psychotherapy for LGBT patients.

Other hypotheses posit different causes for the association between exposure to stigma and poor mental health. The *selection hypothesis* holds that psychopathological behavior causes the individual to experience increased stigma (Bailey 2020). The *rejection sensitivity hypothesis* suggests that some LGBT people experience increased rates of rejection anticipation that mediate the expression of mental illness in vulnerable individuals. This hypothesis may be compatible with the minority stress theory from a developmental perspective, given that it has been established that childhood exposure to stress increases the long-term risk for psychopathology (Baams et al. 2020). The means by which this occurs could include epigenetic, posttraumatic, and other mechanisms operating during development. Understanding possible causes of increased risk for mental disorders can help inform patient case formulations and appropriate psychotherapeutic plans.

An *intersectional perspective* is one in which awareness of other domains of identity, such as race/ethnicity, interact with sexual orientation and gender experience in any given individual to influence physical and mental health. For example, various ethnic groups may hold culturally inflected understandings of sexuality and gender as well as different norms and values regarding LGBT people. Furthermore, human gender and sexual development tends to be socially organized into "sexual scripts," or patterns (a different sense of the term *sexual scripts* refers to the intrapsychic organization of sexual fantasies). Psychotherapists and their supervisors must know how sociodemographic factors such as race/ethnicity and acculturation affect LGBT individuals' developmental norms, identity, access to social supports, coming out, and other variables that can influence mental health.

Psychotherapy Adaptations for LGBT Patients

The concepts defined in the previous section provide the basis for appropriate adaptation of standard psychotherapy interventions to the LGBT population. As cross-cutting developmental and mental health risk issues, developmental experiences such as identity concealment and mental health risk factors such as stigma may be a relevant focus of different psychotherapeutic modalities.

For example, cognitive-behavioral therapy (CBT) might focus on depressogenic or anxiogenic cognitions salient to the LGBT population, such as those related to rejection anticipation and reality-testing of fears of nonacceptance. In focusing on these cognitions, the CBT therapist would need to consider a patient's real experiences of anti-LGBT stigma, the patient's ability to evaluate these and navigate social safety, and the patient's developmental experiences affecting self-esteem and social anxiety. A well-known manualized adaptation of CBT for sexual minority men is John Pachankis's ESTEEM (Effective Skills to Empower Effective Men) protocol (Pachankis et al. 2015). This 10-session intervention assumes that mood and anxiety symptoms are understandable responses to minority stress, and that early and ongoing minority stress can lead to the development of maladaptive cognitions and behavioral strategies. There is some preliminary evidence that the ESTEEM protocol may be especially helpful for sexual minority men who carry strong negative beliefs about being gay or bisexual.

Interpersonal therapy, which may be framed around depression related to difficulty with role transitions, might be adapted to LGBT patients, given the salience of such transitions for these individuals—coming out or (in the case of transgender patients) social gender transition or surgical or endocrine sex reassignment (Pachankis 2018). Psychodynamic psychotherapy with LGBT patients may need to pay particular attention to issues related to the developmental impact on character defenses of gender-nonconforming expression in middle childhood and its effect on gender-based self-esteem. This process may entail monitoring by supervisor and supervisee of transference/countertransference with special attention to the impact of this developmental experience on the patient's experience of the therapist and the therapist's experience of the patient. The psychodynamic therapist may also consider how a patient's unique life course experiences have affected that patient's personality structure.

We remind the reader that consideration of these cross-cutting issues should take place in the context of a full, appropriate diagnostic assessment and case formulation.

Clinical Competence: Basic Skills for Supervisors of Psychotherapy With LGBT Patients

It is important that psychotherapists and their supervisors consider how a particular patient may have been affected by the developmental experiences reported by many nonheterosexual and transgender people. These experiences can lead these individuals to "feel different" and cause peers and/or family to react in stigmatizing ways. Psychotherapists and supervisors are advised to keep abreast of the research on sexual and gender development and their relation to mental health needs in arriving at a case formulation, psychotherapeutic goals, and a treatment plan for LGBT patients.

Whether therapists treating LGBT patients should disclose their own sexual orientation is an important consideration that is beyond the scope of this chapter but has been extensively discussed elsewhere. There are a variety of perspectives on this issue and no one correct answer to the question of whether a therapist should or should not disclose their sexual or gender identity to a patient. Patients might wish to know this about their therapist for a variety of reasons. LGBT psychotherapists and their supervisors must assess whether disclosing this information is in a patient's best interest and in furtherance of a psychotherapeutic treatment plan. In some situations, especially in supportive psychotherapies, serving as a role model could be helpful for LGBT patients. In other situations, such as in more exploratory psychodynamic psychotherapies, reflecting on what a patient thinks or the meaning of a patient's question about the therapist's identity could be a fruitful exploration, and therefore requires that the therapist abstain from revealing this information, at least for a while. Such possibilities must be weighed against the risk that a patient could misinterpret abstinence as shame-based identity concealment in the therapist, with negative ramifications. Psychotherapists and their supervisors must carefully evaluate such issues on a case-by-case basis.

Vignettes Illustrating Treatment Principles and Key Psychotherapy Skills

Each of the vignettes that follow illustrate one or more of the Learning Goals listed at the beginning of this chapter. For convenience, these goals are shown again in Table 15–1.

Vignette 1: Sexual Repression and Anxiety (Learning Goals 2 and 4)

Mr. S, a 30-year-old white cisgender male graduate student, sought out psychotherapy for panic disorder after an unsuccessful combination treatment consisting of CBT and pharmacotherapy. He had grown up in a very close-knit Catholic family that espoused highly negative views about homosexuality. Despite identifying as straight, Mr. S reported no history of normative dating experiences and no clear sexual/romantic desires or fantasies about women. He hesitantly complained of external pressure from his mother to finally "settle down" and "start a family." The therapist, a gay man, found himself surprised by Mr. S's self-identification, having assumed that he was gay, and wondered to himself whether his conservative

Table 15–1. Learning goals for supervision of psychotherapy with LGBT patients

1. Identify unique developmental experiences of lesbian, gay, bisexual, and transgender (LGBT) patients in domains of sexual orientation, gender identity, and gender expression (e.g., nonconforming childhood gender expression, impact of stigma, being "in the closet" versus "coming out").

2. Describe basic ways in which psychotherapy might require adaptation for LGBT patients in light of these unique experiences (e.g., for patients with identity concealment, rejection anticipation, family nonacceptance).

3. Describe basic ways in which unique experiences of LGBT patients, supervisees, and/or supervisors might affect the supervision of psychotherapy (e.g., anticipation of gaps in understanding, shame, disclosure conflicts).

4. Identify ways in which these unique experiences could influence transference, countertransference, and parallel processing among patient, supervisee, and supervisor (e.g., identifications, therapist/supervisor values, normative models).

religious background had arrested a process of exploring sexual fantasies and identity.

The therapist began a course of panic-focused psychodynamic therapy (Busch et al. 2012). Using Mr. S's symptoms as a lens and engaging the patient's curiosity, the therapist explored the meanings surrounding the episodes of panic. Mr. S's panic attacks often emerged at the gym, where he reported comparing his body with the bodies of other men, and fixating on aspects of their bodies. Mr. S also experienced anxiety around an "intense" friendship with an "out" gay man. Gradually, the therapist made bids for reflection as to why these contexts appeared to foment panic—what difficult feelings might be arising? The therapist additionally interpreted an approach-avoidance dynamic discernible in Mr. S's interactions with his gay friend; he suggested that something about the intensity of his feelings for his friend was intolerable, with panic serving as an injunction preventing them from meeting. Mr. S eventually "came out" to his therapist, which was a watershed moment demarcating total remission of his panic symptoms. The therapist's tactful exploration of Mr. S's repressed sexual feelings—ultimately through material Mr. S himself brought to therapy—was critical to his treatment.

Takeaway Points for Vignette 1

- Therapists' countertransferential reactions to a patient's LGBT identity should be noted and carefully reflected upon. At times such reactions may contain insight into the patient's experiences vis-à-vis their sexual orientation and gender, while at other times these reactions may reflect stereotypes and/or stigmas held by the therapist.

- Despite overall improvements in the status of sexual and gender minorities in society, significant aspects of sexual and gender identity may still be repressed, avoided, or unarticulated.
- Because conflicts surrounding sex, sexuality, and gender may manifest as or contribute strongly to a patient's symptoms, identifying and helping the patient to tolerate or resolve these conflicts may be important for resolving symptom disorders.

Vignette 2: New Same-Sex Attraction and Identity Confusion (Learning Goals 1 and 2)

Ms. L, a 19-year-old from a Mexican immigrant family, is a first-generation community college student. Having been consistently attracted to males previously, she experiences an unexpected sexual attraction to a female classmate in the context of their friendship. She senses that her friend feels the same. Ms. L is highly ambivalent, thinking she may be in love but feeling distressed about what this attraction means about who she is, what her family will think, and what her future will be. She seeks counseling.

The therapist's evaluation yields a diagnosis of major depressive disorder, mild severity. Ms. L expresses a preference for psychotherapy rather than pharmacotherapy. In light of scant adaptations of depression-specific psychotherapies to LGBT populations that are generalizable to this patient's case, the therapist seeks consultation from a supervisor familiar with LGBT mental health. The supervisor explains that female and male sexual orientations may differ, with female sexuality being more relationally dependent. She advises the therapist to explore what Ms. L's current attraction means in the context of her personal values, family relationships, culture, and assimilation. The therapist helps Ms. L to tolerate uncertainty about the future and to test evidence about family relationships without idealization or devaluation in order to assess risks and benefits of disclosure of the relationship.

Takeaway Points for Vignette 2

- Attraction/fantasy, behavior, and identity are separate domains of sexual orientation.
- These domains may be congruent or incongruent, and may be associated with identity concealment, the meanings (both psychodynamic and psychosocial) of which must be examined and understood.
- Sexual identity may change in some individuals over time; such change is more likely to occur in women.
- Facilitating an individual's adaptation to their sexual orientation is a valid goal of treatment.

Vignette 3: Self-Stigmatization Manifesting as a Transference Distortion (Learning Goal 4)

Mr. H, a 25-year-old cisgender gay male graduate student, presented with complaints of anxiety and difficulty establishing an intimate relationship.

The referral source told the therapist that the patient had asked for a gay male therapist. Although Mr. H himself had not mentioned this request when they started therapy, the therapist thought it was understood. The therapy proceeded with Mr. H focusing on his dating experiences, which tended to be short-lived. He was always insecure about his dates' interest in him, and was rejection-sensitive.

One day, 6 months into the therapy, Mr. H abruptly said to the therapist, "I'm wondering if you're gay." Surprised, the therapist responded, "I thought you came to me because of that." Mr. H replied, "Yes, but you seem too normal, too well-adjusted." This line of exploration opened up a deep-seated internalized homophobia that the patient had kept to himself. The therapy was then able to access a "gut level" feeling of inferiority within Mr. H related to being gay. As the therapy advanced, Mr. H was able to resolve the negative views of being gay that he had kept hidden. It emerged that, in parallel with the patient's sensitivity to rejection, Mr. H subtly devalued any man he dated in a way that doomed any potential relationship.

Takeaway Points for Vignette 3

- Political advances have not totally removed aspects of societal stigma regarding homosexuality, and such views can be present in seemingly well-adjusted gay people and can affect their social and interpersonal functioning, as well as their self-esteem.
- Internalized homophobia can have a negative impact on intimate relations unless the person resolves their underlying idealization of the "straight world."
- Cognitive learning may not be enough to resolve a person's internalized homophobia. The patient in this vignette needed to have an affectively charged experience of his negative feelings about homosexuality within the therapy before he could move beyond them.

Vignette 4: Trauma and Gender Identity; Impact of Underlying Personality Traits/Structure on Lived Experience (Learning Goals 1 and 2)

Ms. Z, a 27-year-old white transgender lesbian woman, presented for treatment of PTSD following a sexual assault. In this attack, she had been followed into a bar restroom by a man, who proceeded to force himself upon her. Ms. Z was terrified she would be murdered if he discovered she had a penis. When he attempted to put his hand down her pants, she tricked him into leaving by promising him sex later. In the aftermath of this traumatic experience, Ms. Z found herself battling conflicting feelings of anger and aggression mixed with guilt, wariness, and mistrust. This incident exacerbated her experience of conflicted, opposing emotions in relation to her girlfriend. For example, she sometimes described their relationship in an idealized way, but at other times indicated that she felt trampled upon and unable to say no to her girlfriend's wishes.

An important part of the treatment was to understand the intersections between Ms. Z's gender identity and the meanings of her trauma. It became clear that she viewed anger as being a dangerous, distinctly "male" emotion that she should not have. The therapist drew attention to how Ms. Z imagined that her girlfriend would be extremely hurt if Ms. Z were ever to disagree or be angry with her. Ms. Z had reported the attempted rape to the police, who purportedly did not take it seriously, even going so far as to suggest that because she had a more stereotypically "masculine" build, she should have been able to fend off her assailant. This remark reinforced Ms. Z's preexisting sense that anger was incompatible with her identity. In fact, it seemed that in Ms. Z's mind, the act of feeling or expressing anger would somehow symbolically "undo" her transition, "revealing" her as male. The therapist also observed that the alternative response of abnegating her aggression, even if it made Ms. Z feel more "feminine," led to her feeling walked upon and anxiously vigilant about her presentation in her daily life. This work helped Ms. Z to name and resolve her conflictual fantasy that she should have been capable of fighting off her rapist, while facilitating her acceptance of her aggressive wishes, reducing her feelings of guilt and blame.

* * *

This vignette shows the interactions among symptoms, experiences of life, and underlying personality structure. By the latter, we refer to the degree to which psychological forces, especially affects of a loving/affiliative nature and affects of an assertive/aggressive nature, have been integrated into a complex, interrelated fabric, in contrast to a situation in which an aspect of psychological life remains at odds with a person's experience of themselves. In this case, Ms. Z was not comfortable with aggressive feelings. Multiple factors could converge to result in her uneasiness in relation to this part of her emotional world, including 1) the internalization of a stereotyped view that assertiveness/aggression cannot be acceptable in a woman and 2) the likely association in her mind of aggression with traumatizing figures. The resulting rejection of any assertiveness/aggression in her subjective experience limited Ms. Z's range of emotional and interpersonal effectiveness and depth. By helping Ms. Z see that aggressive feelings are not necessarily associated with abusive behavior, her therapy helped Ms. Z broaden her range of emotional experience and interpersonal relatedness. This vignette illustrates that the specific experiences of a transgender patient, or of any other sexual minority patient, may ultimately connect with the universal issues of possible psychological conflict around internal emotional states.

Takeaway Points for Vignette 4

- LGBT individuals are at higher risk of exposure to major traumas, including child abuse and rape.
- Transgender individuals may deal not only with stigma regarding their transgender identity, but also with stereotypes and ideals about their transitioned gender.

Vignette 5: Adolescent Nonbinary Gender Identity, Anxiety, and Developmental Conflict (Learning Goals 1, 2, 3, and 4)

Ken, a 15-year-old Asian American high school student assigned male at birth, had been experiencing a sad, fearful mood, a drop in grades, and school avoidance following initiation of mandatory physical education. Previously uncomfortable in rough-and-tumble play, preferring female friends, and frequently teased, Ken had confided a nonbinary gender identity to their mother. The school avoidance triggered family conflict, with the mother supporting home schooling and the father insisting that Ken face their fears and return to school.

The school referred Ken to a mental health care program, where they began treatment with a trainee in supervision. Forging an alliance around Ken's goals of overcoming fear and restoring academic functioning, the therapist used cognitive-behavioral techniques such as graded exposure to anxiety-provoking imagery and stimuli, evidence-testing, and reframing of anxiogenic cognitions. Ken responded well.

The clinical alliance deepened, and Ken displayed increasing curiosity about the psychological underpinnings of their anxiety. The therapist and the patient began to explore associations and dreams psychodynamically. Conflicts over adolescent separation and individuation emerged, including regressive dependency wishes, idealization of the maternal relationship, and projection of hostility onto others, and interfered with the patient's ability to accurately assess social situations and cope with real transphobia. Ken responded to clarification and interpretation with insight and relief, admixed with moments of regression when under stress. During those times, Ken would appear more anxious and dependent, and the psychotherapist would appear less engaged in treatment and supervision.

The supervisor noticed these changes in the supervisee, which suggested an apparent loss of confidence in his own ability—and, although reticent to acknowledge it, loss of faith in the supervisor's ability—to empathize with Ken and understand culturally salient issues. The supervisor clarified a parallel process in the supervision, involving regressed, guilty, and passive-aggressive defenses that the patient was manifesting.

This intervention freed the therapist to address the maladaptive psychological defenses of the patient, who subsequently declared a nonbinary gender identity and a new name—"Kit"—to peers. Kit recovered their premorbid functioning, with a return to excellent school performance, enhanced social skills, and new friendships, and is now free of clinically significant anxiety or school phobia.

Takeaway Points for Vignette 5

- Gender expression and gender identity (i.e., gender experience) are unique developmental domains.
- People with noncisgender identities experience the same range of psychological problems and mental health conditions as the general population.

- Psychotherapy with LGBT patients requires a comprehensive case formulation that encompasses social and emotional development, sexual and gender development, empirical diagnosis, and cultural competence.
- A psychodynamic formulation includes awareness of defense mechanisms that could potentially affect social competence and achievement of developmental milestones. However, transgender and gender-nonbinary identity is not associated with any specific psychodynamic profile.

Conclusion

The reasons for which patients seek psychotherapy are as varied among LGBT populations as they are among the general population. Consequently, LGBT patients may benefit from the same range of psychotherapeutic treatments (with the same requirements for supervision) as those used with other patient populations. Furthermore, LGBT people often have additional needs relating to their unique developmental and interpersonal experiences. These experiences include feeling different, being exposed to stigmatization, wrestling with the dilemma of whether to come out, and dealing with other unique stressors that can affect self-esteem. For these patients, their LGBT status may either be an explicit focus of treatment or be entirely incidental to their chief complaint. Regardless of a patient's reason for seeking therapy, the same psychotherapies applicable to all patients, when appropriately adapted to the unique needs of the individual, can be equally helpful to LGBT patients. Both trainee psychotherapists and their supervisors can benefit from bearing in mind the unique developmental experiences of LGBT people in domains of sexual orientation, gender identity, and gender expression. By remaining mindful of these unique experiences, which result in unique needs, therapists and supervisors can adapt their techniques accordingly, monitor their influence on the psychotherapeutic countertransference and supervisory relationship, and enhance the quality of psychotherapeutic care provided to LGBT individuals.

References

Adelson SL; American Academy of Child and Adolescent Psychiatry (AACAP) Committee on Quality Issues (CQI): Practice parameter on gay, lesbian, or bisexual sexual orientation, gender nonconformity, and gender discordance in children and adolescents. J Am Acad Child Adolesc Psychiatry 51(9):957–974, 2012 22917211

American Psychiatric Association: Diagnostic and Statistical Manual of Mental Disorders, 3rd Edition. Washington, DC, American Psychiatric Association, 1980

American Psychiatric Association: Diagnostic and Statistical Manual of Mental Disorders, 4th Edition. Washington, DC, American Psychiatric Association, 1994

American Psychiatric Association: Diagnostic and Statistical Manual of Mental Disorders, 5th Edition. Arlington, VA, American Psychiatric Publishing, 2013

Baams L, Kiekens WJ, Fish JN: The rejection sensitivity model: sexual minority adolescents in context. Arch Sex Behav 49(7):2259–2263, 2020 31664554

Bailey JM: The minority stress model deserves reconsideration, not just extension. Arch Sex Behav 49(7):2265–2268, 2020 31853696

Bailey JM, Zucker KJ: Childhood sex-typed behavior and sexual orientation: a conceptual analysis and quantitative review. Developmental Psychology 31(1):43–55, 1995

Bayer R.: Homosexuality and American Psychiatry. New York, Basic Books, 1981

Busch FN, Milrod BL, Singer MB, Aronson AC: Manual of Panic Focused Psychodynamic Psychotherapy—eXtended Range (Psychoanalytic Inquiry Book Series, Vol 36). New York, Routledge, 2012

Cabaj RP: Working With LGBTQ Patients. Washington, DC, American Psychiatric Association, n.d. Available at: https://psychiatry.org/psychiatrists/cultural-competency/education/best-practice-highlights/working-with-lgbtq-patients. Accessed August 30, 2021.

Drescher J, D'Ercole A, Schoenberg E: Psychotherapy With Gay Men and Lesbians: Contemporary Dynamic Approaches. New York, Harrington Park Press, 2003

Drescher J, Schwartz A, Casoy F, et al: The growing regulation of conversion therapy. J Med Regul 102(2):7–12, 2016 27754500

Friedman RC, Downey JI: Sexual Orientation and Psychoanalysis: Sexual Science and Clinical Practice. New York, Columbia University Press, 2002

Hines M: Brain Gender. Oxford, UK, Oxford University Press, 2004

Institute of Medicine, Committee on Lesbian, Gay, Bisexual, and Transgender Health Issues and Research Gaps and Opportunities: The Health of Lesbian, Gay, Bisexual, and Transgender People: Building a Foundation for Better Understanding. Washington, DC, National Academies Press, 2011

McEwen BS, Gray JD, Nasca C: 60 years of neuroendocrinology: redefining neuroendocrinology: stress, sex and cognitive and emotional regulation. J Endocrinol 226(2):T67–T83, 2015 25934706

Meyer IH, Frost DM: Minority stress and the health of sexual minorities, in Handbook of Psychology and Sexual Orientation. Edited by Patterson CJ, Augelli AR. New York, Oxford University Press, 2013, pp 252–266

Pachankis JE: The scientific pursuit of sexual and gender minority mental health treatments: toward evidence-based affirmative practice. Am Psychol 73(9):1207–1219, 2018 30525805

Pachankis JE, Hatzenbuehler ML, Rendina HJ, et al: LGB-affirmative cognitive-behavioral therapy for young adult gay and bisexual men: a randomized controlled trial of a transdiagnostic minority stress approach. J Consult Clin Psychol 83(5):875–889, 2015 26147563

Pachankis JE, McConocha EM, Reynolds JS, et al: Project ESTEEM protocol: a randomized controlled trial of an LGBTQ-affirmative treatment for young adult sexual minority men's mental and sexual health. BMC Public Health 19(1):1086, 2019 31399071

United Nations Human Rights Council: Practices of so-called "conversion ther-
    apy": Report of the Independent Expert on protection against violence and dis-
    crimination based on sexual orientation and gender identity (A/HRC/44/53).
    01 May 2020. Available at: https://documents-dds-ny.un.org/doc/UNDOC/
    GEN/G20/108/68/PDF/G2010868.pdf?OpenElement. Accessed August 20,
    2022
World Health Organization: International Classification of Diseases, 11th Revi-
    sion. Geneva, World Health Organization, 2019

16

Psychotherapy Supervision for the Treatment of Substance Use Disorders

Kimberly R. Stubbs, M.D.
Yi-lang Tang, M.D., Ph.D.

KEY LEARNING GOALS

- Understand how to help supervisees conceptualize and approach substance use disorders.

- Differentiate among various evidence-based psychotherapeutic strategies for providing comprehensive treatment for substance use disorders.

- Identify the components of supervision that may improve clinical outcomes in patients with substance use disorders.

SUBSTANCE USE and substance use disorders (SUDs) are ubiquitous. In DSM-5 (American Psychiatric Association 2013), SUDs are defined as "a problematic pattern of substance use leading to clinically significant impairment or distress." SUDs affect a person's brain and behavior and may impair the person's ability to control the use of particular substance(s).

Many factors contribute to the onset and continuation of SUDs, including 1) the nature or pharmacological properties of the substance; 2) individual factors such as genetics, personal predispositions, and personality characteristics; and 3) environmental factors such as the availability and accessibility of certain substances, childhood experiences, and social and cultural influences.

The mainstream view of SUDs is that they are diseases of the brain affecting multiple neurobiological circuits, including those involved in reward and motivation, learning and memory, and inhibitory control over behavior. Addiction can be conceptualized as chronic changes in the brain systems that mediate the experience and anticipation of reward, and in higher-order systems that underlie judgment and cognitive control (Volkow et al. 2016). These changes lead to three recurring stages: binge and intoxication, withdrawal and negative affect, and preoccupation and anticipation (or craving). Each stage is associated with the activation of specific neurobiological circuits and consequential clinical and behavioral characteristics (Koob and Volkow 2010). Alternatives to the brain disease model often highlight the social and environmental factors that contribute to addiction, as well as the learning processes that translate these factors into negative outcomes (Heilig et al. 2016). Learning theories based on both classical and operant conditioning principles have a strong influence on the current understanding of SUDs and treatment interventions. These principles help explain why certain stimuli trigger cravings even after an extended period of abstinence (classical conditioning) or how rewards and punishments promote or suppress certain behavior (operant conditioning). Psychodynamic approaches to SUDs are thought to be most effective as part of a comprehensive treatment plan. Substance use behavior is often addressed as a defensive strategy for coping with negative feelings or mood states, such as depression, helplessness, anger, or hostility or as a means of gaining a sense of self-control. The self-medication hypothesis is based on the idea that people engage in substance use behavior not because they seek the euphoric feelings ("high") but rather to relieve negative feelings or change an uncomfortable emotional state (Khantzian 1985, 1997). Although this explanation makes intuitive sense, research data do not yet support this hypothesis (Blume et al. 2000).

When treating a patient with a suspected SUD, therapists should keep the following general considerations in mind:

Intoxication and withdrawal. Patients who present with intoxication or signs of withdrawal will need to be managed in a medical setting to ensure their physical safety. These individuals have a reduced ability to meaningfully engage in therapeutic interventions. Supervisors can remind supervisees to watch patients for symptoms of intoxication or withdrawal.

Resistance and relapse. Supervisors can help trainees manage the characteristic challenges associated with lack of motivation, denial, and resistance to change by providing appropriate patient education, confronting patients' denial, and attending to their own negative countertransference. Supervisors can encourage trainees to

- Conceptualize "resistance" as a challenge to the therapeutic process rather than as a patient characteristic.
- Foster an empathic environment in which any "lapse" or "relapse" can be openly discussed within the therapy session rather than mislabeled as a treatment failure.
- Re-evaluate treatment goals, motivation, and progress toward change as the patient fluctuates between different stages of change (Prochaska and Prochaska 2020) during treatment.
- Consider using other treatment supports such as self-help groups and/or medication to promote better outcomes.
- Watch for and address expected frustration that follows chronic or recurrent relapses in the patient.

Harm reduction versus abstinence approach to treatment. Supervisors can help prepare supervisees to discuss the differences between abstinence and harm reduction approaches. In abstinence-based treatment, patients are expected to abstain completely from all substances of abuse (nicotine often not included). Patients who do not commit to abstinence may easily escalate their substance use or develop an addiction to another substance. Harm reduction focuses on reducing the negative consequences of SUDs. This approach recognizes that abstinence may not be realistic for all patients, and that any change that reduces the harm associated with substance use can be valuable (Tatarsky 2003). In recent years, the evidence base supporting harm reduction approaches has grown (Klein 2020).

Family involvement. The relationships between patients' families and patients' SUDs are complex and often bidirectional. Familial factors (e.g., genetics, childhood maltreatment, parental substance use, parenting styles) can influence risk of SUDs while having a family member with an SUD often negatively impacts family structures and functions. Supervisors can help supervisees consider whether family involvement in treatment might enhance patient outcomes.

Monitoring of adherence and the role of urine drug screens. One of the hallmark behaviors of patients with an SUD is dishonesty about their substance-using behavior. Drug testing may play an important role in SUD diagnosis and treatment (Jarvis et al. 2017). Urine drug screens serve as a valuable tool for documenting progress, identifying the use of unprescribed or unreported substances, detecting adherence to pre-scribed medications, assisting clinical assessment, and guiding treatment planning. Supervisors should discuss with supervisees the risks and benefits of repeated drug testing and how to manage the implied lack of trust.

Co-occurring personality disorders and PTSD. The co-occurrence of personality disorders and SUDs seems to involve shared vulnerabilities and risk factors. These common genetic and sociocultural factors are particularly applicable to interactions between addiction and antiso-cial personality disorder and borderline personality disorder. Comorbidity between SUDs and PTSD is equally common. A growing body of research data supports the efficacy of integrating the treatment of SUDs with that of PTSD (Berenz and Coffey 2012). Supervisors can help supervisees look for these common comorbid conditions and con-sider modifying treatment to address them.

A major principle guiding the treatment of SUDs is that interventions must be individualized. This means considering what level of treatment is required for a particular patient. Options for treatment include routine or specialized outpatient treatment, intensive outpatient programs, partial hospitalization, residential treatment, or medical/psychiatric inpatient care. For all patients with SUDs, the treatment plan should address any associated medical, psychological, social, vocational, and legal problems. Because an in-depth discussion of the American Society of Addiction Medicine (ASAM) guidelines for determining the appropriate level of care is beyond the scope of this chapter, we will limit our focus to patients re-ceiving psychotherapy for a general psychiatric condition who have been identified as also having an SUD.

Supervision of Evidence-Based Treatment Modalities

Once a potential SUD has been discovered in a supervisee's therapy pa-tient, the supervisor can initiate a discussion addressing the following questions: 1) Does the patient need referral to a specialized addiction pro-gram? 2) If the patient is remaining in therapy, which evidence-based ap-proach(es) should be used? Supervisors can help supervisees select the most appropriate treatment approach.

- *Motivational interviewing* (MI) or *motivational enhancement therapy* (MET) is best suited for patients who are ambivalent about changing their substance use behavior or who focus on the negative consequences of change. In cases where the patient is truly committed to change, other approaches may be more appropriate and beneficial.
- *Cognitive-behavioral therapy (CBT) for SUD* is best suited for patients who are ready to make active changes. This "harm reduction" approach allows therapists to work incrementally with patients toward their self-selected goals, thereby promoting autonomy.
- *Contingency management* (CM) is most useful in the treatment of cocaine or methamphetamine use disorder. CM can also be incorporated into other psychosocial treatments such as group counseling and/or CBT.
- *Twelve-step facilitation* (TSF) assists patients who are considering participation in 12-step-based programs such as Alcoholics Anonymous (AA). The ideal candidates for TSF have a pre-existing interest or experience in the 12-step approach. TSF seems less effective in patients who have acute or serious comorbid medical or psychiatric illness, who have extreme opioid and/or cocaine use disorders, who are unemployed, and/or who have no family support.

In the subsections that follow, we demonstrate ways that supervisors and supervisees can incorporate these approaches into psychotherapy.

Motivational Interviewing or Motivational Enhancement Therapy

Motivational interviewing is an effective modality for fostering a patient's intrinsic motivation for changing a variety of behaviors, including alcohol use disorder and illicit drug use (Lundahl et al. 2010).

Vignette 1

> Mr. K is a 35-year-old man being treated with psychotherapy for generalized anxiety disorder. Mr. K discloses that he received a driving while intoxicated (DWI) charge. He is embarrassed about this charge and is concerned that it may negatively affect his employment. Additionally, Mr. K mentions his wife's concerns about his alcohol use. He feels that his wife's attention to his alcohol use is unwarranted. He has no intention of discontinuing or decreasing his alcohol use. The supervisor and the supervisee decide to use MI/MET techniques to explore Mr. K's perspectives on his alcohol use.

The supervisor can help build the trainee's skills in use of MI techniques, which include 1) asking permission before offering advice, 2) making affirmations, and 3) emphasizing the patient's autonomy. The supervisor can ask about the trainee's interventions—for example, "Before providing psychoeducation on the effects of alcohol, how did you ask for the patient's permission?" When discussing how to provide genuine affirmations, supervisors can help supervisees reflect on aspects of their patients that they appreciate. Emphasizing patient autonomy in the MI/MET format involves exploring options for change as well as the option of sustaining current SUD behavior. The mnemonic OARS can be used to remember the following clinical skills: Open-ended questions, Affirmations, Reflections, and Summaries.

Patients who are in the *precontemplation stage* (Prochaska and Prochaska 2020) are not considering change. Creating ambivalence about change brings them one step closer to actual change. Supervision at this stage involves guiding the trainee to adopt an empathic stance and minimize confrontations about the patient's resistance to change or "denial." One strategy in the precontemplation stage is to respond to patients with more reflections than questions in order to elicit the patient's underlying thoughts and beliefs.

The *contemplation stage* is characterized by patient ambivalence and resistance to change. The supervisor may provide guidance by discussing ways in which resistance may appear in the context of therapy and strategies for "rolling with resistance." In this stage of therapy, the supervisee's goal is to elicit the patient's reasons for maintaining the status quo while developing rationales in favor of change.

Vignette 1 (continued)

Mr. K: Well, to be honest, I really think my wife is blowing my alcohol use out of proportion. I don't drink any more than my friends do, and I report to work every day and take care of the family financially. I don't know why she is so hard on me about drinking.

Supervisee: Has anyone else expressed a concern about your drinking?

Mr. K: My primary care provider mentioned that some of my liver tests were abnormal, but that only happened once, and when he rechecked the labs, they were normal again. I think it was after the holidays, and the abnormal labs were just a fluke. I haven't had a problem since.

Supervisee: It sounds like you feel that your doctor's and wife's concern about your alcohol use is unsubstantiated.

Mr. K: Yeah, and alcohol helps me relax. It helps my anxiety, and I'm not giving that up.

Based on the information provided, Mr. K is likely in the precontemplation stage. During this stage, the supervisor notes that empathically engaging the patient in considering change is essential. Supervisors may want to emphasize the difference between *engaging* the patient and attempting to "convince" the patient or provide "advice." Supervisors may challenge supervisees to think of some open-ended questions that might engage the patient in a conversation about change.

Study evidence suggests that MI sessions preceding another treatment may enhance treatment retention, behavioral change, and outcomes (Bien et al. 1993; Burke et al. 2003; Hettema et al. 2005). If a supervisee identifies a patient as being in the preparation or action stage of change, the therapy could transition to a more action-oriented modality, such as CBT.

Cognitive-Behavioral Therapy

Vignette 2

> Ms. M is a 22-year-old graduate student who presents to the university counseling center because of "binge drinking" that has resulted in blackouts and hospitalizations. Ms. M has made previous attempts to moderate her alcohol consumption, and her longest sobriety period was 4 months. In addition to alcohol use, Ms. M reports occasional use of marijuana and cocaine. Ms. M's last alcohol use was approximately 72 hours prior to the current outpatient evaluation. After establishing the patient's safety, the therapist begins an in-depth analysis of the patient's substance use behavior and its impact.

Substantial scientific evidence supports the efficacy of CBT-based approaches for the treatment of SUDs. CBT theories emphasize how an individual's environment, temperament, and learning processes influence their SUD behavior and rely on the concept of reinforcement. Guiding supervisees through a CBT approach provides the opportunity for reviewing important principles such as classical conditioning, operant conditioning, and modeling, and may include reflecting on the pharmacological and social reinforcements that influence early substance use. Reviewing these psychological principles will help the trainee focus therapy on identifying and modifying cognitive distortions and reinforcing adaptive behaviors. An important theme that emerges when supervising a CBT case is that person–environment interactions influence initiation, maintenance, and change of SUD behavior. Supervision is best focused on CBT techniques that may alter the person–environment interaction as a way of changing behavior.

Encouraging an immediate change in the patient's substance use is a good starting point for the trainee therapist. It is difficult to foster the development of insight and problem-solving skills without an initial reduction in substance use. After a period of abstinence or reduced substance use, the focus can shift to maintaining the changes. The supervisor can lead a "functional analysis" of the environmental and person-specific factors that influence the patient's substance use. This analysis, a core component of the CBT treatment model, involves investigating skill deficits, emotional states, and environments that may "trigger" or reinforce a patient's substance use. The supervisor assists the supervisee in using the functional analysis to gauge progress and identify persistent behaviors.

Next, the supervisor helps the supervisee develop techniques and strategies to change the factors associated with substance use. Skills training and relapse prevention techniques help the patient develop strategies for coping with future high-risk situations. Concomitant concerns, such as relationship difficulties or psychiatric comorbidities, may also be addressed, although the primary focus should be on changes related to the substance use. Supervisors may need to help supervisees refocus the treatment if they find that the attention frequently shifts to non-substance-use content.

Vignette 2 (continued)

Ms. M: I've been to a couple of AA meetings in the past, but I didn't get much out of them. It just wasn't for me. I don't think I want to give up alcohol completely. Alcohol is such a big part of my social life. I just want to moderate my drinking.

SUPERVISEE: Do you mind telling me more about the connection between alcohol and your social life?

Ms. M: I'm in a very stressful graduate program, and my classmates and I like to get together and celebrate after academic milestones. It's the way I de-stress and connect with my peers. I have quite a bit of social anxiety, and alcohol really helps me loosen up.

SUPERVISEE: I am hearing you say that there are some social and emotional benefits that are connected to your alcohol use. Perhaps we can explore those further, along with some of the disadvantages of your alcohol use.

An early supervision target in a CBT treatment is solidifying the collaboratively selected short-term and long-term goals. Greater commitment from the patient to a specific goal increases the likelihood of reaching it. The use of worksheets may be helpful when there is ambivalence about change, and supervisors can encourage supervisees to help patients identify the advantages and disadvantages of continuing substance use versus becoming abstinent. The supervisor may also discuss strategies for challenging patient thoughts and beliefs about alcohol use (e.g., developing alternative activities to cope with negative emotions and improve relaxation).

Contingency Management

Vignette 3

> Ms. N, a 44-year-old woman with stimulant use disorder (cocaine), returns to her therapist after discharge from an intensive outpatient program (IOP) for substance use. As part of the patient re-intake evaluation, the supervisee notes that although Ms. N has participated in rehabilitation programs—including residential treatment for stimulant use disorder—in the past, she has left programs prematurely. Ms. N's last treatment was a short stay in a residential program, which she left against medical advice (AMA) after 14 days. The supervisor works with the supervisee to develop a treatment plan for Ms. N.

CM is based on the principles of operant conditioning, which posits that all behaviors can be shaped or changed when the appropriate rewards and negative consequences are either provided or withheld. CM is rooted in the following assumptions:

1. Behaviors are shaped by their consequences; behaviors will be more likely to occur when they are positively reinforced and will be less likely to occur when they are disincentivized or punished.
2. Substance use is an operant behavior that is motivated and maintained by the biologically reinforcing effects of drugs, which include euphoric subjective effects and/or relief from withdrawal symptoms.
3. Substance use can be modified by manipulating environmental factors, such as peer pressure.
4. Enhancing the positive consequences of substance abstinence by providing alternative sources of reinforcement will result in a decrease in substance use.

How does CM work? Patients receive a reward for meeting a preset treatment goal or receive a negative consequence if they do not meet the mutually agreed-upon goal. In CM, SUD patients receive incentives (often in the form of cash, a voucher, or another prize) that are contingent upon their treatment attendance and/or verified negative drug testing results. This differs from the life experience of SUD patients, in which rewards for abstinence are often unpredictable, intangible, or remote (e.g., employment, relationship, financial situation). CM creates an environment in which drug/alcohol abstinence or another desired behavior is met with more predictable, more tangible, more salient, and more immediate rewards (reinforcers). The ideal treatment goal is that patients will continue the desired behavior (such as abstinence) even after the CM program ends.

Supervisors can help supervisees implement CM treatment by helping them to

1. Identify the target behavior.
2. Choose an appropriate reinforcer.
3. Reduce the time period between the target behavior and the delivery of the reward or consequence. Shorter delays between target behavior and incentive delivery are associated with improved efficacy.
4. Develop a plan to effectively monitor the accurate and systematic delivery of consequences.

CM is one of the most effective treatment approaches for directly addressing SUDs, especially stimulant use disorders (Bentzley et al. 2021). CM also has strong empirical support as an adjunctive intervention to improve treatment attendance in other psychosocial treatments (e.g., group treatment) and to improve medication adherence.

Vignette 3 (continued)

After discussion with his supervisor, the supervisee and Ms. N agree on a voucher-based CM approach and begin discussing its implementation.

> Ms. N: I can agree that cocaine use has caused me a lot of problems. But I smoke marijuana occasionally as well, and that's never been a problem for me. It helps me to sleep mostly. Is marijuana use going to affect my vouchers?
>
> Supervisee: That's an excellent question. We've spent some time discussing some of the negative consequences that you've experienced related to your cocaine use. Perhaps we can discuss some of the pros and cons of making a change with your marijuana use. Do you have any reasons for not changing at this time?

As this vignette demonstrates, polysubstance use is common, and supervisors may need to work with supervisees to identify sequential strategies that require progressively more difficult abstinence goals. Supervisors should ensure that supervisees understand the basic CM concepts of positive reinforcement, negative reinforcement, positive punishment, and negative punishment as well as their effects on a target behavior. Some evidence suggests that voucher programs can improve abstinence rates when combined with MET or CBT (Budney et al. 2000, 2006). Supervisors can encourage supervisees to conduct regular reassessments of patient progress and incorporate other evidence-based therapeutic modalities into the treatment as needed.

Twelve-Step Facilitation

Vignette 4

> Mr. X is a 62-year-old man with alcohol use disorder and major depressive disorder who currently receives medication and psychotherapy. The supervisor and the trainee discuss the advantages of Mr. X attending AA meetings. Mr. X has avoided AA because of deep feelings of shame and guilt surrounding his alcohol use. Mr. X does not have any close family or friends. His feelings of isolation and loneliness have been identified as "triggers" for continued alcohol use.

TSF treatments are a set of semistructured therapies designed to help people abstain from substance use by encouraging their active participation in AA or another 12-step mutual-help programs. Basic assumptions behind TSF include the following: 1) SUD is a multifaceted illness influenced by medical, social, emotional, and spiritual factors; 2) abstinence is the best way to address the problem; 3) emotional and spiritual growth is a critical recovery process; 4) participation in a mutual-help group will assist patients in achieving and sustaining recovery; and 5) because patients often have barriers to participating in 12-step groups, directly addressing these obstacles can facilitate participation and recovery.

Although there are several types of TSF interventions, they all emphasize patient engagement and participation in 12-step groups. The assumption is that participation leads to better outcomes (Nowinski and Baker 2017). A recent comprehensive meta-analysis of 27 published studies showed that AA/TSF interventions have benefits similar to those of other treatments (i.e., MET, CBT) on all drinking-related outcome measures; this study also found AA/TSF to be superior to CBT in maintaining continuous abstinence and remission (Kelly et al. 2020).

In TSF, therapists help patients accept the nature of the diagnosis of alcohol use disorder and help them commit to a 12-step program. Therapists work with patients collaboratively to track their attendance and other related activities (e.g., finding a sponsor, working the steps, acceptance of psychotropic medications). TSF also focuses on discussing common themes in 12-step literature and meetings, such as spirituality, the concept of a higher power, and the meaning of surrender.

Supervisors can help supervisees work with concepts unique to TSF, such as spirituality and the problem of powerlessness. A discussion during supervision might address the issue of religiosity versus spirituality. Supervisees may encounter patient resistance to the TSF approach from the misconception that a 12-step-oriented treatment is a religious program. In fact, the idea that there is a "power greater than the self" may be redefined as becoming more open to outside help. Supervisees may also have difficulty conceptualizing the core concept of powerlessness. Supervisors can review the nonmodifiable genetic and biological factors that influence addiction, and emphasize that while patients may lack power over a substance, they can take responsibility for addictive behaviors and make better choices to promote their own recovery.

Conclusion

Despite the wide range of therapies and techniques used to address SUDs, most of these modalities share certain fundamental principles. For patients to become active participants in therapy, therapists must address patient ambivalence and resistance. Growing evidence points away from the utility of confrontation and toward the benefits of bolstering the patient's own motivational resources. Supervisors play a key role in illuminating how trainees' implicit biases or countertransference can affect treatment. The importance of empathy and a positive therapeutic relationship cannot be overstated. Supervisors can encourage unconditional positive regard, empathy, and genuineness as necessary conditions for positive change (Rogers 1957). Therapeutic interventions may directly address substance use or may focus on helping patients to recognize high-risk situations, thoughts, and emotions. Many behavioral approaches encourage identifying the contingency or relationship between substance use and a reinforcer. A focus on building and maintaining positive social supports is central to 12-step approaches and may also be useful as an adjunct to other treatment modalities. Collaborative and comprehensive treatment is essential to address the medical and psychiatric comorbidities that often complicate SUD treatment. Supervisors and supervisees may need to learn more about these evidence-based treatments of SUDs.

Additional Resources

Galanter M, Kleber HD: Psychotherapy for the Treatment of Substance Abuse. Arlington, VA, American Psychiatric Publishing, 2011

Miller WR, Rollnick S: Motivational Interviewing: Helping People Change, 3rd Edition. New York, Guilford, 2012

Velasquez MM, Crouch C, Stephens NS, DiClemente CC: Group Treatment for Substance Abuse: A Stages-of-Change Therapy Manual, 2nd Edition. New York, Guilford, 2016

Walters ST, Rotgers F (eds): Treating Substance Abuse: Theory and Technique, 3rd Edition. New York, Guilford, 2012

References

American Psychiatric Association: Diagnostic and Statistical Manual of Mental Disorders, 5th Edition. Arlington, VA, American Psychiatric Publishing, 2013

Bentzley BS, Han SS, Neuner S, et al: Comparison of treatments for cocaine use disorder among adults: a systematic review and meta-analysis. JAMA Netw Open 4(5):e218049, 2021 33961037

Berenz EC, Coffey SF: Treatment of co-occurring posttraumatic stress disorder and substance use disorders. Curr Psychiatry Rep 14(5):469–477, 2012 22825992

Bien TH, Miller WR, Boroughs JM: Motivational interviewing with alcohol outpatients. Behavioural and Cognitive Psychotherapy 21(4):347–356, 1993

Blume AW, Schmaling KB, Marlatt GA: Revisiting the self-medication hypothesis from a behavioral perspective. Cognitive and Behavioral Practice 7(4):379–384, 2000

Budney AJ, Higgins ST, Radonovich KJ, Novy PL: Adding voucher-based incentives to coping skills and motivational enhancement improves outcomes during treatment for marijuana dependence. J Consult Clin Psychol 68(6):1051–1061, 2000 11142539

Budney AJ, Moore BA, Rocha HL, Higgins ST: Clinical trial of abstinence-based vouchers and cognitive-behavioral therapy for cannabis dependence. J Consult Clin Psychol 74(2):307–316, 2006 16649875

Burke BL, Arkowitz H, Menchola M: The efficacy of motivational interviewing: a meta-analysis of controlled clinical trials. J Consult Clin Psychol 71(5):843–861, 2003 14516234

Heilig M, Epstein DH, Nader MA, Shaham Y: Time to connect: bringing social context into addiction neuroscience. Nat Rev Neurosci 17(9):592–599, 2016 27277868

Hettema J, Steele J, Miller WR: Motivational interviewing. Annu Rev Clin Psychol 1:91–111, 2005 17716083

Jarvis M, Williams J, Hurford M, et al: Appropriate use of drug testing in clinical addiction medicine. J Addict Med 11(3):163–173, 2017 28557958

Kelly JF, Abry A, Ferri M, Humphreys K: Alcoholics Anonymous and 12-step facilitation treatments for alcohol use disorder: a distillation of a 2020 Cochrane Review for clinicians and policy makers. Alcohol Alcohol 55(6):641–651, 2020 32628263

Khantzian EJ: The self-medication hypothesis of addictive disorders: focus on heroin and cocaine dependence. Am J Psychiatry 142(11):1259–1264, 1985 3904487

Khantzian EJ: The self-medication hypothesis of substance use disorders: a reconsideration and recent applications. Harv Rev Psychiatry 4(5):231–244, 1997 9385000

Klein A: Harm reduction works: evidence and inclusion in drug policy and advocacy. Health Care Anal 28(4):404–414, 2020 33079317

Koob GF, Volkow ND: Neurocircuitry of addiction. Neuropsychopharmacology 35(1):217–238, 2010 19710631

Lundahl BW, Kunz C, Brownell C, et al: A meta-analysis of motivational interviewing: twenty-five years of empirical studies. Research on Social Work Practice 20(2):137–160, 2010

Nowinski J, Baker S: Twelve-Step Facilitation Handbook: A Therapeutic Approach to Treatment and Recovery, 2nd Edition. Center City, MN, Hazelden Publishing, 2017

Prochaska JO, Prochaska JM: Enhancing motivation to change, in The ASAM Essentials of Addiction Medicine, 3rd Edition. Edited by Herron AJ, Brennan T, American Society of Addiction Medicine. Philadelphia, Wolters Kluwer Health/Lippincott Williams & Wilkins, 2020, pp 354–459

Rogers CR: The necessary and sufficient conditions of therapeutic personality change. J Consult Psychol 21(2):95–103, 1957 13416422

Tatarsky A: Harm reduction psychotherapy: extending the reach of traditional substance use treatment. J Subst Abuse Treat 25(4):249–256, 2003 14693253

Volkow ND, Koob GF, McLellan AT: Neurobiologic advances from the brain disease model of addiction. N Engl J Med 374(4):363–371, 2016 26816013

17

Supportive Psychotherapy Supervision in the Acute Care Setting

Annabel C. Boeke, M.D.[*]
David Veith, M.D.[*]
Alison E. Lenet, M.D.
Deborah L. Cabaniss, M.D.

KEY LEARNING GOALS

- Understand that supportive psychotherapy and supportive psychotherapy supervision can be provided outside of the traditional outpatient clinic.

- Appreciate the many advantages of supervision of hospital-based psychotherapy: seeing the patient with the trainee, obtaining collateral information on the patient from the hospital team, and offering real-time feedback to trainees on their therapy skills.

- Recognize three common steps of supervision in acute care settings: learning about the patient, setting goals, and working with the patient to take action on these goals.

---

[*]These authors contributed equally to this work.

ALTHOUGH PSYCHOTHERAPY training primarily takes place in outpatient settings, fundamental psychotherapy principles can be readily applied in acute care settings such as the inpatient unit (Rosnick 1987), the consultation-liaison (CL) service (Nash et al. 2009), and the emergency room (ER) (Fauman 1983). In these settings, patients frequently present with acutely compromised psychological functions that are clear targets for supportive interventions, making these clinical environments ideal for supportive psychotherapy supervision.

Acute Care Settings: The Perfect but Underutilized Place to Begin Psychotherapy Supervision

Given the high clinical acuity of patients, rapid turnover of trainees and patients, and competing clinical priorities, acute care services might not seem to be an ideal setting for psychotherapy supervision. However, several features of acute care services make them an advantageous setting for beginning psychotherapy training. Many characteristics of acute care settings lend themselves well to supervising trainees in supportive psychotherapy and may actually provide supervisors with opportunities not available in outpatient settings. For example, supervisors can offer real-time feedback on a trainee's therapeutic skills that can be implemented with the patient the same day. Unlike typical outpatient clinics, acute care settings allow opportunities for trainees and supervisors to examine patients' interactions with others (e.g., staff, other patients) and to observe how they use defense mechanisms in acutely stressful situations. Residents usually rotate on acute care services before moving to outpatient settings, and supportive psychotherapy can be conceptualized as a core skill set that provides the foundation for learning other psychotherapies (Plakun et al. 2009). Additionally, surveys of psychiatry residents have documented that trainees want to learn psychotherapy skills on inpatient units (Lonergan et al. 2020) and in the consultation-liaison setting, where patient acuity makes navigating countertransference of both psychiatric and medical teams a high priority.

Despite this potential, acute care settings are rarely used for psychotherapy education. Blumenshine et al. (2017) found that psychiatry residency program directors expressed interest in using acute care settings for supportive psychotherapy supervision but cited time and supervisor experience as major barriers. Few models exist for teaching psychotherapy in non-outpatient settings (Hunter et al. 2007; Jiménez and Thorkelson

2012; Lonergan et al. 2020; Stein and Jacobo 2013). In addition, there may not be room in an already-crowded curriculum for a formal course on psychotherapy in acute care settings.

However, incorporating supportive psychotherapy supervision into acute care services is less difficult than one might think. Many clinicians who work in these settings use supportive psychotherapy with their patients and can be empowered to teach it to their trainees. The confidence and enthusiasm of supervisors can go a long way toward improving a trainee's understanding of supportive psychotherapy and the valuable role it plays in the treatment of a wide range of patients.

The Supervisory Frame in Acute Care Settings

The supervisory frame in acute care settings is quite different from that in outpatient settings. Supervisors should adapt the supervision to the tempo and resources of the clinical situation. Here are a few guidelines:

- *See the patient with the trainee.* Supervisors should consider whether some degree of direct supervision is feasible. Seeing patients together is an efficient use of time on busy services, and direct observation of trainees' psychotherapy skills is enormously helpful for trainees.
- *Keep sessions short.* Busy services call for efficient supervision. Five to 10 minutes of supervision after a clinical encounter may be just enough. Time constraints require supervisors to be focused and clear. Saying "Let's take a few minutes to discuss the psychotherapeutic goals and techniques" indicates to trainees that this aspect of teaching is in fact psychotherapy supervision.
- *Talk where you can.* Ideally, the setting would be private and free from distractions. However, in acute care settings, the only available space might be a crowded workroom.
- *Set appropriate goals.* Goals for the supervision will depend on the experience and training stage of the supervisee. For example, senior psychiatry residents may benefit from more advanced goals, such as addressing a medical team's countertransference on the CL service or incorporating family members into a therapeutic strategy on an inpatient unit. In contrast, a medical student may want to learn how to conduct a basic assessment of a patient's current mental status and psychological functioning, or basic psychotherapeutic techniques that may be transferable to other specialties and settings.

Three-Step Supportive Psychotherapy Supervision for Inpatient, Consultation-Liaison, and Emergency Room Settings

Clinicians working in acute care settings may find the "3-Step Supportive Psychotherapy Manual" (Cabaniss 2015; included as an appendix to this chapter) helpful for supervision. This manual was designed to focus supervision of supportive psychotherapy in acute care settings and to address barriers of time and supervisor experience. It can also help supervisors understand that much of what they do already is psychotherapy, enabling them to become more aware of their interventions and helping them to more explicitly supervise trainees.

The three steps in this manual are as follows:

1. *Learn about the patient.* In this step, the supervisor helps the trainee to efficiently gather information about the patient's current psychological functioning. This task includes assessing a patient's sense of self, relationships, reality testing, judgment, defense mechanisms, coping skills, and other factors.
2. *Set goals.* The supervisor then helps the trainee to focus on a reasonable psychotherapeutic goal, developed collaboratively with the patient.
3. *Work together to take action on goals.* Finally, the supervisor helps the trainee to forge an alliance with the patient, set a frame, and choose specific supportive techniques to help the patient make progress toward the chosen goal.

Once supervisors are familiar with the 3-Step Manual, they can use it to help focus supervision and treatment in any acute care setting. Although the manual is particularly helpful when all three steps are followed, using any of the steps can be helpful for supervision. In the following subsections, we provide practical examples of supportive psychotherapy supervision in inpatient, CL, and ER settings.

Supportive Psychotherapy Supervision on Inpatient Units

Busy psychiatric inpatient units pose many challenges to psychotherapy education. Trainees often have large caseloads of acutely ill patients. Some patients might be hospitalized involuntarily, a circumstance that could negatively affect the therapeutic alliance. These factors, coupled with rapid patient turnover, might make an inpatient unit seem poorly suited for psychotherapy education (Greenberg and Borus 2014).

However, inpatient units provide unique opportunities for psychotherapy supervision. Supervisors and trainees working in inpatient settings can observe how a patient functions throughout the day to see which defenses are employed in real time (Silver et al. 1983). Inpatient supervisors can also directly observe their trainees interacting with patients and can offer detailed feedback. Finally, psychiatric inpatients are almost inevitably suffering from some level of emotional distress and impairments in functioning (Stein and Jacobo 2013), offering clear psychotherapeutic targets for trainees to address.

Specific Suggestions for Supervisors on Inpatient Units

- *Utilize interprofessional input.* Inpatient supervisors can encourage trainees to use nursing reports and multidisciplinary rounds to develop a broader perspective on patients, how they interact with others, and what defenses they use (e.g., splitting). These perspectives can be harder to elicit during outpatient psychotherapy sessions (Rosnick 1987).
- *Identify countertransference reactions.* Supervisors should be attuned to trainees' countertransference reactions. These reactions may be easier to miss in outpatient settings, where supervisors learn about patients only through the filter of trainees' reports. Supervisors can observe patterns that emerge in trainees as they respond to various situations and patients. This information may allow supervisors to provide valuable feedback and to better anticipate some of the challenges that trainees may face in psychotherapy with future patients.
- *Model use of supportive therapy techniques.* Supervisors can conduct sessions with patients while trainees are present and afterward explicitly point out specific supportive psychotherapy techniques they used during these observed sessions.

Using guidance provided in the 3-Step Manual (Cabaniss 2015; see chapter appendix), supervisors can help trainees identify psychotherapeutic goals for patients soon after they are admitted, implement supportive interventions, observe the in vivo effects of the interventions, and make further adjustments as needed.

Case Vignette: Inpatient Unit

Dr. Stewart, a postgraduate year 1 (PGY-1) psychiatry resident, is presenting the case of his patient, Mr. Ruben, to his psychotherapy supervisor, Dr. Park, an attending psychiatrist on an inpatient unit:

> Mr. Ruben is a 38-year-old man with a history of major depressive disorder who was admitted after a suicide attempt via an overdose

of diphenhydramine. He was at his baseline level of functioning until 8 weeks ago, when he was fired from his "dream job" as a programmer at a prestigious tech company. Since then, he has experienced low mood and difficulty sleeping. He has been isolating himself and has spent most of his time watching TV alone. On the day Mr. Ruben was brought to the ER, his friend had come to his house to look for him because Mr. Ruben hadn't answered his phone in several days. Upon discovering Mr. Ruben passed out next to a suicide note and an empty bottle of diphenhydramine, the friend called an ambulance. When I interviewed him this morning, Mr. Ruben showed psychomotor slowing and was tearful. He was perseverative on the topic of his psychiatric admission being "yet another in a string of failures," and he repeatedly referred to himself as "an unemployed loser." Overall, Mr. Ruben meets criteria for a major depressive episode.

The dialogue below illustrates how Dr. Park (Supervisor) might conduct psychotherapy supervision with Dr. Stewart (Trainee) over the course of the week.

Day 1

Supervisor: Let's think about how we can help Mr. Ruben while he is hospitalized. Along with adjusting his medications, we can use supportive psychotherapy. Given the severity of his symptoms, we may have more than a week to work on specific goals and gauge the effects of our interventions. What do you see as his primary difficulty right now?

Trainee: It seems like he's really down on himself in light of his being let go from his "dream job."

Supervisor: I agree—it sounds like he has significant deficits in self-esteem regulation. Aside from your own interview, was there any information from other sources, like the nursing report, that may point toward additional problems?

Trainee: The nurse working with him reported that Mr. Ruben has spent almost the entire weekend in his room and that he hasn't participated in groups. The only person he's reached out to since he's been here is his mother.

Supervisor: It sounds like he has difficulty reaching out to others when he's in crisis. When you interviewed him, did you notice any particular strengths?

Trainee: Yeah, I did—he's personable and relates well to people. He was apparently excelling at work before being let go. It's interesting—he sees losing his job as a personal failure, but it actually sounds like his entire department was restructured, and he got unlucky.

Supervisor: That's an interesting point. Given what we know about his deficits and strengths, what's a concrete goal for Mr. Ruben over the next few days?

TRAINEE: The thing that stood out to me was his low self-esteem. I could remind him of his recent accomplishments at work and challenge the misconception that he was let go because of his performance.

SUPERVISOR: Great idea. You can have him discuss other times when he felt capable or handled a situation well. It's also important to build a good alliance with him and normalize some of the apprehension he might be feeling about the hospital environment.

Day 4

SUPERVISOR: How are things with Mr. Ruben?

TRAINEE: He's still depressed, but today his affect was a bit brighter. Also, for the first time, he said that losing the job was just bad luck—he even said it was "their loss" for letting him go.

SUPERVISOR: It sounds like his self-appraisal is more in line with his actual abilities, and his self-esteem is improving. Another problem we identified was his tendency to self-isolate when he's in crisis—any thoughts on how we might address this as we approach discharge?

TRAINEE: He's mentioned having many close friends, but it sounds like he didn't let them know how much he was suffering. They clearly care about him—one even made a home visit when he didn't answer his phone!

SUPERVISOR: So, it sounds like the supports are there. What would you suggest?

TRAINEE: I could encourage him to be open with his friends about his feelings and help him practice what he might say to them if he feels depressed again. That way, he could have a plan to reach out if he is in another crisis situation.

SUPERVISOR: Great idea—his interpersonal skills are a strength, and bolstering his support system might help future episodes be less severe. Nice job!

Supportive Psychotherapy Supervision on a Consultation-Liaison Service

Providing psychotherapy on a medical unit involves logistical and clinical challenges. Privacy is often limited by visiting family members, medical staff, or the presence of other patients in shared rooms. Medically hospitalized patients often have a combination of fatigue, delirium, and physical limitations that may interfere with communication. At times, trainees must also help patients navigate issues inherent in the hospital environment, such as conflicts between the patient and the primary team.

Despite these challenges, CL services provide an excellent environment for trainees to learn supportive psychotherapy. Trainees have the opportunity to observe patients during an acutely stressful event—a medical hospitalization—and learn about their coping skills. In some cases, trainees may also be able to directly witness the benefits of their psychotherapeutic interventions in terms of improved medical outcomes (Griffith and Gaby 2005; Rozensky 2006). Furthermore, the additional work of liaising with the treatment team provides trainees with an extra opportunity for using supportive psychotherapy techniques, as well as the possibility of teaching these techniques to others, further consolidating their learning.

Specific Suggestions for Supervisors in the Consultation-Liaison Setting

- *Think outside the box.* Supervisors can help trainees understand the need for a more flexible frame in this setting and can suggest specific strategies to overcome logistical hurdles, such as bringing a chair to the patient's room or seeing patients outside of hours when other teams are making their rounds. Likewise, it may be appropriate to help the patient assume a more comfortable position for the interview or to ask a nurse to administer a dose of pain medication to the patient prior to the therapy visit. Trainees who have recently been immersed in the world of outpatient therapy may initially be uncomfortable adapting the treatment frame in this way (Nash et al. 2009; Solomon et al. 1980).
- *Clarify the trainee's role.* Supervisors can help trainees clarify their role in the patient's care, taking into account both the primary team's experience and the patient's experience of the specific problem that prompted the team to request a psychiatric consultation. When these perceptions are in conflict, the issue can be discussed in supervision. Psychiatry residents who have fresh memories of being the intern on an internal medicine team, for example, may feel a conflict between the goals of the primary team and the goals of the patient. Framing the objective of CL psychotherapy as an effort to help the patient adapt to the stress of illness and hospitalization will help residents to navigate this conflict (Hunter et al. 2007; Perry and Viederman 1981; Teitelbaum 1985–1986).
- *Involve the medical/surgical team.* Members of the medical team, including nurses, nursing aides, and physical therapists, can provide valuable information on the patient's functioning. When appropriate, supervisors can encourage trainees to involve other staff in working toward the patient's therapy goals. For example, trainees can enlist the help of nurses, occupational therapists, speech therapists, and other care providers in creating a daily schedule for a depressed patient who

is struggling with behavioral activation during a prolonged hospitalization.

Using the three-step approach (Cabaniss 2015; see chapter appendix), supervisors can implement supportive psychotherapy techniques to assist trainees in the direct care of the patient, as well as to navigate interpersonal dynamics with medical teams. Goals can be adjusted on the basis of patient factors (e.g., length of hospitalization, comfort level, illness prognosis).

Case Vignette: Consultation-Liaison Service

Dr. Gupta, a PGY-2 psychiatry resident, is presenting the case of his patient, Mr. Connolly, to his psychotherapy supervisor, Dr. Klein, an attending psychiatrist on a CL service:

> Mr. Connolly is a 58-year-old man with a medical history of idiopathic pulmonary fibrosis and no psychiatric history. He was hospitalized for a unilateral lung transplant 2 months ago and has experienced numerous complications since then. Psychiatry was consulted for suicidal ideation after Mr. Connolly told the transplant team resident that he'd "rather kill [him]self than spend one more day in this damn hospital." The team expressed frustration that the patient was "not engaged" with components of his treatment, including physical therapy. When I talked to Mr. Connolly, he reported feeling hopeless and overwhelmed about being in the hospital for so long. He denied any suicidal ideation, and explained that he made that statement out of frustration after he'd waited for hours to receive his pain medication. I think that he meets criteria for an adjustment disorder with depressed mood.

The dialogue below illustrates how Dr. Klein (SUPERVISOR) might conduct psychotherapy supervision with Dr. Gupta (TRAINEE) over the next few days.

Day 1

> SUPERVISOR: Mr. Connolly sounds like someone who could benefit from bedside supportive psychotherapy. What do you think?
>
> TRAINEE: Maybe, but I'm not sure how that would work practically. It's hard to imagine doing real therapy in the hospital.
>
> SUPERVISOR: You don't actually need an office to do therapy—all you need is a patient, a therapist, a frame, and a shared goal of improving the patient's mental health. The first step is learning about the patient. What do you think is the most challenging aspect of this situation for Mr. Connolly?

TRAINEE: I think it's hard for him to be so dependent on other people in the hospital. He was the chief of his fire station—he described himself as "Mr. Fix-It" to me. I saw the end of his physical therapy session yesterday, and he can't even walk on his own right now.

SUPERVISOR: It sounds like Mr. Connolly's job was important to his sense of self. It would be helpful to learn more about other aspects of his identity and psychological functioning.

TRAINEE: Well, he seems proud of his children, but says he never was able to spend enough time with them. In terms of his defense mechanisms, it sounds like he generally relies heavily on isolation of affect and sublimation. He said that when he lost a member of his crew to a bad fire a few years ago he dealt with it by "buckling down and working twice as hard." That's part of what makes this situation difficult for him—he can't use work to deal with his feelings now.

SUPERVISOR: I would try to figure out other strategies he's used to handle stressful situations in the past; that may help the two of you understand how he can navigate his challenges now. Once you've had a chance to learn more about him, you should try to establish one or two specific goals to work on together.

Day 2

SUPERVISOR: How did it go with Mr. Connolly yesterday?

TRAINEE: It was hard to get started; we got interrupted by consultants twice. At one point, I even had to hoist him up and readjust his pillow! I probably shouldn't have done that—some of my outpatient supervisors have told me that even a handshake with a patient is too much. But he just looked so uncomfortable sliding down the bed.

SUPERVISOR: It's great that you noticed that—making sure the patient is physically comfortable at the start of the session helps establish an alliance and minimizes distractions. Sometimes in CL psychiatry, we have to be more flexible with the frame, although there are still things you can do to establish it, such as scheduling your visits in advance for less busy times of day.

TRAINEE: Other than the interruptions, I think it went OK. He said that the way he expressed his frustration was a bit extreme, but he's tired of feeling like a "useless lump" in the hospital, and he wanted the team to understand where he's coming from.

SUPERVISOR: Terrific. He wants to feel understood by his team, and maybe wants to regain his sense of self, despite being a patient. How would you work on those goals with him?

TRAINEE: It might help to discuss connecting with other aspects of his identity while he's here. For example, he said that when

> his wife left him, listening to music helped him get through. When I suggested he spend some time compiling his favorite songs to share with his daughter, his eyes lit up.
>
> SUPERVISOR: Great idea. I might also consider some joint problem solving or role-play for specific situations in the hospital, like if he is in pain or if he feels his team is not understanding him. Better communication with the team might help him regain some of the sense of control he has lost.

Supportive Psychotherapy Supervision in the Psychiatric Emergency Room

Clinical work in the emergency setting is fast-paced and busy, and psychotherapy may not be seen as a priority. Trainees commonly evaluate patients and either discharge or admit them within the same day, which limits their clinical contact to one or two interactions. The physical environment of the ER can also be challenging, with little privacy, noises from monitors and other patients, and a wide variety of presentations and acuity in the patient population. Because patients may be acutely intoxicated or agitated, the safety of the trainee needs to be prioritized.

In addition to the inherent challenges of ER work, there are challenges to the frame of the supervision itself. With increases in shift work, a supervisor may have only one shared shift with a trainee, which can make it more difficult to observe the trainee over multiple interactions with various patients and develop rapport within the supervision.

Despite the many challenges involved in conducting and supervising psychotherapy in the ER, there is also an opportunity to discuss the potential benefits of brief psychotherapeutic interventions such as safety planning (Stanley and Brown 2012) and to make explicit what the trainee is already doing that is consistent with supportive psychotherapy.

Specific Suggestions for Supervisors in the Psychiatric Emergency Room Setting

- *Think about safety.* Supervisors can discuss safety concerns and how these concerns might affect where and how trainees conduct their interview(s) with patients.
- *Be efficient.* Supervisors should be mindful of time constraints and streamline their supervision sessions with trainees, limiting the focus to one or two teaching goals per session. They may ask trainees whether there are specific topics they would like to learn more about, such as evaluating patients, thinking of appropriate goals with them, or using specific supportive psychotherapy techniques. Supervisors can incor-

porate psychotherapy supervision into discussions of other aspects of the patient's care, so that trainees can save time and understand how the psychotherapy fits into a patient's overall medication management and disposition planning.

Using the 3-Step Manual (Cabaniss 2015; see chapter appendix), supervisors can work with supervisees to quickly identify and incorporate an appropriate psychotherapy goal into the patient's care.

Case Vignette: Psychiatric Emergency Room

Dr. Allen, a PGY-3 psychiatry resident, is presenting the case of his patient, Ms. Zhou, to his psychotherapy supervisor, Dr. Cruz, during the overnight shift in the Psychiatric ER:

> Ms. Zhou, a 27-year-old student with bipolar I disorder, was brought to the ER by her sister because of increasingly erratic behavior. Ms. Zhou is in the process of finishing her thesis and forgot to pick up her lithium refill last week. The sister notes that Ms. Zhou isn't sleeping much, is irritable, and has even started accusing her roommate of stealing her thesis ideas. Ms. Zhou speaks quickly, has circumstantial and overinclusive speech, and expresses paranoia about her roommate, but she seems to have a good understanding of what is happening. She acknowledges that she is having some manic symptoms. She is not agreeable to psychiatric admission because of her thesis deadline, but she is willing to restart her lithium, work on getting more sleep, and see her outpatient providers more frequently. There are no acute safety concerns.

The dialogue below illustrates how psychotherapy supervision might proceed between Dr. Cruz (Supervisor) and Dr. Allen (Trainee) in this setting.

> Supervisor: Now that we have a plan for Ms. Zhou's medication and disposition, let's take a couple of minutes to make a plan for the psychotherapy. She won't be your patient for much longer, but you can still use supportive psychotherapy techniques in the ER to help her achieve at least one of her goals. Even brief interventions can have an impact! Let's think about which areas of Ms. Zhou's psychological functioning are most impaired and figure out a reasonable goal from there. What do you think?
>
> Trainee: Well, she's paranoid about her roommate, so her reality testing is somewhat impaired. I did wonder about her judgment with stopping the medication, but she has pretty good insight and agreed to come to the ER with her sister to get help. I guess I was most struck by the impact on her executive functioning. She's really struggling

with how to juggle everything—her treatment, her thesis, and her roommate.

SUPERVISOR: I agree. So, let's focus on the goal of helping her plan the next steps for re-entering her life. How might you discuss this with her?

TRAINEE: Maybe I can work with her to make a written schedule of the coming week. It could include her appointments, medication times, when she would like to be in bed by, and also some breaks during the day. In terms of the paranoia toward her roommate, maybe we can come up with a plan about what she can say or do if she is feeling suspicious again. She can write down her ideas now, so that in the heat of the moment she can have something to look at. But I really don't know how to help with the thesis—that just sounds like a stressful situation!

SUPERVISOR: It does sound stressful—and I think acknowledging that can be helpful for your alliance with Ms. Zhou. Figuring out what to do about her thesis sounds like a larger issue; perhaps you can encourage her to talk about that with her outpatient providers. Where do you feel safe meeting with her, and for how long?

TRAINEE: I'll use the interview room. I don't have acute safety concerns, and I think it would be helpful for her to be in a less stimulating environment. Because her thinking is a little circumstantial, I'll probably need about 10 minutes.

SUPERVISOR: Sounds like a good plan. Let me know how it goes.

Conclusion

Although acute care settings may not seem to be an ideal environment for psychotherapy supervision, they lend themselves well to the use of supportive psychotherapy and offer unique opportunities for psychotherapy supervision. Through use of the three-step approach introduced in this chapter and included in the chapter appendix, supervisors can efficiently incorporate discussions of supportive psychotherapy techniques into the work they are already doing to help trainees understand that these techniques are applicable for a wide variety of patients and settings.

References

Blumenshine P, Lenet AE, Havel LK, et al: Thinking outside of outpatient: underutilized settings for psychotherapy education. Acad Psychiatry 41(1):16–19, 2017 27283018

Cabaniss DL: 3-Step Supportive Psychotherapy Manual. 2015. Available to members of the American Association of Directors of Psychiatry Residency Training (AADPRT) at: https://www.aadprt.org/training-directors/virtual-training-office. Accessed August 22, 2022.

Fauman BJ: Psychiatric residency training in the management of emergencies. Psychiatr Clin North Am 6(2):325–334, 1983 6351038

Greenberg WE, Borus JF: Focused opportunities for resident education on today's inpatient psychiatric units. Harv Rev Psychiatry 22(3):201–204, 2014 24802727

Griffith JL, Gaby L: Brief psychotherapy at the bedside: countering demoralization from medical illness. Psychosomatics 46(2):109–116, 2005 15774948

Hunter JJ, Maunder RG, Gupta M: Teaching consultation-liaison psychotherapy: assessment of adaptation to medical and surgical illness. Acad Psychiatry 31(5):367–374, 2007 17875621

Jiménez X, Thorkelson G: Medical countertransference and the trainee: identifying a training gap. J Psychiatr Pract 18(2):109–117, 2012 22418401

Lonergan BB, Duchin NP, Fromson JA, AhnAllen CG: Skills-based psychotherapy training for inpatient psychiatry residents: a needs assessment and evaluation of a pilot curriculum. Acad Psychiatry 44(3):320–323, 2020 31828674

Nash SS, Kent LK, Muskin PR: Psychodynamics in medically ill patients. Harv Rev Psychiatry 17(6):389–397, 2009 19968453

Perry S, Viederman M: Adaptation of residents to consultation-liaison psychiatry, I: working with the physically ill. Gen Hosp Psychiatry 3(2):141–147, 1981 7250694

Plakun EM, Sudak DM, Goldberg D: The Y model: an integrated, evidence-based approach to teaching psychotherapy competencies. J Psychiatr Pract 15(1):5–11, 2009 19182560

Rosnick L: Use of a long-term inpatient unit as a site for learning psychotherapy. Psychiatr Clin North Am 10(2):309–323, 1987 3110749

Rozensky RH: Clinical psychology in medical settings: celebrating our past, enjoying the present, building our future. Journal of Clinical Psychology in Medical Settings 13(4):343–352, 2006

Silver D, Book HE, Hamilton JE, et al: Psychotherapy and the inpatient unit: a unique learning experience. Am J Psychother 37(1):121–128, 1983 6846663

Solomon S, Saravay SM, Steinberg H: Supervision in liaison and consultation psychiatry. Gen Hosp Psychiatry 2(4):294–299, 1980 7461447

Stanley B, Brown G: Safety planning intervention: a brief intervention to mitigate suicide risk. Cognitive and Behavioral Practice 19(2):256–264, 2012

Stein MB, Jacobo MC: Brief inpatient psychotherapeutic technique. Psychotherapy (Chic) 50(3):464–468, 2013 24000872

Teitelbaum ML: Doubts about being of value: an important aspect of countertransference in consultation-liaison psychiatry. Int J Psychiatry Med 15(4):329–333, 1985–1986 3830941

APPENDIX

3-Step Supportive Psychotherapy Manual[*]

Much of what we do with patients all day is psychotherapy. When we do things like help patients to make sense of their experience, set personal goals, feel better about themselves, cope with stress, and get along better with others, we are doing psychotherapy. So, it's probably just a new way to think about what you are already doing! And it doesn't have to take a lot of time. Here's a 3- step manual to help you make psychotherapy part of what you do in every patient interaction. You can do all three steps in a single encounter with a patient.

The kind of psychotherapy we're talking about is supportive psychotherapy, which helps people improve their functioning. It's very well suited for acute or short-term clinical situations, as well as for settings in which you are less likely to do intensive or long-term psychotherapy (such as community clinics). Most mental health providers are engaged in supportive psychotherapy with patients without even knowing that they are doing it. This short guide is designed to you to more effectively use supportive psychotherapy in your interactions with patients.

Before you start—consider—what is psychotherapy?
To be psychotherapy, you need

- A patient
- A mental health provider
- Talking
- A frame (the parameters of the therapy, such as where you will meet, for how long, and what the fee will be)
- The shared goal of improving the patient's mental and emotional health

This can be easily done in these settings and can be enormously helpful to patients.

---

[*] 3-Step Supportive Psychotherapy Manual. Copyright © 2015, Deborah L. Cabaniss, M.D. All rights reserved.

STEP ONE – LEARN ABOUT THE PATIENT

When you meet patients, you are going to learn about them. To best help them with their function, you want to learn

- What's happening right now?
- What's causing them the most difficulty?
- How have they handled crises in the past?

Important functions to learn about include

- Sense of self
- Relationships with others
- Ways of coping with stress and strong feelings
- Thinking and decision making
- How they spend their time (working and playing)

Even while you are getting this information – which you can do in a short initial encounter – you are beginning the psychotherapy. Remembering these essential questions will help you learn about the patient:

- Who are the most important people in your life now and how are you getting along with them?
- Tell me about a time that you feel like you handled a crisis well.
- What are the things that you are most proud of in your life?
- How can I most help you now?

After talking to the patient, take a few minutes to review the patient's functioning and to think about how you and the patient together could work to improve it.

STEP TWO – SET GOALS

Find out what the patient wants to work on and help them create a realistic goal to work on right now. Although patients may have many goals, here are 6 basic psychotherapy goals that can be useful for patients in any settings and clinical situation:

1. Understanding one's own feelings and feeling understood by others
2. Making sense of what brought them to treatment
3. Mobilizing adaptive coping skills to deal with current problems
4. Maintaining self-esteem in the face of current problems
5. Getting along with other people
6. Planning for the short-term future (ongoing treatment and re-entry to their lives)

Next, take a few minutes to choose together one or two goals that make sense and are meaningful for this patient now

STEP THREE – WORK TOGETHER TO TAKE ACTION ON THE GOAL

There are three basic skills that you need for any psychotherapy:

1. **Making an alliance** – To conduct psychotherapy, the patient has to trust that you are trying to help them. You can help to develop this trust by introducing yourself and trying, from the first time you meet, to show the patient that you are interested, that you understand, and that you can see things from his/her point of view (empathy). Being friendly, restating things that the person tells you, making good eye contact, and instilling hope are all ways to do this. There's always a way to instill hope, even when the situation is dire; for example, you can help someone to view their voluntary admission as the start of better self-care, or to think about a serious illness as a moment to really connect to family members. You have information to get, but making good eye contact rather than writing notes is key.

2. **Setting the frame and establishing boundaries** – No matter where you see patients you need to set a frame together – this includes

   - Where you will meet
   - When you will meet
   - How long your meetings will be
   - How many total meetings you will have
   - Whether there will be a fee

   The frame is different in different settings – could be a 10 minute conversation in front of a nurses' station on an inpatient unit or a 15 minute conversation at the bedside on a medical service. Think about the best frame for this patient, considering the capacity and needs of the patient and discuss so that you can decide upon a mutually agreed upon plan.

3. **Empathic listening** – Try to listen in order to understand the patient's point of view. This could be very different from your point of view. Periodically check that you're on the right track by saying things like, "So it sounds like what you're feeling is…" or "Let me see if I'm understanding what you're trying to say…"

Take a few moments to think about your strategies for making an alliance, what frame makes sense in this situation, and how to listen empathically.

Now you're ready to go!

When you see the patient, talk together about

- **Goals** – ask about what they would like to work on, share what you're considering and why, and reach a mutually agreed upon decision.
- **The frame** – discuss the frame that you've thought of so that the patient knows your recommendation about when you'll be meeting and for how long. Discuss and reach a mutually agreed upon decision.

You can use the following basic psychotherapy techniques to help you achieve the 6 major psychotherapeutic goals for these settings:

1. **Encouraging the patient to talk about feelings** – Simply talking about feelings can be very therapeutic. You can also help people to name their feelings, validate their feelings, feel that their feelings are understandable, and begin to understand why they might be having those feelings.

2. **Helping the patient to tell the story of the current situation** – This is already part of what you do when you take a history. Re-stating it in a linear form can help the patient to make more sense of what happened. This can be very organizing and therapeutic to a patient in crisis.

3. **Encouraging the patient to discuss ways they have coped with past difficulties** – This can help you to encourage use of coping strategies that are already strong and to try to modify or discourage less adaptive coping strategies. Encouraging patients to talk about their lives, particularly things that they think that they have done well, can give you information about strengths that you might not otherwise see in the patient in acute crisis. Once you have some sense of these, you and the patient can think together about how to apply them to the current situation.

4. **Highlighting strengths and past accomplishments** – You don't only want to hear about the crisis – you want to hear about the whole person, particularly things that the person has done well and is proud of. Reminding the patient of these strengths is key to maintaining self-esteem during the crisis. Praise and encouragement are important supportive psychotherapy interventions that can help you to achieve this goal.

5. **Learning about key relationships and role play** – Learning about the key relationships in the person's life will help you to know 1) upon whom the person can rely and 2) strengths and challenges that the person has in interpersonal relationships. Problems with relationships –

either with family members and/or with members of the treatment team – are often central to the crisis. Practicing new ways of relating to these key people during this time, including role-play with you, is a good way of addressing this. "Let's think together about how to ask for help from the nurse next time she comes…."

6. **Talking about next steps** – One of the most important roles for psychotherapy in these settings is connecting the person to ongoing treatment and helping the person to re-enter his/her life. Helping the person who has burnt bridges save face is important, as is building a bridge to the outpatient treatment team. Simple techniques, such as carefully planning out the first day after discharge (writing a list together) can be very organizing. Focusing on short-term rather than long-term goals is key here.

Consider discussing your plan with a peer or supervisor.

REMEMBER – You are always a psychotherapist!

Most of your work with patients in clinical settings is psychotherapy. Psychotherapy doesn't just happen in outpatient offices during 45-minute sessions. So, when seeing patients, take a few minutes to think about how patients are functioning and how you might help them improve their function in the face of current problems. Your patients will benefit and you will be doing psychotherapy!

18

Supervision of Cognitive-Behavioral Therapy

Donna M. Sudak, M.D.
Evgenia Royter, D.O.

KEY LEARNING GOALS

- Recognize that supervision of cognitive-behavioral therapy (CBT) generally has a structure that parallels the processes of CBT.

- Focus CBT supervision to increase adherence to CBT principles and provider competence in CBT.

- Include active learning techniques and practice of therapy skills.

IN THIS CHAPTER we briefly review the evidence supporting supervision as a practice to ensure the skillful delivery of cognitive-behavioral therapy (CBT), describe the components of supervision that promote efficiency and effectiveness, and pose questions for future research. We hope that the material presented will promote further inquiry into the evaluation of supervision in other forms of psychotherapy. Despite the widespread tradition of psychotherapy supervision and its place as the "gold standard" for the dissemination of psychotherapeutic interventions by trainees, there exists surprisingly little empirical evidence for its effectiveness in training competent CBT therapists (Alfonsson et al. 2017). The "dose" of supervision and the "active ingredients" needed to enhance the outcomes of patients with psychiatric disorders are similarly unclear. *Adherence* in this context means "Is it CBT?" *Competence* means "Is this CBT that is custom-tailored to the needs and conceptualization of a particular patient, and is it efficiently delivered?" CBT supervision is time-consuming and resource-intensive, prompting the need for further examination to determine whether supervision is the best means of attaining fidelity to a treatment model and better outcomes for patients. One foundational principle that underlies any effective CBT supervision is that therapists in training must possess the basic psychotherapy skills common to all treatments—that is, the capability to form a good therapeutic alliance with and develop an empathic connection to the patient. If these skills are not present, supervisors must teach them first. CBT relies on a strong therapeutic bond that incorporates the concept of "collaborative empiricism"; the therapist and the patient work as a team of co-investigators to understand and solve the problems of the patient. Supervisors must make certain that supervisees can employ relational skills that allow for such a collaboration with a wide range of different types of patients.

Evidence for the Efficacy of Supervision in Cognitive-Behavioral Therapy

Numerous recent reviews and chapters regarding CBT supervision speak to the relative paucity of research supporting its efficacy. This lack of data limits our understanding of the mediators and moderators of effective supervision and diminishes our capacity to enhance efficiency and disseminate best practices. Existing CBT supervision competency frameworks and standards have been developed by expert consensus (Milne and Dunkerley 2010) but lack firm support in the literature. The lack of access to high-quality CBT that is faithful to the model increases the importance of determining the essential elements that produce competent CBT clinicians. CBT is generally taught to therapists with some form of didactic training followed by supervision with feedback to improve adherence. The practice of providing short, intensive didactic workshops with little to no subsequent supervision (i.e., "train and hope" [Beidas and Kendall 2010]) has not been effective in increasing the numbers of qualified CBT practitioners. The following review of the literature examines the benefits of supervision and explains why supervision is vital to CBT training.

One of the first empirical studies to show the benefit of supervision on CBT practice was conducted by Alfonsson et al. (2020) in a single-case experimental design. Six therapists were provided with clinical supervision using a CBT competency-based protocol. Therapist scores on the Cognitive Therapy Scale—Revised (Blackburn et al. 2001) significantly increased during the phase of the study devoted to supervision. Another case study of training with 16 weeks of "model-consistent CBT supervision"—in which the CBT model was employed as a framework for supervision, and self-practice was included as a key component—showed significant improvement in adherence to CBT protocols and competence, as measured by standardized rating scales (Waltman 2016). *Adherence* in this context denoted that the therapist was following the standard protocols for CBT for a particular disorder (e.g., using behavioral activation and thought recording for patients with depression). *Competence* meant that the therapist provided treatment of an individual patient skillfully within the framework, as measured by the standard scales used to rate therapist performance in CBT (e.g., the Cognitive Therapy Rating Scale [CTRS]; Young and Beck 1980).

A study conducted to evaluate which components of supervision are needed to keep clinicians working within CBT protocols recruited 78 clinicians who worked with patients with substance use disorders (Sholomskas et al. 2005). Clinicians were randomly assigned to one of three groups: 1) CBT manual-based learning alone, 2) review of the manual and interactive web-based training, or 3) review of the manual along with a didactic seminar followed by supervision of casework. Assessments were completed before training at baseline, 4 weeks postbaseline after exposure to web training/didactics, and 3 months after posttraining (including supervision). There were no significant differences among the groups at baseline. Outcomes were primarily measured by assessing the clinician's ability to demonstrate key CBT techniques, which included explaining the CBT rationale for treatment and performing a functional analysis of 1) drug use, 2) coping with cravings, and 3) automatic thoughts. CBT clinicians were videotaped in a role-play exercise that was later reviewed and rated—via the Yale Adherence Competence Scale (YACS; Carroll et al. 2000)—by independent individuals who were blinded to the treatment conditions. YACS is a general standard system used to evaluate therapist adherence that measures the extent to which the therapist covered an intervention and the skill with which the intervention was delivered. The results posttraining showed that the group with supervision had significantly greater improvement in adherence and skill compared with the manual-only group (Sholomskas et al. 2005).

Whereas the Sholomskas et al. (2005) study looked at the power of supervision to reinforce a therapist's use of CBT principles and approaches, a study by Schoenwald et al. (2009) examined the relationship between supervisor/therapist adherence to a treatment protocol and patient outcomes 1 year posttreatment. The findings showed that supervisors who focused on adherence to the therapy protocol increased the adherence of therapists to the protocol, which resulted in improved outcomes in their patients. This study highlighted the importance of supervision in obtaining better patient outcomes (Schoenwald et al. 2009).

Some efforts have been made to measure the long-term impact of supervision. Liness et al. (2019) published results of a study in which therapist competence and patient outcomes were assessed at the beginning of training, at the end of training, and 12 or more months posttraining. Assessment of audio-recorded trainee therapy sessions using the Cognitive Therapy Scale—Revised showed that 100% of trainees achieved competence during training, and 84% demonstrated continuing competence posttraining (Liness et al. 2019). In addition, clinical outcomes were examined and showed significant improvement across all measures at follow-up, despite an increase in the complexity of patient presentations at follow-up. A positive trend was found between therapist competence and clinical outcomes, but the results failed to reach statistical significance. It was difficult to draw conclusions due to the small sample size and lack of a control group. However, resulting positive trends in this study show the need for more studies targeting competence–outcome relationships (Liness et al. 2019).

Rakovshik et al. (2016) examined the effects of internet-based CBT training with and without supervision to assess the utility of supervision. Sixty-one therapists were randomly assigned to one of three groups: 1) internet-based training with a consultation worksheet (IBT-CW), 2) internet-based training with CBT supervision via Skype (IBT-S), and 3) a control group that received the training materials after the data were collected ("delayed training" [abbreviated as DT]). CBT skills were evaluated at baseline, midway through the study, and at the completion of training via competency ratings of recorded therapy sessions. The IBT-S group showed significantly increased CBT competence posttraining compared with the IBT-CW group and the DT control group (Rakovshik et al. 2016). No significant differences in competency ratings were found between the IBT-CW group and the DT group. This shows that effective CBT supervision may occur in situations where traditional, in-person training is not available (Rakovshik et al. 2016).

In a meta-analytic review, Zarafonitis-Müller et al. (2014) examined the relationship between therapist competence and adherence to protocols and patient outcomes. Although therapist competence had a positive effect on patient outcomes, adherence to protocols did not produce significant differences in patient outcomes. This finding indicates a need for a greater emphasis on therapist competence during training. Another systematic review, by Alfonsson et al. (2018), examined the effects of supervision on therapist competence and patient outcomes in CBT. The study authors noted that the relatively limited existing data indicated that supervision may have benefits on the competence of novice clinicians, but that effects on clinical outcomes are unclear. They also did not find sufficient evidence to distinguish between the effects of different types of supervision (e.g., in-person vs. standard delayed).

An attempt to identify key components of CBT supervision by Weck et al. (2017a) led to an empirical randomized controlled pilot study of 19 therapist–patient dyads in two groups—one in which therapists received competence feedback and the other in which they did not (control group). Feedback was given at intervals across a course of treatment by clinicians blinded to study conditions who used the CTRS to rate work samples. Therapists in both groups received regular supervision, but only those in the competence feedback group received written qualitative and quantitative feedback. Results showed a larger increase in CTRS-measured competence in the competence feedback group compared with the control group (Weck et al. 2017a).

Finally, cost-effective training is necessary for effective dissemination. Measurement of therapist adherence and competence by independent raters is preferable, although it is costly and labor intensive. One way to address this barrier is to employ subjective reporting of competence utilizing clinician self-reports and supervisor reports. Such reports would be beneficial if they are shown to agree with independent rater reports. Caron et al. (2020) examined the relationships among clinician ratings, supervisor ratings, and independent ratings of clinician competence in a randomized controlled study. Fifty-nine clinicians were randomly assigned to one of two groups: delivering treatment as usual (TAU) or conducting CBT for pediatric anxiety. Supervisors rated clinician competence after each supervision session, and clinicians completed a self-assessment of confidence after each therapy session. The clinician self-report was designed to align with supervisor ratings of competence but was not a true rating of self-reported competence. The independent raters used audio recordings to rate clinician competence. The results showed accuracy discrepancies among clinician ratings, supervisor ratings, and independent ratings of clinician competence. Clinicians and supervisors in the TAU group overestimated clinician competence, which is consistent with findings in previous studies. However, in the CBT group, clinicians overestimated competence and CBT supervisors underestimated competence in comparison with the independent raters. Given the inconsistency of these results, implementation of the "gold standard" of independent observer ratings is recommended until a more standardized approach is developed for training and feedback by supervisors (Caron et al. 2020).

Distinctive Features of Cognitive-Behavioral Therapy Supervision

Historical Development

The development of CBT supervision parallels the development of CBT provision in many ways (Liese and Beck 1997; Padesky 1996). In the early stage of CBT clinical supervision, descriptive accounts of supervisory sessions became the model for CBT supervisors who wished to work within a structured framework. Such accounts describe clinical supervision with core components that mirrored the structure of therapy, focusing on questions regarding patient management and conceptualization followed by feedback and homework. As CBT practice became more widely disseminated, guidelines were developed for CBT supervision, and competency frameworks were disseminated (American Association for Marriage and Family Therapy 2014; American Psychological Association 2015; Borders et al. 2011; Falender et al. 2004; Roth and Pilling 2008). Milne and Reiser (2017), among others, described the development of a model for supervision that integrated available evidence with expert consensus and evidence from other fields of dissemination and training to further refine the initial descriptive model. Several frameworks for CBT supervision were created by synthesizing details of supervision performed during CBT efficacy trials (Roth and Pilling 2008; Roth et al. 2010). Despite these efforts, no current model for CBT supervision has been fully researched and shown to be the most effective.

Parallel Structure of Therapy and Supervision

The structured nature of CBT supervision has been promulgated as a way to model and inculcate the elements of a CBT session, but there are other reasons behind the structure. The structure of both CBT and CBT supervision is designed to facilitate learning. The parallel structure of therapy and supervision is an inherently logical outgrowth of a fundamental principle of CBT—that is, that therapy (and supervision) involves learning something new in an efficient and durable way. Direct observation, role-play, and feedback are core interventions that facilitate the growth of the supervisee and the retention of supervisory learning. Unfortunately, data obtained from a wide variety of supervisors indicate a suboptimal use of these interventions in supervisory practice (Townend et al. 2002; Weck et al. 2017b). Dorsey et al. (2018) found that direct observation, role-play, and feedback accounted for less than 25% of the time spent in supervision. Studies such as these point to the variable quality of the supervisory experience and the need for further standardization and training for supervisors (Dorsey et al. 2018).

Activities of the Effective CBT Supervisor

Many activities of the CBT supervisor are similar to those of good supervisors in any tradition. Given that supervision promotes learning in the context of a relationship, the supervisor prioritizes the relationship with the supervisee, and socializes the supervisee into supervision with an eye toward bonds, tasks, and goals. Examples of information needed to facilitate a supervisory bond, set learning goals, and prioritize the most useful tasks include the background and culture of supervisees, their experience with specific types of therapy, and their learning goals. Supervisors may use case conceptualization/formulation of the supervisee to most effectively target interventions and plan the supervision. Of critical importance is specific information about a supervisee's prior CBT training. If supervisees' knowledge of CBT has been confined to lectures alone, extensive training will be required within supervision, because supervisees will not have had sufficient practice to implement CBT skillfully. Practicing of CBT skills through role-play within the supportive environment of supervision and having the corrective experience of receiving focused, performance-based feedback are critical to therapist development. Until the trainee has the ability to deploy the skills needed to treat patients, more evocative supervision is inappropriate.

Attitudes about and experience with CBT therapy differ among supervisees. Many trainees will have had little experience with CBT supervision, or will have had supervision consisting only of a general report of the events of therapy from the prior week, with instructions intoned by the wise supervisor across the room. Socialization of trainees to a model that incorporates principles of adult learning and prioritizes efficiency will often be needed. An explicit discussion of learning goals and incorporation of those goals into a contract for supervision underscores the importance of the relationship, activates prior learning, and promotes a commitment to the work of supervision. Such a contract should also address the framework of supervision (time, place, and so forth) and the expectations regarding session recordings and should include emergency contacts and a description of what to tell patients about supervision. The evaluative component of supervision produces significant anxiety in many trainees. The supervisor and the supervisee should discuss the methods and frequency of evaluation and should include these details in the supervision contract.

An important consideration in forming a supervisory alliance is fostering trust between the supervisor and the supervisee. Failure of trainees to disclose significant therapy details or the limits of their knowledge because of a lack of trust in the supervisor is a well-known impediment to supervision (Ladany et al. 1996). Nondisclosure in supervision may lead to ineffective supervision at best, or suboptimal patient care at worst. The development of trust between supervisor and supervisee can be facilitated in several ways. Supervisors should express genuine interest in their supervisees and in their learning and should provide praise appropriate to supervisees' performance. Supervisors should review evaluation requirements, the evaluative measures to be used, and the frequency of evaluation. Finally, an open discussion of cultural differences between supervisor and supervisee must occur, along with a discussion of the supervisee's comfort in navigating such differences with patients. Open and honest dialogue about race, culture, ethnicity, and gender is essential for fostering a relationship that allows for discussion of difference with the supervisor and the supervisee's patients.

Supervisees need to understand how supervision sessions will proceed. Once the supervisor is confident that the supervisee can capably perform patient assessments, there is little value in spending supervision time reviewing the patient's history. This is not to say that the history is unimportant. It is crucial. What is not needed is an oral retelling of the history. Instead, the supervisee may provide written summaries and case conceptualizations prior to the session for the supervisor's review, with questions or missing data subsequently clarified during supervision. Often the need to write a case formulation and history in advance helps the supervisee to clarify questions about the patient and to determine what data are missing. Supervision then begins with a discussion of the questions the supervisee has about the patient and how to proceed with therapy. The supervisee's provision of materials in advance enhances efficiency and gives the supervisee and the supervisor an opportunity to reflect on the case conceptualization and what information might be missing. Supervisees may need to be taught how to frame questions for the supervisor. Such critical thinking about patients is key to learning self-supervision. Supervisors hope to instill a spirit of inquiry and humility within their supervisees that will ultimately assist them in their efforts to help patients make changes in their lives. Such values will also assist supervisees in navigating necessary changes in therapy when it is not proceeding as expected.

Encouraging Recording

CBT supervision is highly reliant on evaluation of recorded therapy material and subsequent discussion of events within the session. Items to discuss are collaboratively prioritized by the supervisor and the supervisee in conjunction with learning goals. Many supervisors find it extremely challenging to obtain recordings from supervisees. Supervisees frequently experience significant anxiety when facing the tasks of obtaining the patient's permission to record and providing recordings for the supervisor's review. This trepidation is perfectly understandable and may be mitigated by several activities of the supervisor.

When possible, clinic policy may establish recording as standard for every patient and supervisee, so that the burden of negotiating for consent is removed from the supervisee. This practice is likely to make recording routine and facilitate the reviewing of sessions by the supervisor–supervisee dyad. Even when the clinic already requires recording, teaching trainees the process for obtaining informed consent around recording is valuable. Supervisors may remind supervisees of the rationales for recording, examine supervisees' beliefs about recording, and engage supervisees in rehearsing, in the less-threatening role-play format, the process of asking patients for consent to record. Role-playing how to ask for consent to record with increasingly difficult patients or scenarios the supervisee fears allows the trainee to begin to develop a fluent repertoire of responses. For example, if a supervisee is particularly anxious about encountering a patient who has concerns that the supervisee is recording because he or she lacks sufficient experience to conduct the treatment, the supervisor and the supervisee can develop and practice a series of responses to this concern. When possible, supervisors should provide recordings of their own work with patients (particularly when there have been challenges) to help defuse supervisees' anxiety.

Another aspect of recording that may require troubleshooting is the technical task of obtaining reasonable-quality recordings in an unobtrusive manner that maintains patient privacy. Clear instruction (preferably including handouts) on how to transfer and remove downloaded files electronically should be provided in supervision. A "test run" of recording equipment with another person prior to using it with patients will help ensure that any recording is of good quality. Even when recordings are not being used for supervision, recording should be done at every session to reduce anxiety and to normalize the practice.

Finally, recordings that amplify and enrich supervision reinforce the value of this method of collecting data about therapy. Supervisors should incorporate a review of recordings at every session. Supervisees may cue up segments that illustrate aspects of their therapy sessions about which they feel particularly proud or have specific questions, until they are fully comfortable with the process. (For further information on the use of recordings in supervision, see Chapter 9, "Using Process Notes and Audio and Video Recordings in Psychotherapy Supervision.")

Role-Play

Role-play is a cornerstone of CBT training. Bearman et al. (2013) found that engaging in role-play in supervision was associated with an increased frequency of therapists trying new skills with patients. Because CBT training is so variable, it is often necessary to use role-play in supervision to assist the supervisee in mastering basic skills. When used to build therapists' skills, role-play practice should involve a range of patient difficulty and should mirror the variety of patients that the supervisee sees. Once mastery of the fundamental interventions of CBT is attained, role-play may be used to practice particular aspects of patient care that the supervisee finds to be a challenge. For example, a supervisee who is avoiding exposure-based interventions because of fears that the patient may have a panic attack in session may practice varying scenarios where patients have panic during the session to develop a sense of mastery in approaching such work. Reverse role-play, wherein the supervisor plays the part of therapist, may similarly enhance learning, especially when followed by an additional role-play with the supervisee playing the part of the therapist, allowing for incorporation of ideas stimulated by the practice role-play. Smartphone recordings of role-plays in supervision allow supervisees to review and reflect on the role-play experience and may enhance their learning.

Feedback

We believe that performance-based feedback is the cornerstone of skill training and the development of expertise. The CBT supervisor uses feedback wisely. Several principles regarding providing feedback must be kept in mind as supervision proceeds:

1. Make careful and specific observations of supervisee performance and pick one or two specific areas to target with feedback at each supervision session.

2. Provide feedback that indicates what has been performed well before providing any corrective feedback. This may help diminish supervisees' anxiety and increase their receptivity to corrective feedback.

3. When providing corrective feedback, be clear and specific. Model skills that are needed and then ask supervisees to practice those skills. Provide feedback on supervisees' practice efforts and assign a related activity for supervisees to practice in the week to come.

Supervisors must balance the learning needs of the supervisee and the clinical needs of the patient. For example, if supervisees are having significant difficulty with several elements of their therapy sessions with patients, such as setting an agenda and finding a focus, supervisors have the difficult tasks of sustaining supervisees' ability to attend to feedback and also determining which skills must be improved quickly in the service of supervisees' patients. Maintaining the delicate balance of support and challenge, while keeping patient welfare at the forefront, is a test of skill for supervisors. (For more information on feedback in supervision, see Chapter 6, "Practical Methods That Foster Supervisor Growth.")

Effective Action Planning

Similar to the process in therapy with patients, material learned in a supervision session will need to be deliberately practiced in order to become a regular part of a supervisee's repertoire. It is important to devise a meaningful method for reviewing and implementing the learning that occurs in supervision. Ideally, such assignments will include reflection and focused practice. The supervisor should model the practice of giving specific, written, collaboratively designed tasks that logically follow from the supervision session. Supervisors must also make certain that each assignment is reviewed at the next supervision session. For example, if a supervisee is working on setting agendas in a timely fashion, the supervisor may ask the supervisee what kind of exercise might be useful for practicing this skill in the coming week. The two of them may then design a form in which the supervisee can set the agendas for several patient therapy sessions in the upcoming week, as well as noting the time when each was set. The supervisor and the supervisee can then use the CTRS to rate this effort at the next supervision session.

Inculcating the Habit of Lifelong Learning and Expertise Development

Supervision that teaches a process of continual self-evaluation and reflection, coupled with progress monitoring and deliberate practice, may lead to better patient outcomes and the development of expert performance. The focused training program Self-Practice/Self-Reflection is one way to enhance competence in CBT (Bennett-Levy 2006). Several studies have supported the efficacy of this method in leading to superior patient outcomes. Chow et al. (2015) demonstrated that therapists who engaged in self-reflection, reviewed recordings of their work, deliberately attempted to improve their empathic responses to patients, and took time to consider treatment planning had patient outcomes superior to those of therapists who did not engage in such activities. Teaching supervisees to use validated instruments to assess patient progress, to evaluate the strength of the therapeutic alliance, and to monitor their own fidelity to therapy protocols shows trainee therapists how to obtain data they can use for self-reflection and self-improvement. Supervisees should be taught how to use such data to construct personal improvement plans, using checklists, coaching, and feedback so that they may continually refine and improve their skills.

Future Directions and Areas for Inquiry

As we have noted, there is limited research examining the specific aspects of supervision that most significantly affect therapist adherence to CBT protocols and patient outcomes. At least one study (Dorsey et al. 2017) has highlighted the lack of research focused on identifying the most salient interventions and determining how to maximize their use via supervision. Studying these factors would help ensure that CBT supervision is both efficient and impactful. There is also a need to evaluate the benefits and pitfalls of teletherapy supervision and virtual supervision.

References

Alfonsson S, Spännargård Å, Parling T, et al: The effects of clinical supervision on supervisees and patients in cognitive-behavioral therapy: a study protocol for a systematic review. Syst Rev 6(1):94, 2017 28490376

Alfonsson S, Parling T, Spännargård Å, et al: The effects of clinical supervision on supervisees and patients in cognitive behavioral therapy: a systematic review. Cogn Behav Ther 47(3):206–228, 2018 28929863

Alfonsson S, Lundgren T, Andersson G: Clinical supervision in cognitive behavior therapy improves therapists' competence: a single-case experimental pilot study. Cogn Behav Ther 49(5):425–438, 2020 32213046

American Association for Marriage and Family Therapy: Approved supervision designation: Standards Handbook. 2014. Available at: https://aamft.org/AAMFT/ENHANCE_Knowledge/Approved_Supervisor_Resources/Supervision/Supervision.aspx?hkey=f3fe9160-efbc-490e-b6f7-7a493fa47632. Accessed January 7, 2021.

American Psychological Association: Guidelines for clinical supervision in health service psychology. Am Psychol 70(1):33–46, 2015 25581007

Bearman SK, Weisz JR, Chorpita BF, et al; Research Network on Youth Mental Health: More practice, less preach? The role of supervision processes and therapist characteristics in EBP implementation. Adm Policy Ment Health 40(6):518–529, 2013 23525895

Beidas RS, Kendall PC: Training therapists in evidence-based practice: a critical review of studies from a systems-contextual perspective. Clin Psychol (New York) 17(1):1–30, 2010 20877441

Bennett-Levy J: Therapist skills: a cognitive model of their acquisition and refinement. Behavioural and Cognitive Psychotherapy 34(1):57–78, 2006

Blackburn I-M, James IA, Milne DL, et al: The revised cognitive therapy scale (CTS-R): psychometric properties. Behavioural and Cognitive Psychotherapy 29(4):431–446, 2001

Borders LD, DeKruyf L, Fernando DM, et al: Best practices in clinical supervision. Association for Counselor Education and Supervision. April 22, 2011. Available at: https://acesonline.net/wp-content/uploads/2018/11/ACES-Best-Practices-in-Clinical-Supervision-2011.pdf. Accessed January 7, 2021.

Caron EB, Muggeo MA, Souer HR, et al: Concordance between clinician, supervisor and observer ratings of therapeutic competence in CBT and treatment as usual: does clinician competence or supervisor session observation improve agreement? Behav Cogn Psychother 48(3):350–363, 2020 31806076

Carroll KM, Nich C, Sifry RL, et al: A general system for evaluating therapist adherence and competence in psychotherapy research in the addictions. Drug Alcohol Depend 57(3):225–238, 2000 10661673

Chow DL, Miller SD, Seidel JA, et al: The role of deliberate practice in the development of highly effective psychotherapists. Psychotherapy (Chic) 52(3):337–345, 2015 26301425

Dorsey S, Pullmann MD, Kerns SEU, et al: The juggling act of supervision in community mental health: implications for supporting evidence-based treatment. Adm Policy Ment Health 44(6):838–852, 2017 28315076

Dorsey S, Kerns SEU, Lucid L, et al: Objective coding of content and techniques in workplace-based supervision of an EBT in public mental health. Implement Sci 13(1):19, 2018 29368656

Falender CA, Cornish JA, Goodyear R, et al: Defining competencies in psychology supervision: a consensus statement. J Clin Psychol 60(7):771–785, 2004 15195339

Ladany N, Hill CE, Corbett MM, Nutt EA: Nature, extent, and importance of what psychotherapy trainees do not disclose to their supervisors. Journal of Counseling Psychology 43(1):10, 1996

Liese BS, Beck JS: Cognitive therapy supervision, in Handbook of Psychotherapy Supervision. Edited by Watkins CE Jr. Chichester, West Sussex, UK, Wiley, 1997, pp 114–133

Liness S, Beale S, Lea S, et al: The sustained effects of CBT training on therapist competence and patient outcomes. Cognitive Therapy and Research 43(3):631–641, 2019

Milne DL, Dunkerley C: Towards evidence-based clinical supervision: the development and evaluation of four CBT guidelines. The Cognitive Behaviour Therapist 3(2):43–57, 2010. Available at: https://doi.org/10.1017/S1754470X10000048. Accessed August 16, 2022.

Milne DL, Reiser RP: A Manual for Evidence-Based CBT Supervision. Chichester, West Sussex, Wiley-Blackwell, 2017

Padesky CA: Developing cognitive therapist competency: teaching and supervision models, in Frontiers of Cognitive Therapy. Edited by Salkovskis PM. London, Guilford, 1996, pp 266–292

Rakovshik SG, McManus F, Vazquez-Montes M, et al: Is supervision necessary? Examining the effects of internet-based CBT training with and without supervision. J Consult Clin Psychol 84(3):191–199, 2016 26795937

Roth AD, Pilling S: Using an evidence-based methodology to identify the competencies required to deliver effective cognitive and behavioural therapy for depression and anxiety disorders. Behavioural and Cognitive Psychotherapy 36(2):129–147, 2008

Roth AD, Pilling S, Turner J: Therapist training and supervision in clinical trials: implications for clinical practice. Behav Cogn Psychother 38(3):291–302, 2010 20367895

Schoenwald SK, Sheidow AJ, Chapman JE: Clinical supervision in treatment transport: effects on adherence and outcomes. J Consult Clin Psychol 77(3):410–421, 2009 19485583

Sholomskas DE, Syracuse-Siewert G, Rounsaville BJ, et al: We don't train in vain: a dissemination trial of three strategies of training clinicians in cognitive-behavioral therapy. J Consult Clin Psychol 73(1):106–115, 2005 15709837

Townend M, Iannetta L, Freeston MH: Clinical supervision in practice: a survey of UK cognitive behavioural psychotherapists accredited by the BABCP. Behavioural and Cognitive Psychotherapy 30(4):485–500, 2002

Waltman SH: Model-consistent cognitive behavioral therapy supervision: a case study of a psychotherapy-based approach. J Cogn Psychother 30(2):120–130, 2016 32755911

Weck F, Kaufmann YM, Höfling V: Competence feedback improves CBT competence in trainee therapists: a randomized controlled pilot study. Psychother Res 27(4):501–509, 2017a 26837800

Weck F, Kaufmann YM, Witthöft M: Topics and techniques in clinical supervision in psychotherapy training. The Cognitive Behaviour Therapist 10:E3, 2017b

Young JE, Beck AT: Cognitive Therapy Scale Rating Manual, Revised Draft. 1980. Available at: https://beckinstitute.org/wp-content/uploads/2021/06/CTRS-Full-Documents.pdf. Accessed March 23, 2022.

Zarafonitis-Müller S, Kuhr K, Bechdolf A: [The relationship between therapist's competence and adherence to outcome in cognitive-behavioural therapy—results of a meta-analysis] (in German). Fortschr Neurol Psychiatr 82(9):502–510, 2014 25177902

PART IV

Challenges in Psychotherapy Supervision

19

The So-Called Difficult Supervisee

Allison Cowan, M.D., DFAPA

KEY LEARNING GOALS

- Recognize that challenging situations in psychotherapy supervision often stem from a strain on the supervisory alliance, a lack of focus on the work of supervision, the topics being discussed, or a failure to discuss difficult topics.

- Focus on maintaining the alliance and attending to the tasks of supervision to improve the effectiveness of supervision and patient outcomes.

Dr. Ragland [*texts supervisor*]: Hi. Running late. Got slammed on the inpatient unit.
Supervisor: Hi! See you when you get here.
Dr. Ragland: Actually, is it okay if we skip today? There's so much going on here.
Supervisor: I have this time set aside for your psychotherapy supervision because it's important. If you can't make it let me know. I can also offer you a time to reschedule if that would work better for you.
Dr. Ragland: Oh okay. Never mind. I'm on my way.
[*Dr. Ragland was able to make it to psychotherapy supervision 15 minutes late.*]

This vignette represents one of the many difficulties in psychotherapy supervision. The supervisor has set the expectation that supervision, like psychotherapy, should occur regularly and within the expected frame. When the trainee suggested changing the frame, the supervisor reinforces the importance of supervision, while demonstrating flexibility.

* * *

A systematic analogy can be drawn between the process of psychotherapy and that of psychotherapy supervision (Milne 2006). Some of the most important factors in both psychotherapy and psychotherapy supervision are the real relationship between patient and therapist, the shared creation of expectations, and the participation in healthy actions (Wampold and Budge 2012). These factors are not only analogous, they are interrelated. DePue et al. (2016) found that ratings of the supervisor–supervisee relationship showed positive contributions to the therapist–patient therapeutic alliance. Supervisees who rated their supervisory relationship highly were also more likely to rate their therapeutic alliance with the patient highly (DePue et al. 2016).

A strong supervisee–supervisor relationship can lead to a stronger connection and feeling of efficacy when working with patients. Rapport and client focus are factors in the supervisory relationship that are mirrored in the therapeutic relationship. The "good enough" psychotherapy supervisor deliberately enhances rapport by being active and patient, a good listener and team player, focused and flexible, curious and respectful, and empathic. The good-enough supervisor also focuses the supervision by working with the supervisee to

- Prioritize and appreciate the importance of supervision.
- Create goals for supervision.
- Synthesize clinical material into comprehensible patterns.
- Connect theory and clinical material.
- Create comprehensive formulations.
- Choose psychotherapy interventions based on those formulations.
- Connect interventions to patient progress and outcomes.
- Develop increasing assurance and autonomy.

This approach will help supervisors focus on improving the outcome of supervision. It is easy to blame supervisees for challenges in supervision, when instead these challenges are often the result of external events or a dynamic within supervision. In this chapter, we consider issues encountered with supervisees who are frequently absent or tardy, nondisclosing, timid, unengaged, and overly confiding.

The Frequently Absent or Tardy Supervisee

(Continuing from the previous vignette after Dr. Ragland comes to the office for supervision)

DR. RAGLAND: Sorry, I'm late. I'm glad you got my text that I was running behind.

SUPERVISOR: I'm glad you're here. It's good to see you.

DR. RAGLAND: Yeah, we were just really slammed, and I was trying to get things finished up before coming over. I thought that maybe, since not a lot has happened with my patient since our last supervision, we didn't need to meet.

SUPERVISOR: It sounds like it was a big effort to make it over to this building, especially when you had so much work that felt more pressing.

DR. RAGLAND: Yes! Exactly! You know they really get after you if you don't get the orders entered on time. Besides, you always seem so chill. I also thought that you maybe had stuff you'd rather be getting done, too, you know. Like if we didn't have supervision, you would be glad to have some extra time, too.

SUPERVISOR: Hmm, maybe a couple different things are going on here. You were very busy this morning and trying to catch up. I wonder if you also thought I'd appreciate it if you canceled.

DR. RAGLAND: Yes—I'm always glad when people cancel because it gives me a little extra time.

SUPERVISOR: What if I looked forward to seeing you and to our supervision?

DR. RAGLAND: Wow. I never considered that. I mean, really? You do?

SUPERVISOR: Yes. I do. I'm wondering if being late is connected to how you are feeling about our supervision. What's it like for you to have to make time to come here? How are you feeling about what we do in here?

In this vignette, the supervisor gently reinforces the frame of supervision and suggests alternative viewpoints on cancellations to the supervisee. Dr. Ragland assumed that the supervisor viewed spending time with supervisees as burdensome. In making this assumption, Dr. Ragland may be projecting his own feelings—either about doing therapy or about engaging in supervision—onto the supervisor. The supervisor uses this opportunity to question Dr. Ragland about the supervision and to draw attention to the role that this enactment may play in supervision.

* * *

In working with supervisees who are frequently tardy or absent, it is important to determine the primary cause for their tardiness or absence. The first step is ensuring that the supervisee has been appropriately informed of the need for a supervisory framework. If the supervisory frame has not been effectively described or established, the supervisor can initiate a discussion about this topic, as demonstrated below:

> SUPERVISOR: I don't know that I've ever talked about my expectations for us in here. I'm sorry I haven't brought this topic up until now, but I think we can discuss it now. I think it is most helpful for us to meet every week at the same time for the same amount of time—just like in psychotherapy. This time is important to me, and I hope it's important to you, too. How does that sound?

*   *   *

Other factors cited for absences and tardiness are anxiety, feelings of inadequacy, avoiding shame, withdrawal from the process of supervision, avoidant attachment style, and difficulty with time management (Hahn 2001; Rosenbaum 1953; Watkins 1995). When supervisees are in a training program, other possibilities include difficulties with being assertive when they need to leave their current rotation to come to supervision, lack of interest in psychotherapy, and previous negative experiences in supervision. Resistance to discussing real or perceived errors in patient cases or disagreements with the supervisor can lead to avoidance of supervision. Gentle probing of these possibilities can help strengthen the supervisor–supervisee relationship by building honesty, trust, and rapport:

> SUPERVISOR: Dr. Banks, I notice that you've had some trouble making it to our sessions. We moved to this time so that you'd be able to make it over from the hospital. I notice that hasn't worked. How are you doing?
>
> DR. BANKS: I know, I know! I'm so sorry! I just couldn't ask my attending to leave. She just kept talking and talking, and I was trapped there. I was watching the clock the whole time, and I knew I had to leave, but I couldn't find the right time to say something.
>
> SUPERVISOR: Ah, okay. What do you imagine your attending would have said if you let her know you had psychotherapy supervision?
>
> DR. BANKS: I guess I assumed my attending would be mad at me for asking. But because I didn't even ask, I don't know what she would have said. Maybe my attending was busy and distracted, too. I didn't think of that. Okay, I'll try it next time.

This supervisor helped the supervisee reflect on possible causes for not leaving her workplace on time.

*   *   *

Self-reflection on the part of the supervisor is also important. If the supervisor has modeled laxity surrounding attendance or timeliness, the supervisee may be reflecting this.

> SUPERVISOR [*calling a supervisee who was 15 minutes late*]: Hi, Dr. Canby, I had you down for supervision now.
>
> DR. CANBY: Oh, sorry. I'm headed there now. I didn't think it would be a huge deal if I was late. I can still meet for an hour after I get there.
>
> SUPERVISOR: I'm glad you're on your way. I have only the next 30–35 minutes, so when you get here, let's make the most of that time.
>
> DR. CANBY [*after arriving*]: Yeah, sorry. We just hadn't been meeting regularly so I guess it just slipped my mind.
>
> SUPERVISOR: Yes. I'm sorry I did have to miss last week for urgent patient care, and we planned on not meeting the week before that due to a scheduling conflict. I could see where it felt like I didn't think our meeting regularly was important. Let's make sure this time really does work best for both of us, and we can both make an effort to prioritize supervision.

Here the supervisor acknowledges previous issues with establishing and keeping the frame. Dr. Canby and the supervisor then continue to discuss timeliness and attendance with the understanding of the roles each will play.

> DR. CANBY: Sorry, I'm late again.
>
> SUPERVISOR: I'm glad you made it. This might be a good time for us to go over our roles and expectations again—that we'll meet weekly, at the same time, and talk over relevant issues in therapy and in supervision.

A supervisor operating in a "good enough" fashion can reduce supervisees' anxiety, shame, and self-doubt; increase supervisees' identity development; and help build a sense of efficacy and competence (Watkins et al. 2015). When appropriate, acknowledging and discussing external contributing factors can also be helpful (Enlow et al. 2019).

The Nondisclosing Supervisee

Supervisee nondisclosure in psychotherapy supervision is not uncommon, and its frequency has been inversely correlated with the strength of the supervisory alliance (Gibson et al. 2019). Studies indicate that trainees also may withhold or refrain from disclosing clinical material during supervision (Hutman and Ellis 2020). Outright lies are typically treated differently from nondisclosure or withholding of information and should be reported to the appropriate clinical and educational supervisor.

> Ms. Pardo, a patient being treated by the supervisee, Dr. Dunn, had abruptly stopped coming to therapy. The supervisor and Dr. Dunn agreed that Dr. Dunn would contact Ms. Pardo to discuss the situation. A few weeks later, Dr. Dunn stated that he had terminated with Ms. Pardo. The

supervisor subsequently received a message from the clinic that Ms. Pardo wanted to get back into therapy but had not been able to get in touch with Dr. Dunn to reschedule. Ms. Pardo reported that there had been no contact from Dr. Dunn.

> Supervisor: I got a message that you hadn't called Ms. Pardo back?
> Dr. Dunn: Yikes, okay. No, I didn't. I didn't want to tell you. I didn't think she was appropriate for psychodynamic psychotherapy. I didn't want to see her anymore, and I didn't know how to say that, so I didn't call her back. I worried you'd be mad, so I didn't mention it.
> Supervisor: Oh. I didn't know you felt that way. I'm sorry I made you feel like you couldn't be upfront with me. I want to understand more about why you don't want to work with Ms. Pardo and also understand how we can work so you feel comfortable sharing all of the clinical material with me?

Supervisees are more likely to withhold important information when they are either particularly anxious or have had previously negative supervisory experiences (Mehr et al. 2010). Nondisclosures during supervision often indicate a weaker supervisory alliance (Gibson et al. 2019; Hutman 2015) and have specifically been attributed to difficulty talking with supervisors about the supervisory relationship; supervisees may fear hurting the supervisor's feelings or be reluctant to share their perceptions of the supervisor's competence (Reichelt et al. 2009). Being a "good enough" supervisor means fostering a positive supervisory alliance, bringing the same nonjudgmental stance that therapists bring to psychotherapy, and showing a warm curiosity about the reasons behind any nondisclosures.

> Supervisor [the next week]: I was thinking about our difference of opinion on Ms. Pardo's case. I thought you were working well with her. I didn't understand how uncomfortable you felt.
> Dr. Dunn: Yes. I've been thinking about it, too. I felt stuck between your expectations for me to work with her and not wanting to share with you my feelings.
> Supervisor: That makes sense. I'm sorry I didn't see it before. Thank you for telling me.

Here the supervisor acknowledges their mistake, which allows Dr. Dunn to be more forthcoming about their own discomfort. Exhibiting composure and humility allows the supervisor to demonstrate "good enough" supervising by modeling how to reflect on a conflict and openly address what has not been said.

*   *   *

While nondisclosure might stem from a variety of sources, such as anxiety, forgetfulness, or misunderstanding, occasionally supervisees will engage in behavior that is intentionally deceitful.

> SUPERVISOR: How is it going with your patient who wanted to move from weekly sessions to once-a-month sessions? Were you able to discuss with them what we'd talked about?
>
> DR. EVANS: Yes. It's fine now. They're still coming to appointments weekly.

[Later the supervisor discovers that Dr. Evans's patient quit treatment some time ago.]

> SUPERVISOR *[at the next supervision]*: I thought you said that your patient was coming in weekly? I looked, and the patient has quit altogether.
>
> DR. EVANS: You must have misunderstood what I said.
>
> SUPERVISOR: I have a different experience, and I'm concerned that we have had this level of misunderstanding. Could you help me understand what is going on?

Intentional deceit or lying may reflect a variety of underlying issues in the supervisory relationship:

- Lying in supervision may "function both as an expression of and a defense against the trainee's own retaliatory impulses" toward the supervisor or as a way to set a boundary when not feeling safe to have a discussion in supervision (Hantoot 2000, p. 182).
- The specter of shame in psychotherapy supervision should also be attended to. Previous strains or ruptures in the working alliance and negative supervisory experiences could also be formulated as shaming experiences contributing to nondisclosure (Yourman 2003).
- Supervisees can withhold information that might make the supervisor dislike a patient, especially if the supervisee likes the patient. This can also be observed in clinical case presentations, where trainees may withhold information from the group that they worry would turn the group members against the patient.
- Supervisees may withhold information as a manifestation of parallel process. For example, patients who repeatedly lie to their therapists create a dynamic of deception that therapists may then unconsciously reenact with supervisors.

If lying persists, it may represent a deeper rupture in the relationship or a more severe character pathology on the part of the supervisee. Discussion with leadership in the residency training personnel may be warranted in terms of professional sanctions. If the basic foundational trust has been breached, the only recourse may be to end the supervision.

The Incurious Supervisee

A trainee, Dr. Frost, has been in supervision for several months. His supervisor notices that Dr. Frost struggles to bring topics for discussion into supervision, does not seem curious about his patients' inner lives, and generally gives advice to patients rather than using more psychodynamic interventions such as active listening and reframing of content.

SUPERVISOR: So tell me what's going on with your patient.

DR. FROST: She's fine.

SUPERVISOR: Okay, great! In my notes from our last week's supervision, you had talked with her about her relationship with her parents. What has transpired?

DR. FROST: Oh, we didn't talk about that this week.

SUPERVISOR: Okay. What did you talk about in session?

DR. FROST: Her job is stressful, but she said she tried the journaling I suggested.

SUPERVISOR: Could you tell me a little more about the job situation?

DR. FROST: Her boss is mean to her.

SUPERVISOR: Oh, interesting. What connections can you make with her upbringing?

DR. FROST: I hadn't thought about it.

SUPERVISOR: That's fine. We can do it now. Last week you said that her parents had very high expectations for her that she felt like she never lived up to. Is that similar to what's going on at work?

DR. FROST: Not really. It's more that her boss criticizes her for no reason.

SUPERVISOR [gently]: And that is in no way familiar to how she talked about her family?

DR. FROST: Maybe? I guess.

Supervisors can use the supervisory process to model the work that is expected to happen in psychotherapy. In this vignette, the supervisor attempts to help Dr. Frost make connections between historical information and present issues. The supervisor also models curiosity for Dr. Frost, hoping that he will become curious about the dynamics of his patient's symptoms.

*   *   *

When confronted with an incurious or unengaged supervisee, a supervisor can use the same techniques that they would use with a patient to encourage psychological mindedness. Hall (1992) defined psychological mindedness as the interest in and ability for "reflectivity about psychological processes, relationships, and meanings…, across both affective and intellectual dimensions" (p. 131). Developing empathy and curiosity in a supervisee is one goal of a good-enough supervisor. If a supervisee continues to manifest a lack of curiosity in both therapy and supervision, the supervisor can try engaging the supervisee in role-play and practicing with clinical vignettes.

Supervisee mental health issues can also contribute to disinterest in or apathy toward the complexity of their patients' inner lives. Determining whether a supervisee is inhibited or withdrawn because of a current or past experience of shame in supervision and then working through that state can help build resilience to shame (Lane 2020). Specific techniques include acknowledging personal vulnerability and gentle inquiry to explore and validate feelings of shame in the context of the supervisory working alliance (Lane 2020).

The Anxious Supervisee

Timidity or anxiety in supervisees may have many root causes. Therapists might have a temperament that is more reserved, lack confidence in their clinical skills, or disagree with the interventions suggested by the supervisor. The anxious supervisee might lack motivation, a sense of autonomy, or self–other awareness (McNeill et al. 1992). Supervisors should match supervisory interventions to the functional level of the trainee.

> Supervisor: Your patient hasn't paid the bill for the last three sessions. What did they say when you talked to them about it?
> Dr. Graham: I haven't brought it up yet.
> Supervisor: I thought you were going to say something last week?
> Dr. Graham: I was. But I was a little nervous about what I was supposed to say. I know that you think I should, but I feel so weird asking for money. And it seems rude. What if they quit because of it?
> Supervisor: That sounds like something that we should talk over. You have some mixed feelings about talking about the money with your patient and you have some concerns that this would be received as rude, but you also have to handle the bill. That puts you in a bit of a bind.
> Dr. Graham: I guess. I want to do what you told me, but I don't want to be weird—you know, like asking them for money. The last time I did this, the patient said I only cared about the money. I don't want to lose this patient!

This supervisee appears to be functioning with a high level of anxiety, low efficacy, and low independence. Suggested supervisory interventions include structured support and education to enhance supervisees' sense of efficacy in treatment (Stoltenberg 1997). Encouraging discussion of roadblocks or other hindrances and ascertaining the supervisee's understanding of the need for an intervention can generate a conversation about the symbolism of an unpaid fee and the therapist's reluctance to bring up the topic of money. This could also lead to discussions about supervisees paying for supervision (if they are) or the value of supervision.

* * *

More advanced trainees will need a different level of intervention. In the next vignette, the trainee, Dr. Knox, has previously demonstrated exquisite sensitivity to making others uncomfortable. To avoid this anxiety, he often avoids potentially conflictual topics.

> Dr. Knox: Remember last week when I mentioned how my patient Ms. Oliver was discussing her complicated feelings toward her boss and her parents? This week she used some of those same words to describe her feelings about me. So I said, "Ms. Oliver, that is so interesting. I've noticed that sometimes you talk about your manager and me in the same way. I wonder if I make you angry sometimes, like she does?" But I guess I must have missed the mark, because she said that wasn't it at all.
>
> Supervisor: That's a great observation you made. I think you're on the right track. I wonder if you might be correct with your observation even if your patient may not have been ready to talk it over. What do you think?
>
> Dr. Knox: She is very reluctant to be critical of anyone, so I could see that she would not want to feel like she was criticizing me.

This supervisee is able to make connections and is taking steps toward independence and increased self-efficacy. They also are able to bring topics to supervision in an effort to lead the discussion both with the supervisor and with the patient, with some residual anxieties about their abilities.

The Oversharing Supervisee

> Dr. Norton [entering the supervisor's office]: Hi, How are you? My sister came into town last night and we went out and got really drunk. So, I'm really feeling it today!
>
> Supervisor: Oh. Are you feeling well enough to do your clinical work and have supervision now? Do we need to reschedule?
>
> Dr. Norton: Oh, haha, no, this happens all the time!
>
> Supervisor: Dr. Norton, I have to say I'm a little worried about some of the things you've told me. Are you okay?

Most of the vignettes presented so far have highlighted the importance of rapport between the supervisor and the supervisee. In this vignette, however, the key to addressing the supervisee's oversharing is for the supervisor to keep the focus on the tasks of supervision. Some supervisees can mistake the supervisory relationship for one of friendship or clinical treatment rather than that of an educational, mentoring experience. Another important consideration is that supervisees who overshare with their supervisors might also be oversharing with their patients.

> Dr. Norton: I told my patient I'm not going to be there next week because of my trip to Cancun.
> Supervisor: How did your patient take that?
> Dr. Norton: He laughed and told me to have fun, to not do anything he wouldn't do.
> Supervisor: I wonder what he meant by that?
> Dr. Norton: Oh, he didn't mean anything by it.
> Supervisor: Okay. Did you mention to your other patients where you were going?
> Dr. Norton: Yeah, I told all of them. I feel bad keeping secrets from them.
> Supervisor: This is very interesting to me.
> Dr. Norton: I feel bad for abandoning them. I feel like they should know, even if it makes them mad.
> Supervisor: Did someone get mad at you?
> Dr. Norton: You remember Ms. Wood? She said it was a waste of money and that I'd be better off paying my student loans. And that she didn't know if she'd be able to keep coming. Oh, no. That's probably something, right?
> Supervisor: Let's keep talking about it. Leaving your patients for vacation seems to be difficult for you.

Dr. Norton's conflicted feelings about leaving her patients for vacation has led her to overshare with her patients. The supervisor can encourage Dr. Norton to consider the impact of this oversharing on the patient and remind the trainee that not all feelings need to be acted upon. The supervisor can explore Dr. Norton's conflicted feelings while encouraging appropriate and professional boundaries in the therapeutic relationship. The supervisor should be watchful for other possible episodes of oversharing and should intervene with a balance of advice-giving and nonjudgmental curiosity, provided that the situation does not call for greater action. (For ethical issues that might arise in supervision, see Chapter 5, "Ethical Issues in Psychotherapy Supervision.")

Difficult Conversations

Both supervisors and supervisees can have difficulties raising issues in supervision and in therapy that may be emotionally laden or charged. Avoidance of discussions about race, health care disparities, religion, gender identity or expression, discrimination, microaggression, disabilities, and socioeconomic differences is commonplace and can impair the supervisory alliance, leading to difficulties in both supervision and patient care. Speaking the unspoken is a cornerstone of psychotherapy, and modeling willingness to engage in fraught conversations for supervisees can be a fruitful way to deepen supervision.

> In the following vignette, a trainee, Dr. Mota, opens the floor for discussion, and the supervisor engages with the content.
>
> > Dr. Mota: My patient was talking about how glad he is that I understand him. He said that when he was talking about microaggressions at work, he knew he didn't have to explain it to me.
> > Supervisor: Oh, that's so important. I don't know that you and I have ever talked about microaggressions in general, or microaggressions at work. What has it been like for you at the clinic? And what has it felt like in here? I hope you would be able to let me know if I've said or done anything that has made you feel uncomfortable.
> > Dr. Mota: Gosh, um. Thanks for asking. I feel good that my patient feels connected to me. But also, it's tricky because he doesn't know that our backgrounds are pretty different. So, it's like we're similar but have divergent life stories. I feel better now that I know we can talk about it here.

A supervisor whose stance reflects cultural humility can strengthen the supervisory working alliance, even when there have been missed opportunities to discuss race, culture, and other aspects of social identity.

Conclusion

Challenges in supervision often reflect problems in the quality of the relationship between psychotherapy supervisor and supervisee. Like the therapist–patient relationship, this relationship is one of the most powerful tools for change. A challenging supervisee often indicates a strain or turbulence in the supervisory working alliance, a lack of focus, or a failure to discuss a difficult topic. Strengthening the relationship and maintaining the focus promote better outcomes in supervision and in therapy, reduce supervisee anxiety, and encourage supervisee independence, efficacy, and curiosity.

Additional Resource

McNeill BW, Stoltenberg CD, Romans JS: The integrated developmental model of supervision: scale development and validation procedures. Professional Psychology: Research and Practice 23(6):504–508, 1992

References

DePue MK, Lambie GW, Liu R, Gonzalez J: Investigating supervisory relationships and therapeutic alliances using structural equation modeling. Couns Educ Superv 55(4):263–277, 2016

Enlow PT, McWhorter LG, Genuario K, Davis A: Supervisor–supervisee interactions: the importance of the supervisory working alliance. Training and Education in Professional Psychology 13(3):206–211, 2019

Gibson AS, Ellis MV, Friedlander ML: Toward a nuanced understanding of nondisclosure in psychotherapy supervision. Journal of Counseling Psychology 66(1):114–121, 2019

Hahn WK: The experience of shame in psychotherapy supervision. Psychotherapy: Theory, Research, Practice, Training 38(3):272–282, 2001

Hall JA: Psychological-mindedness: a conceptual model. Am J Psychother 46(1):131–140, 1992 1543250

Hantoot MS: Lying in psychotherapy supervision: why residents say one thing and do another. Acad Psychiatry 24(4):179–187, 2000

Hutman H: Supervisee nondisclosure: do supervisors' multicultural competence and the supervisory working alliance matter? Unpublished doctoral dissertation, Department of Educational and Counseling Psychology, State University of New York at Albany, 2015 [ProQuest Dissertations Publishing No. 3736285, 2015]. Available at: https://www.proquest.com/openview/eec35b2fefeaea322c25c7597dcae0bc/1?pq-origsite=gscholar&cbl=18750&diss=y. Accessed April 30, 2022.

Hutman H, Ellis MV: Supervisee nondisclosure in clinical supervision: cultural and relational considerations. Training and Education in Professional Psychology 14(4):308–315, 2020

Lane WB Jr: Integration of shame resilience theory and the discrimination model in supervision. Teaching and Supervision in Counseling 2(1), Article 4, 2020

McNeill BW, Stoltenberg CD, Romans JS: The integrated developmental model of supervision: scale development and validation procedures. Professional Psychology: Research and Practice 23(6):504–508, 1992

Mehr KE, Ladany N, Caskie GIL: Trainee nondisclosure in supervision: what are they not telling you? Counselling & Psychotherapy Research 10(2):103–113, 2010

Milne D: Developing clinical supervision research through reasoned analogies with therapy. Clinical Psychology & Psychotherapy 13(3):215–222, 2006

Reichelt S, Gullestad SE, Hansen BR, et al: Nondisclosure in psychotherapy group supervision: the supervisee perspective. Nordic Psychology 61(4):5–27, 2009

Rosenbaum M: Problems in supervision of psychiatric residents in psychotherapy. AMA Arch Neurol Psychiatry 69(1):43–48, 1953 12996131

Stoltenberg CD: The integrated developmental model of supervision: supervision across levels. Psychotherapy in Private Practice 16(2):59–69, 1997

Wampold BE, Budge SL: The 2011 Leona Tyler Award Address: The relation-ship—and its relationship to the common and specific factors of psychother-apy. Couns Psychol 40(4):601–623, 2012

Watkins CE Jr: Pathological attachment styles in psychotherapy supervision. Psy-chotherapy: Theory, Research, Practice, Training 32(2):333–340, 1995

Watkins CE Jr, Budge SL, Callahan JL: Common and specific factors converging in psychotherapy supervision: a supervisory extrapolation of the Wampold/ Budge psychotherapy relationship model. J Psychother Integr 25(3):214–235, 2015

Yourman DB: Trainee disclosure in psychotherapy supervision: the impact of shame. J Clin Psychol 59(5):601–609, 2003 12696135

20

Psychotherapy Supervision During Major Life Transitions

Tina Kaviani, M.D.
Adam Brenner, M.D.

KEY LEARNING GOALS

- Recognize that transitions that occur in the life of the patient, therapist, or supervisor might have a sizable impact on therapy or supervision.

- Proactively address in therapy supervision the potential for unexpected medical or personal issues to affect therapy.

- Understand that supervisors are not expected to always have the "right" answers and solutions for the varied ways these issues can present but that productive discussions of such issues can help the trainee explore their thoughts, feelings, and responses.

- Engage in thoughtful discussions of these transitions in supervision to enhance the therapy being provided and the therapist's professional development.

PATIENTS OFTEN present to therapy with emotional turmoil during or following life transitions. Trainee therapists and their supervisors may also experience the stress of life transitions such as pregnancy, divorce, illness, or living through natural disasters. These events in the life of a therapist can have a profound impact on the therapeutic process. If left unexamined, these stressful experiences can result in emotional distancing, empathic failure, or overidentification on the part of the therapist and can ultimately run the risk of rupturing the therapeutic relationship. Supervisors who are attuned to the inevitable impacts of these major life transitions can provide a safe environment for therapists to discuss the ways in which their personal experiences are intersecting with their work with patients. In this chapter we will review common life transitions and how to address them in supervision. Although the focus here is on how to work with a supervisee who is experiencing these events, it is important to remember that supervisors who experience their own major life transitions should consider reengaging in supervision.

Divorce

Divorce is both a common and an enormous stressor. Recent Centers for Disease Control and Prevention (2022) data indicate that for every 1,000 people who marry in the United States, 450 will divorce. The process of divorce includes separating from the spouse, publicly making the separation known, and coping with the many losses that ensue. Some divorces follow a smooth and low-impact course, although this is generally not the case. More often, the stresses involved in the failing relationship, the public divorce process, and the challenges of learning to live as a single person all have profound effects (Johansen 1993).

The divorcing therapist may experience physiological symptoms of stress, such as changes in sleep, appetite, energy, or concentration. Psychological stress is also common. The therapist's self-image may be affected, leading to feelings of either responsibility or abandonment, depending on the reasons for the divorce, as well as questioning of one's worth as a partner or a therapist. Social supports can mitigate these stresses, but sometimes the therapist's community can make things harder. Some therapists may experience criticism from their religious communities, difficulties with the legal system, and loss of support from extended family and friends (Johansen 1993).

Because loss is so central to divorce, the process of coping often follows stages of mourning, which include denial, protest, despair, and detachment. Therapists' need and ability to transition through these stages will have an impact on the therapy they provide (Pappas 1989). When working with supervisees who are divorcing, it is important for supervisors to help them work through the inevitable changes that will affect them and their patients. If the psychological and physiological stresses accumulate to the level of an actual depression, the supervisor's role will include suggesting or referring the trainee for treatment.

It is important for supervisors to be familiar with and ready to discuss the ways that divorce can potentially affect the therapist's clinical work. We focus here on four potential effects: 1) decreased emotional availability, 2) diminished hopefulness for the future, 3) compromised neutrality in listening, and 4) use of a patient as a narcissistic object.

Decreased Emotional Availability

Physiological changes have a direct impact on our availability to our patients. Feeling tired or preoccupied results in limited energy for the patient and difficulty sustaining attention to the patient's material in session. Therapists may cancel or reschedule appointments due to not feeling well or being burdened with divorce proceedings. In session they may be distracted or inattentive, and their listening becomes more concrete, focused on explaining reality rather than on exploring meanings (Johansen 1993). Supervisors can emphasize the time-limited nature of this process and point out the general resilience of therapies that have a solid foundation. Most treatments will tolerate—within limits—the inevitable waxing and waning of emotional presence that is tied up with the therapist's own inner life.

Diminished Hopefulness for the Future

Much of the positive impact of any therapy is derived from the therapeutic factors common to all therapies. A central component is the hope that is engendered in the patient by forming a therapeutic alliance and having a mutually accepted treatment plan. Often, in the face of the patient's resistance and doubts, the therapist supplies the vision of possible change that sustains the work. Loewald (1960) likened this vision to the way that parents simultaneously see their children as they are and as they have the potential to become.

A therapist's divorce can deplete this resource. Therapists may be struggling with disappointment about what their own life has become, and subsequently may doubt what they are capable of in the realms of intimacy, commitment, and so forth. The role of supervisors includes listening to these concerns or bringing them to therapists' attention if they appear unaware of them. Often it will be enough for therapists to have such concerns brought to awareness and normalized. Therapists can then be supported by supervisors in regaining their core position of hopefulness and belief in their patients' capacities for growth.

Loss of Neutrality in Listening and the Potential for Acting Out

Intrapsychic conflicts may have a more direct impact in the form of countertransference, placing the therapist at risk of acting out. As Johansen (1993) noted, "When the patient is considering or processing a divorce, a great many transference experiences are subsequently expected to evolve. When the therapist is getting a divorce[,] we can expect countertransference experiences to appear in the same manner. The question, then, is not whether countertransference experiences will arise, but which ones, when, and with what changes over time" (p. 101).

One common effect of countertransference experiences is that they make it harder to maintain a position of neutrality (Pappas 1989). Therapists may strongly identify with a patient's plight and rather than explore multiple options, may encourage the patient to take a particular course of action. Alternatively, therapists may strongly identify with the patient's spouse or partner, which would color their reactions to the patient. This could lead therapists to subtly or overtly advocate on the spouse's behalf.

Supervision is of great value here. First, supervisors can acknowledge and normalize the inevitability of countertransference, particularly during times of stress in the therapist's life. Such countertransference is not a sign of pathology, weakness, or moral failure, but rather an opportunity for growth for the patient and the therapist (Johansen 1993). If the countertransference has led to enactment, the supervisor can help the therapist explore how to acknowledge this with the patient. The therapist and the supervisor can then explore together the meaning of what occurred. Supervisors should make clear that although supervision can help therapists mitigate the impact of their stress on the treatment, exploring one's own conflicts is a task for personal psychotherapy.

> Patient B has noticed increasing distance between his wife and himself for some time. He describes a recent "friendly lunch" with a female co-worker. Later in the session, he questions his wife's relationship with a male co-worker and wonders whether she is attracted to him. The therapist, who recently went through a painful divorce after learning of his husband's affair, encourages the patient to consider hiring a private investigator. Instead of exploring the patient's possible unconscious projections of his own wishes onto his wife, he takes the patient's anxiety at face value.
>
> The therapist's supervisor helps him to realize that he was projecting his own experience onto the patient. By identifying with the patient, he was unconsciously trying to undo his own traumatic experience of betrayal.

The supervisor then helps the therapist explore how to acknowledge his "out of character" recommendation with his patient. The therapist helped the patient realize that they had both acted on the patient's anxiety rather than allowing for reflection.

Use of the Patient as an Object

Divorce is a process of grieving influenced by the person's environment and what the divorce means to them about themselves, as a person and as a therapist. A person's ability to grieve is affected by their own object constancy and ego strength, as well as their external supports. In circumstances in which any of these are limited, therapists are at risk of using patients as objects to fulfill their own needs (Pappas 1989). For example, a therapist may turn to a patient for appreciation and admiration in order to relieve feelings of guilt and shame. Therapists should view patient appreciation with the same neutral interest and curiosity as any other reaction on the part of patients. But when therapists are feeling especially fragile or unsupported in their personal life, it can be tempting to draw on a patient's positive transference to fill the void. Supervisors should help therapists to be aware of this slippery slope and to monitor themselves for any steps down it.

> Patient X notices that the wedding band has been missing from her therapist's hand over the past few weeks. She mentions her observation and wonders if the therapist is going through a divorce. The therapist, who had been worried about patients learning of his divorce, quickly replies that answering the question would not have a meaningful impact on her treatment, steering the conversation away from the patient's observation.
>
> Here, the therapist, overwhelmed by the negative implications of his personal divorce, avoids allowing the patient to delve into the meaning of the divorce for her. After discussing the encounter with his supervisor, he is able to readdress the topic with his patient, who was able to associate to fears that the therapist would abandon her, much like her mother did after her parents divorced.

Illness

Over the course of their careers, most therapists will experience a planned or unplanned interruption in their work with patients due to an illness or injury. This experience, which will be processed and dealt with in different ways by different therapists, will have different impacts on therapists' patients. The illness or accident and its direct and indirect consequences will have a meaningful effect on the therapeutic process and the patient. Supervisors may want to explicitly inform trainees that known or unexpected medical issues or personal changes are valid topics of discussion in supervision. If possible, such issues are best thought through and discussed well in advance.

There are so many variations in the types of medical situations that interrupt or disrupt therapy that it can be helpful to have some questions in mind. Is the interruption scheduled or unexpected? A therapist may know in advance of a scheduled surgical biopsy, but not of an urgent appendectomy. Will there be changes in the therapist's physical presentation? Some patients undergoing cancer therapy will experience significant weight or hair loss, while others will not have such visible evidence of illness. Similarly, the recovery from some accidental injuries will require a cast or sling, while others will not. Will the condition be time limited, recurrent, or permanent (Grunebaum 1993)? The impact on a patient's treatment of a time-limited infection versus a chronic intermittent inflammatory disease is very different. The specific circumstances will shape the therapists' physical and emotional availability. Supervision can help therapists think through the longer-term implications of illness or treatments and offer guidance on decisions about exactly what should be disclosed.

One critical question is who would be responsible for notifying a therapist's patients in the case of an emergency that leaves the therapist unable to perform this function? Review of the literature reveals that some therapists have had someone leave a note on their office door, while others have relied on colleagues in the community and even spouses to notify patients of their absence. Generally, these are less-than-ideal options and raise concerns regarding confidentiality. This situation highlights the importance of having a current list of patient contacts accessible to an appropriate colleague or administrator in case of an emergency (Counselman and Alonso 1993). Proactive discussions of this scenario can help prepare trainees for such eventualities, as it will be difficult to sort through the emotions during the time of crisis.

On return to practice after a medical leave, the therapist will need to consider what information to share with patients. In cases where the illness or its sequelae are observable and likely to be commented on by patients, it is generally considered good practice to offer some information. The amount of information given should be tailored to the individual patient. A healthier patient would receive less information, while a more primitively organized patient would benefit from more concrete details (Grunebaum 1993). If there is a likelihood that the therapist's condition will lead to more disruptions or absences in the future, it is better to let the patient know of ongoing medical conditions.

As with other questions around self-disclosure, supervisors rarely have "the answer"; rather, they help therapists think through the costs and benefits of various options. Are there aspects of the therapist's condition that are too personal to share? Supervisors can support therapists in defining areas in which their own needs for privacy are paramount. They can then consider how disclosure will affect the patient's therapy. Will not knowing create so much anxiety and confusion in the patient that exploration becomes impossible? Alternatively, will providing information decrease the space for the patient to fantasize and to explore their own thoughts, feelings, and inner world?

The revelation of the therapist's vulnerability and the potential impact on the therapeutic work can lead to feelings of denial, compassion, concern, abandonment, or anger in the patient (Simon 1990). The circumstances will carry different meanings for each patient and will require the therapist to help explore the patient's vulnerabilities within the therapeutic relationship. This can be difficult, because it comes at a time when the therapist's own defenses against helplessness are challenged, leading to feelings of denial, depression, and anger (Grunebaum 1993). If these feelings are left unexamined, therapists risk denial not only of their own fears of helplessness and mortality but also of their patients' fears. In this sense, therapists would be colluding in denial with patients (Counselman and Alonso 1993).

Another important topic for supervision is the appropriate time to return to work following an illness. Considerations include the therapist's desire and need to work. Whether the motivation to return to work is based on financial concerns, the wish to maintain one's identity as a therapist, or guilt over being unavailable to one's patients, some therapists may feel great pressure to resume working (Grunebaum 1993). These factors can contribute to therapists' returning to work too early, ultimately compromising their long-term availability to their patients. These decisions need to be made during a time of vulnerability, and supervision will provide a vital perspective. Supervisors will help therapists remain objective about their own physician's recommendations and will provide support for being patient and ensuring that the eventual return to work is successful.

> While on a planned 2-week vacation, a therapist experienced a sudden loss of vision and unexplained weakness in her legs. Her workup revealed concerns for multiple sclerosis, although the diagnosis was not confirmed. The therapist regained her vision and strength by the end of her vacation and returned to seeing her patients immediately. In therapy sessions, she found herself struggling to concentrate on what her patients were saying, and frequently asking them to repeat themselves. Her supervisor, also noticing her unusual restlessness, questioned how things were going for her

personally. She started by saying that she didn't want to burden the supervisor with her problems, but went on to describe her recent symptoms and hospitalization. The supervisor encouraged the therapist to explore her experience more, and to be curious about ways her stress might be presenting in her work with her patients. From here, they were able to think together about how to support the therapist as she continued to deal with her medical needs while still working with patients.

Pregnancy

In recent decades, there have been increases in the percentage of female psychiatry residents (American Psychiatric Association 2020). One anticipated demographic effect of this change is an increase in pregnancies among these trainees. Additionally, the impact of "invisible pregnancies" (i.e., those involving partners, surrogates, or adoption) is a potential area in which supervisory discussion can offer support and help.

A therapist's pregnancy will have a substantial impact on both patients and the therapist. The pregnant therapist will experience physical and endocrinological changes, activation of unconscious conflicts associated with the pregnancy, and intrapsychic reorganization associated with becoming a parent (Van Niel 1993). Patients will be faced with an obvious and rather provocative insight into their now-pregnant therapist's life. The separate but shared experience of the pregnancy between therapist and patient must be acknowledged and addressed as being meaningful to the therapeutic process within supervision. An invisible pregnancy can similarly affect the therapist's work but can easily go unacknowledged. In this scenario, the role of the supervisor is to help the nonpregnant but expectant therapist to be aware of the emotional impacts of expecting a baby and to explore how these impacts may affect the therapist's work with patients.

The experience of pregnancy can begin well before conception, when a therapist begins to see themselves as ready for parenthood. Supervisees may disclose their hopes and/or plans directly to supervisors or may keep this information private. In either case, they may begin asking supervisors general questions about balancing work and families, or specific questions about how supervisors might structure their practice to accommodate parenthood (Fuller 1987). The months leading up to conception may be a time of considerable stress for the therapist. Some therapists experience prolonged periods of attempting to conceive, with anxieties about the potential to become pregnant or fears of miscarriages. This period can be quite difficult for therapists, especially if they are having difficulty becoming pregnant and are struggling with feelings of defectiveness or inadequacy, which often lead to wishes to hide or deny the stress they are under. Supervisors should be attentive to subtle cues of this prepregnancy phase, encouraging therapists to acknowledge and explore the potential impacts of these experiences on their work with patients.

Upon becoming pregnant, therapists begin to experience physiological and psychological changes. The therapist may develop a preoccupation with her body, possibly feeling poorly, experiencing excitement and/or anxiety and fear surrounding the viability of the pregnancy early on. These experiences can lead to intrapsychic preoccupations in the therapist that may inhibit her ability to think critically about content brought up in session, or may lead to withdrawing from her patients altogether (Van Niel 1993). The therapist begins to publicly announce her pregnancy, and in supervision brings up the topic of when and how to discuss the pregnancy with her patients. She may ask about the appropriate amount of leave to take and how to plan for being absent. In regard to how supervisors should address such questions, it has been noted that most supervisees are hoping to receive specific, uniform "how to" advice, and may find it frustrating to be told that conversations with patients about the therapist's pregnancy and parental leave need to be tailored to individual patients and their needs (Fuller 1987). Supervision is critical as the therapist navigates the different paths; some patients independently may notice her visible changes, while others require being told about the pregnancy by the therapist.

> Patient F's therapist has rescheduled their last two appointments. The patient notices that the therapist appears more tired than usual, distracted, and inattentive. The patient then cancels his next two appointments, stating he has a lot going on at work and can't make it in to see her. The therapist is relieved to have some added time in her schedule, as she is 8 weeks pregnant and not feeling well. When she mentions these absences in supervision, the supervisor encourages her to be curious about the meaning of the patient's cancellations. At their next session, the therapist explores with the patient whether there might have been other possible contributors to his cancellation of their last two appointments. Patient F remembered his father's preoccupation with his special-needs brother. He recalls that he was often forced to take care of himself because his father was busy. Together, Patient F and the therapist were able to explore his fear of burdening his therapist, leading him to cancel the appointments. In supervision, the therapist and supervisor explore potential benefits of her sharing her pregnancy with the patient sooner, given his increasing anxieties related to his father.

Encouraging therapists to inform their patients at 4–5 months into the pregnancy generally allows ample time to discuss the patient's experience of the pregnancy (Shrier and Mahmood 1988). Supervision should be proactive and should focus on a plan for coverage while the therapist is away, as well as a plan to notify patients of an unexpected early absence. Patients should be given a time frame for the therapist's parental leave and should be told how they will be notified when the therapist returns to the office. Supervision should include discussion of the possibility that not all patients will return after a therapist's parental leave.

Supervisors should help pregnant therapists to be attuned to the different ways their patients can respond to their pregnancy. Some will perceive the pregnancy before the therapist discloses the information, others will know of the pregnancy but not acknowledge it, and still others will outright deny it (Fuller 1987). Many patients will initially respond with socially appropriate excitement and congratulatory remarks but will come to experience grief, anger, sexual fantasies, sibling rivalry, and/or fear of abandonment. At a time when therapists are experiencing changing perceptions of themselves and conflicts surrounding the pregnancy, supervisors can help therapists hear their patients clearly and respond to their reactions with curiosity (Van Niel 1993).

> Patient G is a 43-year-old unmarried woman with no children of her own. She expressed outward excitement about the therapist's pregnancy, and commented at every session about how "glowingly beautiful" the therapist looked. She was curious about the gender, other siblings, and how the therapist would manage being a mom and a therapist. The therapist, often perplexed about how to respond to these comments, would often answer the questions, or smile in appreciation of the compliments. Upon return from a 12-week maternity leave, the therapist called and emailed Patient G to inform her of her return. The patient never returned to therapy. After reflecting on this patient in supervision, the therapist was able to see how her own discomfort with the patient's comments about her pregnancy and her new role as a mom prevented her from asking about the meanings of her anticipated motherhood and absence for her patient. Had these been explored, it could have helped maintain the therapeutic relationship.

Upon returning to work, the therapist, whether having personally experienced the pregnancy or supported the pregnancy in their partner or surrogate, may experience sleeplessness, confusion about balancing work and parenthood, and deferment of their own needs. Supervision can provide therapists with an opportunity to become aware of their own conflicts and needs while simultaneously addressing their patients' experiences. Some patients may share excitement and have questions about the gender, name, or details of the delivery and parental leave, while others may express anger at the therapist's absence (Van Niel 1993). Supervisors should again be proactive and inquire about potential conflicts, professional strains, and treatment impacts. As was true before the pregnancy, the response to different patients will be individualized. The supervisor's value is not in providing an algorithm for managing these stressors—that would be impossible. Instead, supervision will provide a safe space for therapists to reflect on their personal experience, integrate this with formulations of their patients, and come to their own decisions about specific issues of work/life balance and clinical management.

Natural Disasters

Natural disasters can have varying impacts on the patient, the therapist, and the supervisor. These experiences can be unique to only one of the three parties, or a shared experience among all of them. As defined by the United Nations Office for Disaster Risk Reduction, a *disaster* is "a serious disruption of the functioning of a community or a society at any scale due to hazardous events interacting with conditions of exposure, vulnerability and capacity, leading to one or more of the following: human, material, economic and environmental losses and impacts" (United Nations General Assembly 2016, p. 13). During these times, calls for therapists may increase, the stress on patients may rise, and the emotional and physical availability of the therapist can be compromised.

Memorable recent disasters in the United States include California wildfires, Hurricane Katrina, Hurricane Ian, the ice storms and electrical shortages that overcame much of Texas in 2021, and the COVID-19 pandemic. These natural disasters resulted in loss of life, damage to homes, damage to community infrastructure and services, psychological trauma, and psychological stress of managing the uncertainties around the aftermath (Cooper 2018). For therapists living through these disasters, the potential for indirect impacts on their work with patients is affected by a few key elements, as detailed below.

The supervisor should consider the magnitude of the event itself, the therapist's degree of exposure, the therapist's preexisting vulnerabilities, and the level of support available to the therapist, both personally and professionally. Having understood the context, the supervisor can then assess the supervisee's levels of stress, support, and coping. Providing a space in which supervisees do not have to justify their own emotional reactivity lays the groundwork for inviting supervisees to acknowledge the ways in which they have been personally affected. Supervisors will often need to be flexible and tolerant of lateness, cancellations, or diminished preparation on the part of supervisees (Adamson 2018). Acknowledging the actual consequences of these natural disasters on therapists opens the door to observing possibilities of a shared experience with the patient or the supervisor, and the ways that it presents in the treatment.

> During an unprecedented ice storm, a therapist's home suffered severe damages from burst pipes following the extreme temperature lows and power outages. As a result, the therapist had to relocate his family while awaiting insurance approval for renovations. Patient S experienced similar woes but is single and is able to stay with a friend as he waits for his condo to be renovated. The therapist felt irritable as the patient explained his situation in a matter-of-fact manner. In supervision, the therapist realized that he had failed to explore the degree of distress the patient was avoiding discussing, and speculated that this oversight might have been tied to the patient's having escaped a house fire during his childhood. The supervisor and the therapist wondered together whether the therapist had been envious of his patient's apparent freedom and flexibility. Perhaps the therapist's discomfort with his own envy had been felt as irritability and had blocked him from helping the patient explore more deeply.

Supervision may be limited or unavailable immediately following an acute disaster due to reallocation of resources of the therapist or supervisor (Adamson 2018). While some disasters occur without warning, others (e.g., hurricanes) may allow some preparation. This highlights the importance of discussing the possibilities of these disasters and shared experiences during ongoing supervision or formal didactic sessions as hypothetical experiences. Once the acute phase of the disaster has passed, it can be valuable to check in with supervisees regarding how they are doing personally, and how their patients are doing, to acknowledge the importance of caring for themselves as well as attending to potential impacts on their clinical work.

Another consideration is the impact of the disaster on supervisors themselves (Bauwens and Tosone 2010). This can easily be overlooked in a supervisor's insistence on being unaffected and fully available to their supervisees during a time of crisis. The ability of supervisors to recognize their own needs during trying times, and to seek their own forms of supervision or support, can be a way of modeling for their supervisees the importance of self-care.

Conclusion

As discussed throughout this chapter, major events in the life of therapists can influence and/or become incorporated into the patient's therapy. Supervisors can help trainees understand that their personal experiences matter and can be discussed in supervision. The supervisor's ability to provide a safe, nonjudgmental space to be curious about the therapist's personal experiences is key to facilitating this trusting communication. Here we have addressed life events such as divorce, pregnancy, illness, and natural disasters, although the list of potential events is much longer. Any of these can contribute to exhaustion or burnout in the supervisor, the supervisee, or both (see Chapter 25, "Addressing Exhaustion and Burnout in Psychotherapy Supervision"). Therapists can learn to apply the same curiosity about how their own life experiences appear in their work with patients, ultimately strengthening the therapy.

References

Adamson C: Trauma-informed supervision in the disaster context. The Clinical Supervisor 37(1):221–240, 2018

American Psychiatric Association: General psychiatry residents by sex 2014–2018 (Table 6), in 2019 Resident/Fellow Census. Washington, DC, American Psychiatric Association, November 2020. Available at: www.psychiatry.org/residents-medical-students/medical-students/resident-fellow-census. Accessed February 2, 2022.

Bauwens J, Tosone C: Professional posttraumatic growth after a shared traumatic experience: Manhattan clinicians' perspectives on post-9-11 practice. Journal of Loss and Trauma 15(6):498–517, 2010

Centers for Disease Control and Prevention: FastStats: Marriage and Divorce. Page last reviewed: March 25, 2022. Available at: https://www.cdc.gov/nchs/fastats/marriage-divorce.htm. Accessed August 22, 2022.

Cooper L: Postdisaster counselling: personal, professional, and ethical issues. Australian Social Work 71(4):430–443, 2018

Counselman EF, Alonso A: The ill therapist: therapists' reactions to personal illness and its impact on psychotherapy. Am J Psychother 47(4):591–602, 1993 8285303

Fuller RL: The impact of the therapist's pregnancy on the dynamics of the therapeutic process. J Am Acad Psychoanal 15(1):9–28, 1987 3570911

Grunebaum H: The vulnerable therapist: on being ill or injured, in Beyond Transference: When the Therapist's Real Life Intrudes. Edited by Gold JH, Nemiah JC. Washington, DC, American Psychiatric Press, 1993, pp 21–50

Johansen KH: Countertransference and divorce of the therapist, in Beyond Transference: When the Therapist's Real Life Intrudes. Edited by Gold JH, Nemiah JC. Washington, DC, American Psychiatric Press, 1993, pp 87–108

Loewald HW: On the therapeutic action of psycho-analysis. Int J Psychoanal 41:16–33, 1960 14417912

Pappas PA: Divorce and the psychotherapist. Am J Psychother 43(4):506–517, 1989 2618943

Rollman BL, Mead LA, Wang NY, Klag MJ: Medical specialty and the incidence of divorce. N Engl J Med 336(11):800–803, 1997 9052662

Shrier D, Mahmood F: Issues in supervision of the pregnant psychiatric resident. Journal of Psychiatric Education 12(2):117–124, 1988

Simon JC: A patient-therapist's reaction to her therapist's serious illness. Am J Psychother 44(4):590–597, 1990 2285082

United Nations General Assembly: Report of the Open-Ended Intergovernmental Expert Working Group on Indicators and Terminology Relating to Disaster Risk Reduction. December 1, 2016. Available at: https://www.preventionweb.net/files/50683_oiewgreportenglish.pdf. Accessed March 12, 2022.

Van Niel MS: Pregnancy: the obvious and evocative real event in a therapist's life, in Beyond Transference: When the Therapist's Real Life Intrudes. Edited by Gold JH, Nemiah JC. Washington, DC, American Psychiatric Press, 1993, pp 125–140

21

Sexual Issues in Psychotherapy Supervision

Alyson Gorun, M.D.
June Elgudin, M.D.
Christian Umfrid, M.D.

KEY LEARNING GOALS

- Recognize that sexual issues may arise in psychotherapy and in psychotherapy supervision and should be discussed.

- Understand that the presentation of sexual issues may be influenced by the gender, race, and sexual orientation of the patient, therapist, or supervisor.

- Model the discussion of sexual issues for supervisees, because some trainees may think it is inappropriate to discuss these issues.

- Be proactive in helping trainees to identify sexual boundary crossings and avoid boundary violations.

THERE IS LIMITED literature examining sexual issues between therapists and patients, and even less about sexual issues between supervisors and supervisees. Yet in one survey ($N=575$), 87% of therapists reported experiencing sexual attraction toward at least one of their patients, and 2.5% of female and 9.4% of male therapists reported sexual contact with a patient (Pope et al. 1986). Clearly, the need for supervision around sexual issues in the patient-therapist dyad is crucial (Pope et al. 2006; Van Rijn 2020).

Sexual harassment also occurs between supervisors and supervisees in academic medicine and psychology training (Brown 1993; Dzau and Johnson 2018). Perpetuating factors include a culture of silence and tolerance around harassment, trainee intimidation, concerns about personal repercussions if trainees report witnessing or experiencing sexual harassment, training in settings where trainees feel isolated, and training in settings that are predominantly male and structured around rank and authority (Bates et al. 2018; Dzau and Johnson 2018; Pope et al. 1979). Sexual harassment can have significant detrimental professional and personal effects, including decreased productivity and performance at work and increased levels of depression and anxiety (Dzau and Johnson 2018).

The presence of eroticism and sexual issues within psychotherapy and supervision may be disturbing to trainees. Certainly, it is unethical, and likely detrimental to trainees, for supervisors to act on these feelings (Ellis et al. 2013). However, when discussed and understood as parallel process, eroticism and sexual attraction within a supervisory relationship may provide critical insight into aspects of the relationship between the patient and the therapist that may have been split off (Greaves 2019). In this chapter we describe issues related to eroticism and sexual boundary crossings/violations that can arise during therapy and supervision and offer practical strategies for managing boundaries, addressing boundary crossings and violations, and using supervision to examine and navigate sexual issues in psychotherapy for the therapist-in-training.

Supervision of Eroticism in the Therapist–Patient Relationship

Dr. Ivan, a third-year psychiatry resident, is treating Mr. Graff with psychodynamic psychotherapy. Mr. Graff, a 34-year-old man who has been married to his wife for 5 years, initially entered treatment for anxiety emerging from their attempts to conceive their first child. Mr. Graff reported having frequent panic attacks and difficulty with erectile dysfunction for the first time in his life, prompting him to seek treatment. Over the course of therapy, it became clear that Mr. Graff struggled with the idea of becoming a father, deepening his relationship with his wife, and committing to having a family.

Mr. Graff has reported feeling distant and emotionally detached from his wife since they started trying to conceive a child; he is embarrassed by his recent inability to maintain an erection during sexual intercourse. In therapy, Mr. Graff has made increasingly frequent comments to Dr. Ivan that he feels understood and cared for by her, and he describes a sense of intimacy and closeness that he had not experienced outside of his relationship with his mother. He longs for this intimacy with his wife. Dr. Ivan has found herself blushing in session, feeling flustered, overly self-conscious, and unsure of how to respond to Mr. Graff. She initially attempted to ignore his flattering and at times flirtatious comments, typically avoiding them entirely and choosing to change the focus to other content in the session.

In supervision, the supervisor noted that Dr. Ivan was often terse and inhibited when discussing Mr. Graff, and also seemed uncharacteristically to lack empathy or curiosity about Mr. Graff's difficulties in his marital relationship. The supervisor described this as a potential negative countertransference and asked Dr. Ivan whether there were other feelings that she was having toward Mr. Graff that she was either denying or intentionally not bringing into supervision. The supervisor also described and normalized the idea of erotic transference/countertransference, and wondered if Dr. Ivan was experiencing this with Mr. Graff. Once her supervisor had brought these concepts into supervision and defined them as common and clinically informative dynamics that may emerge in treatment, Dr. Ivan felt relieved of the shame she had been experiencing about enjoying Mr. Graff's flirtatious comments. Dr. Ivan now had both the vocabulary and the nonjudgmental supervisory space to describe what she was experiencing. Dr. Ivan found that this discussion helped her to organize her thoughts, and noted that her earlier discomfort with the erotic transference and countertransference was alleviated. Dr. Ivan also understood that this experience was appropriate to discuss in supervision.

Supervisors can help provide the critical context and theoretical framework for discussions of eroticism and sexual fantasy in supervision (Charlton 2019). Supervisees early in training often report discomfort with exploring sexualized content in therapy and may believe that such exploration is inappropriate and "off limits" (Heru et al. 2004). Here, Dr. Ivan felt shame about the evolving erotic dynamic with Mr. Graff and responded by becoming inhibited, distant, and detached from her patient in an effort to minimize the erotic feelings. Without the supervisor's help in identifying, labeling, and discussing the erotic dynamic, Dr. Ivan may never have disclosed her uncomfortable feelings, and the treatment may have been negatively affected. The boundaries in psychodynamic psychotherapy may differ from those in other treatment modalities in how they address decisions about personal disclosures and aspects of the therapeutic frame (e.g., frequency and location of meetings). In psychodynamic psychotherapy, exploration of eroticism and sexual fantasy is of significant therapeutic utility, while in other psychotherapy modalities, such an exploratory approach may constitute a boundary crossing between therapist and patient.

In supervision, examination of sexual issues can start with a discussion of the distinction between erotic and erotized transferences, and how eroticism can emerge in the treatment. An *erotic transference* involves the development of loving feelings or sexual fantasies by a patient toward the therapist and represents a reenactment of other important relationships from the patient's present or past. The patient knows that these feelings cannot be fulfilled in reality and is able to continue to work with the therapist productively (Gabbard 2014; Ladson and Welton 2007). Erotic transferences arise in therapy for many reasons; one common reason is to avoid other unconscious material that is more anxiety-provoking and/or difficult to acknowledge. Examples include defending against feelings of aggression, hostility, or envy toward the therapist by limiting affective responses to sexual feelings, or avoiding feelings of dependency by sexualizing the therapeutic relationship (Gabbard 2014). In the vignette, Mr. Graff may have sexualized the therapeutic relationship to avoid talking about his marital conflicts. Supervisors can recommend that supervisees simply comment on what is being experienced in the room and gently reassert boundaries when needed. If there is adequate therapeutic rapport, supervisees can begin to interpret the defensive function of the eroticism and gradually progress toward linking this to prior important relationships in the patient's life (Gabbard 2014).

In contrast to an erotic transference, an *erotized transference* is typically misconstrued by patients as *real* and can lead patients to use the therapy to start a romantic relationship, or to act on their sexual desire for the therapist (Blum 1973). An erotized transference can be particularly challenging to work through, and in some cases may require termination of the therapy (Gabbard 2014; Ladson and Welton 2007).

An *erotic countertransference* is the development of sexual or romantic feelings by a therapist toward the patient. Supervisees may feel shame and guilt related to such countertransferences, especially early on in training and prior to attaining an understanding of their dynamic significance. Early in supervision, supervisors can introduce the topic of erotic countertransference and prompt supervisees to reflect on and learn to recognize the phenomenon. Having the supervisor provide education and initiate an open discussion around erotic feelings in a nonjudgmental and curious manner encourages supervisees to look for and acknowledge this potential dynamic in therapies, and (it is hoped) bring the experience into supervision if it is encountered. Supervisors can help supervisees to better understand the role of an erotic countertransference, which can serve multiple functions in a treatment, including as a defensive process (Gabbard 2014) and as a reflection of the past experiences and needs of the patient, the supervisee, or both.

Erotic countertransferences may present in a variety of ways. Gabbard (2014) identified some of the familiar presentations, noting that the trainee therapist who experiences an erotic countertransference may pull away from the patient as part of their attempts to deny or avoid these perceived "inappropriate" feelings, and may appear to be emotionally detached or indifferent. This response can unintentionally harm the patient and potentially limit the patient's progress in treatment. In another reaction to erotic countertransference, supervisees may project their own sexual feelings onto the patient and experience this as the patient's erotic transference. Alternatively, supervisees may unconsciously encourage a patient's erotic feelings as a way to satisfy their own psychological conflicts and feelings of vulnerability (Gabbard 2014). Although supervisors should refrain from being complicit in a supervisee's denial of such feelings by avoiding discussion of the topic, they should also guard against intruding into supervisees' feelings and underlying conflicts, which carries a risk of boundary crossing within the supervision. If necessary, supervisors can suggest that supervisees discuss the erotic countertransference in their own personal psychotherapy.

Boundary Crossings and Violations Between Therapist and Patient

Therapeutic boundaries include limitations regarding the location of the sessions, therapist self-disclosure, the length of sessions, the payment schedule, acceptance or provision of gifts, and nonsexual physical contact (Gabbard 2009; Syme 2003). As in discussions of sexual fantasies, supervisees need to be provided with a framework for understanding boundary crossings and violations in order to feel comfortable disclosing and discussing such events in supervision. Gabbard (2009) differentiated boundary crossings from boundary violations in their extent, severity, and potential destructiveness to patients and their treatment; *boundary crossings* are noted to be typically isolated events that involve little appreciable harm to patients, whereas *boundary violations* may arise from a pattern of behavior, often involve the therapist taking advantage of the power differential in the relationship, and are more clearly detrimental to patients and their treatment (Gabbard 2009). Any form of sexual contact between a patient and a therapist is deemed unethical by the American Psychiatric Association Principles of Medical Ethics (American Psychiatric Association 2013). Such contact would be categorized as a clear boundary violation, given the inseparable influence of the power differential between therapist and patient and the marked detrimental effect that sexual contact would have on the patient (Gabbard 2009, 2014; Van Rijn 2020).

As Dr. Ivan began to speak more openly to her supervisor about the erotic countertransference, supervision was instrumental in her understanding that her feelings were generated in part by the patient. Dr. Ivan also began to reveal more to the supervisor about her sessions with this patient. In this process, the supervisor discovered that Dr. Ivan had deviated from the treatment frame in a number of ways, including extending her sessions with Mr. Graff far beyond their established session length. Dr. Ivan explained that she had found it difficult to cut him off and end their sessions, because he seemed to need the time, to appreciate her interest in and efforts to understand him, and had felt so helped by her.

The supervisor discussed with Dr. Ivan how the extension of time constituted a boundary crossing. Dr. Ivan was surprised to hear this, since she thought of her flexibility as altruistic and a demonstration that she cared about the patient. She came to understand that her actions were both an enactment of her countertransference and also potentially unhelpful to the treatment frame. The supervisor explained how the boundary crossing was likely linked to the erotic transference/countertransference occurring within the treatment, and provided practical strategies for maintaining boundaries, such as how to end sessions on time. The supervisor discussed the possible defensive function of the erotic transference, including how Mr. Graff's sexualization of Dr. Ivan permitted him to avoid painful marital issues and conflicts around having a child with his wife.

In the vignette, Dr. Ivan had extended the time of her sessions with Mr. Graff. There was no overt harm to Mr. Graff, and Dr. Ivan can explore with Mr. Graff why she may have gone over time, making this a boundary crossing rather than a violation.

The role of the supervisor is to help the therapist understand whether a boundary crossing is due to a psychological conflict within the patient, the therapist, or both parties. When a patient makes overt references to wanting to initiate sexual contact with the therapist, the therapist must clearly tell the patient that any physical contact is not possible, while attempting to explore the meaning of the patient's desire and fantasies. More severely ill patients may not be able to discuss the erotic transference, and should be told clearly and concretely that there is no place for any romantic or sexual relationship between therapist and patient (Gabbard 2014). If the therapist is able to explore the erotic transference with a patient, it is critical to be clear with the patient why and how it is being explored. It is important to maintain an "as if" quality to the exploration and to be clear that it is not reality-based. At times, unclear discussions of erotic transference have led to legal action (Gutheil and Gabbard 1998). If supervisees do engage in sexual conduct with their patients, a formal investigation and disciplinary process should be initiated both within the institution and potentially within the larger professional body (Van Rijn 2020).

Boundary crossings can sometimes appear to be benign. For example, self-disclosure—when done with the intent to help the patient and develop therapeutic rapport and *not* in the service of the therapist's own needs—may be therapeutic under some circumstances; however, this remains controversial in the psychodynamic literature, because self-disclosure may intensify a therapist's personal involvement with the patient, may affect the transference, and could lead to further boundary crossings or violations (Meissner 2002). More modern theories take the position that judicious use of self-disclosure on the part of the therapist is essential to treatment.

Nonsexual physical contact is not typically part of the therapeutic process and may be experienced by the patient as sexual in nature, regardless of the therapist's motives (Gabbard 2009). For this reason, nonsexual physical contact is discouraged and should not be initiated by the therapist. When such contact is initiated by a patient, the therapist's decision around engaging in the contact should be made on the basis of the treatment dynamics, including the context of the nonsexual contact, the presence or absence of an erotic transference, and any relevant cultural factors (Gabbard 2009). In general, the sudden occurrence of any nonsexual physical contact during the course of treatment may signal an unspoken dynamic that requires discussion within the treatment. If there is any suspicion that unconscious or conscious erotic feelings are behind the patient's initiation of physical contact, these contacts should be declined by the therapist and further explored with the patient, as well as in supervision (Gabbard 2009).

Several hypotheses may explain why therapists act on their erotic feelings toward their patients. One involves reenactment of a therapist's own psychological conflicts within the therapeutic relationship and the use of sexual contact as an attempt to resolve these conflicts (Gabbard 2016). For example, some therapists may defend against countertransferential hate by turning it into love (i.e., use reaction formation) or have anger toward authority figures, among other possible conflicts (Van Rijn 2020). Under such circumstances, therapists may falsely believe that they are saving or treating their patients, when in reality they are inflicting great harm (Gabbard 2009; Van Rijn 2020). Therapists with high narcissistic needs may use patients for their own gratification—for example, therapists may distort the dynamics and believe that the patient is sexually interested in them and that a sexual relationship would benefit the patient (Coen 2007). Other therapists, who have historically experienced boundary transgressions in important early relationships, may have difficulty maintaining boundaries in other relationships, including those between therapist and patient. Awareness of these theories may help supervisors decide how to intervene with trainees when boundary crossings and sexualized issues arise in the treatment. Supervisors may want to recommend that trainees discuss these issues in their own personal therapy, while remaining vigilant to the potential for sexual contact and enforcing ethical boundaries to protect the treatment.

It is imperative that supervisors help supervisees to establish appropriate boundaries, maintain these boundaries over the course of treatment, and identify boundary transgressions when they occur. Eventually, supervisees will learn how to independently identify a boundary crossing or a boundary violation and will recognize when extra supervision is needed. Common boundary crossings by early-career therapists include extending the patient's sessions, not charging the patient, and engaging in excessive self-disclosure (Gabbard 2009). While seemingly harmless, such minor boundary crossings can still hold dynamic significance for patient and therapist alike, and can evolve into larger and potentially more harmful or pathological issues over time (Gabbard 2009; Strasberger et al. 1992). Supervision can help identify these instances when they occur (Gutheil and Gabbard 1998).

Eroticism in the Supervisor–Supervisee Relationship

Boundary issues that arise in supervision exist within the subjective emotional experience between the supervisor and the supervisee, the power dynamic inherent in supervision, and the professional and educational structure surrounding the relationship (Charlton 2019). Boundary crossings can occur within the supervisory dyad, just as they can between therapists and patients, and can range from inappropriate self-disclosures to expressions of sexual desire and initiation of physical contact. For example, a supervisor's narcissistic need for validation, admiration, and love can potentially lead to boundary crossings and violations (Charlton 2019). Any sexual feelings and conflicts must not be acted upon and must be closely monitored to prevent harm to the supervisee, the supervisory process, and the therapist's work with patients.

Eroticism that develops between a supervisor and a supervisee can be uncomfortable to discuss. In a study by Heru et al. (2004), psychiatry residents and psychology trainees expressed more discomfort than did their supervisors about discussing sexual topics within supervision. Yet trainees also expressed a preference for talking about erotic feelings in supervision as a preventive measure toward not acting on sexual feelings with patients (Gartrell et al. 1988). Eroticism between a supervisor and a supervisee can even be a learning opportunity when it signals a *parallel process* between the supervisor and the supervisee that mirrors an unconscious erotic dynamic between the supervisee and the patient. In such a case, the supervisee may unconsciously assume the role of patient and/or generate a sexualized dynamic within supervision that echoes the dynamic in the therapy (Greaves 2019).

Supervisors may also want to consider the potential origins of any sexualized feelings within the supervisory relationship and should be keenly aware that their own psychological conflicts may generate erotic feelings (Alfandary 2016; Shadbolt 2020). When these feelings stem from supervisors, they should seek supervision and/or personal psychotherapy. If the sexualized feelings are thought to originate with the supervisee, supervisors are advised to review the situation with an outside supervisor before initiating discussion within the supervision. Such a consultation will facilitate a more objective perspective on the dynamics that may be occurring, including parallel process, and will support supervisors in their interpretation of these dynamics.

Boundary Crossings and Violations Between Supervisor and Supervisee

The supervisor–supervisee relationship is inherently hierarchical, given the differences in academic and professional ranking, status within the professional community, levels of experience, and control over evaluations and professional advancement. This power differential must be taken into account if sexual issues were to arise between a supervisor and a supervisee, as what is consensual or nonconsensual can be difficult to ascertain in the context of such a power imbalance. Some boundary crossings between a supervisor and a supervisee may be unavoidable, given the nature of their professional relationships and their ability to see each other in informal contexts (Ellis et al. 2013). At times, given the personal and exploratory nature of supervision, a supervisor may unconsciously force emotional intimacy upon a supervisee (Ellis et al. 2013; Koenig and Spano 2004). Sadly, in a study of fourth-year psychiatry residents ($N=548$), 4.9% reported that they had been sexually involved with psychiatric faculty members (Gartrell et al. 1988). The idea of "harmful supervision" has been written about extensively, and often involves sexual advances and sexual harassment toward supervisees (Bartell and Rubin 1990; Celenza 2007; Ellis et al. 2013; Lamb et al. 2003). The American Psychiatric Association Principles of Medical Ethics states that sexual involvement between a faculty member or supervisor and a trainee potentially exploits the unequal power dynamic and may be unethical (American Psychiatric Association 2013). A sexual relationship between a supervisor and a therapist can be detrimental to the sense of safety, trust, and respect that allows for learning and may also harm the treatment under supervision.

Intersection of Gender, Sexual Orientation, and Race With Sexual Issues in Supervision

Race, gender, sexual orientation, and cultural factors are often overlooked in supervision and may intersect with sexual issues in the therapeutic encounter. When these factors are discussed openly as part of the supervisory framework, supervisees report a better experience in supervision and an improved supervisor–supervisee relationship (Gatmon et al. 2001). In the supervisory relationship, any discussion of eroticism or self-disclosure by the supervisor should be thoughtfully examined in the context of the supervisor's and the supervisee's gender, sexual orientation, and race, including how these factors may shape the experience of the supervisor or supervisee, and be perceived differently by both.

Differences exist between men and women in regard to comfort with and perceptions surrounding discussions of erotic transference. For example, women and transgender therapists may contend with the fear of being put in physical danger from overtly sexual or physically aggressive male patients (Gabbard 2014; Hobday et al. 2008). One survey of 43 psychotherapy supervisors and 52 trainees found that female respondents were less comfortable with self-disclosure within supervision than were male respondents (Heru et al. 2004). This finding highlights the subjectivity of the supervisory experience, and how it may be influenced by the background (including demographic and cultural factors) of the supervisee. Notably, Gabbard (2014) identified a predominance of prior descriptions of erotic transference being centered on female patients holding erotic feelings toward their therapists, and a pattern of male therapists being advised to use the erotic transference superficially or for their own gratification, instead of as an important dynamic to explore in supervision for the therapeutic benefit of the patient. A therapist's use of a sexualized transference for his or her own self-gratification is unethical (Ladson and Welton 2007).

The patient's sexual orientation may influence the expression of an erotic transference and can generate varying responses in a therapist, depending on the therapist's own sexual orientation, among other factors. The orientation of both therapist and patient in the treatment relationship may influence the transference, the countertransference, how sexual issues are approached with the patient, and even how supervision is conducted and can be most useful (Chui et al. 2018). It is important to note, however, that sexual orientation can be flexible in an erotic and erotized transference and that a heterosexual patient can have homosexual sexual fantasies involving their therapist, or vice versa (Gabbard 2014). Supervisees should be helped to feel comfortable discussing their sexual orientation in supervision should they choose to, in order to consider how their own experiences might unconsciously shape the treatment and the countertransference. If the sexual orientations of the supervisee and the supervisor are discovered to differ, the supervisor is advised to be proactive in discussing issues related to sexual orientation, transference, and countertransference (Hodgson 2020).

Overly intrusive questioning of trainees about erotic countertransference without an appropriate context and without enabling supervisees to maintain their own boundaries, comfort, and privacy can lead to unintentional boundary crossings or violations. Such boundary crossings can also interact with race, gender, and sexual orientation, and it is imperative that supervisors remain sensitive to the unique circumstances faced by each supervisee. For example, a Black female supervisee may have had to contend with the stereotype of the overly sexualized Black woman. Questions about her sexual feelings, especially when not carefully constructed, may be interpreted as supporting that stereotype instead of being understood as an exploration of the therapeutic process. Awareness of the intersectionality of these variables is important to ensure that the supervisor–supervisee relationship remains a safe and supportive one.

Conclusion

Educating trainees on eroticism arising in a treatment can be normalized by introducing terms and concepts early on and modeling a nonjudgmental and exploratory discussion of these ideas. Sexual boundary crossings and violations should be discussed openly so that supervisors can effectively intervene if needed. When sexual issues arise between a supervisor and a supervisee, careful thought must be given to the origin of the sexualization, and outside consultation, personal psychotherapy, and explicit discussion in the supervision can be used to understand and remedy these dynamics. The intersection of race, gender, sexual orientation, and cultural variables is also an essential consideration in discussions on this important, complex, and difficult topic.

References

Alfandary R: Transference-love and institutional involvement in a case of psychotherapy supervision. Psychoanalytic Social Work 23(1):60–71, 2016

American Psychiatric Association: The Principles of Medical Ethics With Annotations Especially Applicable to Psychiatry, 2013 Edition. Arlington, VA, American Psychiatric Association, 2013

Bartell PA, Rubin LJ: Dangerous liaisons: sexual intimacies in supervision. Professional Psychology: Research and Practice 21(6):442–450, 1990

Bates CK, Jagsi R, Gordon LK, et al: It is time for zero tolerance for sexual harassment in academic medicine. Acad Med 93(2):163–165, 2018 29116986

Blum HP: The concept of erotized transference. J Am Psychoanal Assoc 21(1):61–76, 1973 4713717

Brown MD: Sexual intimacies in the supervisory relationship. Unpublished doctoral dissertation, School of Education, Boston College, Newton, Massachusetts, 1993

Celenza A: Sexual Boundary Violations: Therapeutic, Supervisory, and Academic Contexts. Lanham, MD, Jason Aronson, 2007

Charlton RS: Boundaries: management of supervisory roles and behaviors, in Supervision in Psychiatric Practice: Practical Approaches Across Venues and Providers. Edited by De Golia SG, Corcoran KM. Washington, DC, American Psychiatric Association Publishing, 2019, pp 315–322

Chui H, McGann KJ, Ziemer KS, et al: Trainees' use of supervision for therapy with sexual minority clients: a qualitative study. J Couns Psychol 65(1):36–50, 2018 28541059

Coen SJ: Narcissistic temptations to cross boundaries and how to manage them. J Am Psychoanal Assoc 55(4):1169–1190, 2007 18246758

Dzau VJ, Johnson PA: Ending sexual harassment in academic medicine. N Engl J Med 379(17):1589–1591, 2018 30207831

Ellis MV, Berger L, Hanus A, et al: Inadequate and harmful clinical supervision: revising the framework and assessing occurrence. The Counseling Psychologist 42(4):434–472, 2013

Gabbard GO: Professional boundaries in psychotherapy, in Textbook of Psychotherapeutic Treatments. Edited by Gabbard GO. Arlington, VA, American Psychiatric Publishing, 2009, pp 809–827

Gabbard GO: Hysterical and histrionic personality disorders, in Psychodynamic Psychiatry in Clinical Practice, 5th Edition. Arlington, VA, American Psychiatric Publishing, 2014, pp 545–576

Gabbard GO: Sexual boundary violations, in Boundaries and Boundary Violations in Psychoanalysis, 2nd Edition. Washington, DC, American Psychiatric Publishing, 2016, pp 33–58

Gartrell N, Herman J, Olarte S, et al: Psychiatric residents' sexual contact with educators and patients: results of a national survey. Am J Psychiatry 145(6):690–694, 1988 3369554

Gatmon D, Jackson D, Koshkarian L, et al: Exploring ethnic, gender, and sexual orientation variables in supervision: do they really matter? Journal of Multicultural Counseling and Development 29(2):102–113, 2001

Greaves CC: The supervision of countertransference, in Supervision in Psychiatric Practice: Practical Approaches Across Venues and Providers. Edited by De Golia SG, Corcoran KM. Washington, DC, American Psychiatric Association Publishing, 2019, pp 305–314

Gutheil TG, Gabbard GO: Misuses and misunderstandings of boundary theory in clinical and regulatory settings. Am J Psychiatry 155(3):409–414, 1998 9501754

Heru AM, Strong DR, Price M, Recupero PR: Boundaries in psychotherapy supervision. Am J Psychother 58(1):76–89, 2004 15106401

Hobday G, Mellman L, Gabbard GO: Complex sexualized transferences when the patient is male and the therapist female. Am J Psychiatry 165(12):1525–1530, 2008 19047333

Hodgson D: Sexual orientation in the supervisory relationship: exploring fears and fantasies when different sexual orientations are present in the client/therapist and/or supervisory dyad (part 2.3), in Working with Sexual Attraction in Psychotherapy Practice and Supervision: A Humanistic-Relational Approach. Edited By Van Rijn B, Lukac-Greenwood J. New York, Routledge, 2020, pp 134–151

Koenig TL, Spano RN: Sex, supervision and boundary violations: pressing challenges and possible solutions. The Clinical Supervisor 22(1):3–19, 2004

Ladson D, Welton R: Recognizing and managing erotic and eroticized transferences. Psychiatry (Edgmont) 4(4):47–50, 2007 20711328

Lamb DH, Catanzaro SJ, Moorman AS: Psychologists reflect on their sexual relationships with clients, supervisees, and students: occurrence, impact, rationales and collegial intervention. Professional Psychology: Research and Practice 34(1):102–107, 2003

Meissner WW: The problem of self-disclosure in psychoanalysis. J Am Psychoanal Assoc 50(3):827–867, 2002 12434873

Pope KS, Levenson H, Schover LR: Sexual intimacy in psychology training: results and implications of a national survey. Am Psychol 34(8):682–689, 1979 496089

Pope KS, Keith-Spiegel P, Tabachnick BG: Sexual attraction to clients: the human therapist and the (sometimes) inhuman training system. Am Psychol 41(2):147–158, 1986 3963610

Pope KS, Keith-Spiegel P, Tabachnick BG: Sexual attraction to clients: the human therapist and the (sometimes) inhuman training system. Training and Education in Professional Psychology S(2):96–111, 2006

Shadbolt C: The disturbance and comfort of forbidden conversations (sexuality and erotic forces in relational psychotherapy supervision (part 2.2), in Working with Sexual Attraction in Psychotherapy Practice and Supervision: A Humanistic-Relational Approach. Edited By Van Rijn B, Lukac-Greenwood J. New York, Routledge, 2020, pp 115–133

Strasburger LH, Jorgenson L, Sutherland P: The prevention of psychotherapist sexual misconduct: avoiding the slippery slope. Am J Psychother 46(4):544–555, 1992 1443284

Syme G: Dual Relationships in Counselling and Psychotherapy: Exploring the Limits. Thousand Oaks, CA, Sage Publications, 2003

Van Rijn B: Firefighting: managing sexual ruptures and transgressions within counselling and psychotherapy services (part 3.2), in Working with Sexual Attraction in Psychotherapy Practice and Supervision: A Humanistic-Relational Approach. Edited By Van Rijn B, Lukac-Greenwood J. New York, Routledge, 2020, pp 177–194

22

Dealing With Death and Suicide in Psychotherapy Supervision

Michael F. Myers, M.D.

KEY LEARNING GOALS

- Recognize that death of one's patient, whatever the cause, can be one of the most stressful events faced by supervisees in their professional career and presents a major challenge for psychotherapy supervisors.

- Understand that dealing with this potentially devastating event in supervision may require consultation with outside experts and may involve use of specific postvention strategies.

- Appreciate that posttraumatic growth is possible when supervisees feel confident in their supervisor's guidance, clinical maturity, honesty, empathy, and commitment to the process.

Dr. R, a senior psychiatrist at an East Coast medical school, has lost three patients from his private practice to suicide over his lengthy career. "All of these suicides were anxiety-provoking for me, including some sleeplessness and PTSD-type symptoms over the following months." Dr. R has borrowed themes from each of these experiences to enhance psychotherapy supervision of trainees:

1. Using finesse in outreach to the family in the face of hospital lawyers' admonitions,
2. Attending funerals and the healing that ensues,
3. Acknowledging that patients who are determined to kill themselves will employ clever falsehoods,
4. Realizing that some patients are incapable of forming a therapeutic alliance because of their personality deficits, and
5. Lauding the restorative value of posttraumatic growth after suicide.

Surveys have documented that many physicians struggle with and are reluctant to discuss patient death and dying (Caldwell and Mishara 1973). In survey studies, this fear of a patient's death, or "death anxiety," was found to be greatest among physicians who were younger and less experienced (Kane and Hogan 1985–1986); fear was also higher in female than in male physicians and in psychiatrists than in surgeons (Viswanathan 1996). There is evidence that over time, physicians become more proficient in communicating with terminally ill patients and their families about death and dying (Dickinson et al. 1999). It would be helpful if education on this topic were a routine part of psychiatric residency training; however, a 1993 study found that whereas slightly more than half of psychiatry training directors reported offering didactics on death and dying in their programs, only about one-quarter of residents remembered receiving this training (DiMaggio 1993).

It has long been known that losing a patient to suicide is one of the most stressful, if not the most stressful, event in a psychiatrist's career (Gitlin 1999). Because many psychiatrists first encounter a patient suicide during residency, chief residents and program directors have been surveyed over the years about this matter. As recently as 2012, only one in five residency programs reported having a postvention protocol in place to support residents-in-training who experience a patient suicide (Tsai et al. 2012). Residents are at high risk of being traumatized by this experience, in part because of exposure and associated vulnerability in teaching centers, scrutiny via morbidity and mortality rounds, critical incident debriefing, sentinel event and risk management procedures, and litigation fears (Agrawal et al. 2021; Cazares et al. 2015). Posttraumatic growth, including increased personal strength, is facilitated by access to a systematic postvention response, guidelines, and support from colleagues, such as in peer groups of experienced attending physicians and co-residents (Agrawal et al. 2021).

Not all supervisors, even those with a good measure of clinical experience and savvy, are comfortable discussing the deaths of psychiatric patients, especially deaths by suicide, with supervisees. If supervisors have not personally lost a patient to suicide, they may have difficulty empathizing with a trainee's tumultuous state or recognizing the depth of turmoil behind the heavily defended persona. If supervisors have experienced patient suicide but have not fully processed, integrated, and grown from the event, their approach to supervision could be anxious or avoidant, and talking about suicide could easily trigger distressing memories for them. Wrestling with an exaggerated sense of clinical responsibility, they may not have acknowledged or incorporated what Appelbaum (2000) described as patients' roles in their own demise or Bishara's (2016) notion of patients having ultimate sovereignty over their own choices.

Basic trust is central to the supervisor–supervisee relationship, but this tenet is too often aspirational. A "good fit" and a high level of mutual regard in this relationship greatly enhance the likelihood that a grieving supervisee will be able to both reveal and discuss this loss in supervision, with resultant clarity, acceptance, and psychological growth. In some programs, not all resident supervision is one-on-one. Supervisors may be tasked with supervising up to three residents simultaneously, all in the same room and sharing the same weekly hour. This situation introduces even more variables that affect full disclosure and trust. Some residents who have lost a patient might clam up completely, while others might feel enabled and less intimidated in the presence of respected peers.

When One's Patient Dies Suddenly

Upon learning of the unforeseen cardiac death of a beloved psychotherapy patient, Lyss-Lerman (2017) found herself alone and rudderless. Furthermore, she writes that "the literature seemed desperately thin."

> Dr. A, a third-year resident, was following a 50-year-old man with depression and multiple medical problems. She had picked up the patient in July, after the annual transition to a new academic year. Although the patient had been suicidal in the past, his mood was much improved from treatment with antidepressant medication and biweekly 45-minute sessions of supportive psychotherapy. Therapy had been interrupted by hospitalizations for osteomyelitis, diabetes, and an above-the-knee amputation. During one of these hospital admissions, the patient had expressed some discouragement and weariness about his deteriorating medical health and made a statement about looking forward to "joining his grandmother," but a suicide risk assessment was negative, indicating low risk. When the patient did not keep an appointment in November, Dr. A summoned the mobile crisis team. Upon arriving at his home, they were greeted by his

daughter, who had just found him dead. Over the next few days, Dr. A's wish to call the daughter was discussed with her supervisor (the physician of record for the patient), who agreed that such a call would be appropriate. The daughter was told by authorities that her father had died of natural causes. Dr. A felt relieved that she was able to comfort the daughter over the phone about losing her father. A review of the medical chart for quality management and oversight found that it was acceptable and that there was no evidence of error. In discussions with her supervisor, Dr. A wondered whether the patient, given his advancing diabetes and his statement about his grandmother, welcomed death and was ready to die.

Helping the Supervisee Process the Loss

The vignette above concerns the death of a patient being treated by a resident that seems relatively straightforward and uncomplicated. Although the circumstances were sad, there was no evidence that the resident did anything wrong in providing psychiatric care to her patient. Furthermore, her clinical supervisor was the physician of record and provided regular oversight of the resident's treatment of the patient. This individual also bears medicolegal responsibility for the patient's treatment. The discussions between the supervisor and the resident both while the patient was alive and after his death were salutary in helping this resident come to terms with the death of her patient. This type of instruction is the bedrock of all clinical learning in our teaching hospitals.

In a situation of this kind, the role of the psychotherapy supervisor may be negligible. In the vignette, the resident was providing follow-up of the patient's care but was not bringing his case to her weekly supervision. Nevertheless, many residents do—and should feel free to—bring up in supervision any major event that might occur with one or more of their other patients. Although the ability of trainees to bring up situations or events they are dealing with serves many purposes, the most important are probably the following:

1. By speaking of events relating to patients whose treatment is being supervised by someone else, trainees can alert their psychotherapy supervisors to important psychological events in their professional life that may be time-consuming, preoccupying, and potentially destabilizing. Such events may in turn affect trainees' attention to and focus on their long-term psychotherapy patients, and it can be helpful for the supervisor to understand that.

2. Trainees' stories about these events can mobilize additional support from their psychotherapy supervisors. Such support can augment the support that is (one hopes) already being received from the attending of record, but in cases where the support from the latter is perceived

by the resident as lacking or off the mark, the response and empathy from the psychotherapy supervisor will be welcome and perhaps even essential.

Transference Dynamics Associated With the Sudden Death of One's Patient

In other situations, the patient who dies suddenly was one familiar to the supervisor because of the duration of the supervision, although the supervisor may not have met the patient in person. The resident's previous experience with death in their personal and professional life will color how the patient's death is discussed in supervision. Some residents will have suffered losses of key figures in their life even before entering medical school and will have a high level of emotional intelligence on the matter. Indeed, some of these may be "wounded healers" whose losses have in part propelled them into medicine, and perhaps specifically into psychiatry. Nontraditional applicants to psychiatry who are older or who have previous training or certification in other branches of medicine will likely have already experienced losses of patients to death. At the other extreme are residents with minimal experience in their personal life but with some exposure to deaths of patients during their internship year of training. Most residents are in between these two poles. It behooves psychotherapy supervisors to be mindful of the unique and mosaic backgrounds of their supervisees. Some of the transference variables (put into the form of questions) that may arise from the sudden death of a supervisee's patient are as follows:

- What is the degree of responsibility assumed by the resident for this patient's death? Is it excessive? Or the opposite? Something in the middle?
- Does the resident speak or act as if they have failed the supervisor? If so, is this overt and articulated? If not, does the resident's body language suggest guilt or shame?
- How is the resident coping with the loss? Professionally and maturely? Really struggling? Regressed? Cool and detached?
- How much insight and psychological mindedness is the resident displaying? Are they able to compare and contrast their current bereavement with the loss of a parent, grandparent, sibling, friend, or a previous patient?
- What about sociocultural issues? In what way(s) might the resident's reaction to the loss be grounded in their race, ethnicity, gender, gender identity, sexual orientation, age, and other related factors?

- In what ways might the resident's previous losses be shaping their comfort with psychotherapy supervision? Are they fairly open, trusting, transparent? Are they formal and guarded? Are they avoidant?

Content from this list might assist the supervisor in constructing helpful feedback and suggestions for the resident. The scope of potential topics is wide, but intentional discussion can enable reflection, professional growth, and gratitude for the experience.

Countertransference Dynamics Associated With the Sudden Death of a Supervisee's Patient

Like residents, supervisors also have lived unique and varied lives and their previous experiences with death will affect their current response. Some countertransference variables (itemized as above) that may arise from the sudden death of a supervisee's patient are as follows:

- How clear is the supervisor's role here? Does the supervisor feel negligent in any way for the patient's death? Is there any suggestion of vicarious loss?
- What is the supervisor's current and past experience with death in their personal and professional life? What level of maturity is being brought to the supervisory dyadic relationship? How much acceptance is there of patient death in both the trainee's and the practicing psychiatrist's career?
- How knowledgeable is the supervisor about death and dying, both didactically and experientially? Is the supervisor certified in death studies (thanatology) or considering seeking such credentialing?
- What is the attitude of the supervisor toward sharing personal anecdotes about their own exposure to and learning from deaths of their patients? Is disclosure measured and selfless, and distinctly not excessive (i.e., healthy)? Or is the disclosure excessive (indicating working through their own personal grief), with potential embarrassment and awkwardness in the resident?
- What culturally, ethnically, and spiritually informed tenets about death might the supervisor bring to supervision? Does the supervisor have healthy and respectful boundaries regarding the death of patients with supervisees?
- Can the early-career supervisor feel confident in a supervisory knowledge, attitude, and skill set that, despite their relative inexperience, helps the supervisee coping with the sudden death of a patient? Conversely, can the late-career supervisor feel confident in their hard-won

wisdom about the process of psychotherapy, despite perhaps a gap of decades treating the same kind of patient as the trainee?

This list should enable supervisors to think about and reflect upon the awesome responsibility of assisting their trainees in coping with the sudden death of a patient. This content can be enhanced with continued medical education, relationships with colleagues, peer supervision, and personal psychotherapy.

Supporting Supervisees After a Patient's Death: Differing Responsibilities of Psychotherapy Supervision Versus Psychotherapy Treatment

It is essential to safeguard the parameters of the psychotherapy supervisor–supervisee relationship. The death of a patient can be destabilizing for supervisees, and it is good supervisory practice to monitor trainees' response. If it appears that residents have become symptomatic or are showing any behaviors that point to undue inner upset, supervisors should suggest that trainees seek personal treatment. Some residents will already be in treatment (and will have shared this), but that fact does not necessarily indicate that supervisors have no part to play. Simply asking residents whether they are discussing the patient's loss with their own therapist can be fruitful. Surprisingly, or perhaps not surprisingly, some residents will say "No, I didn't want to disrupt the frame." Or, "I'm not sure if my therapist is equipped to help me with this; she's not a physician, she may not get it." Or, "I try to reserve my therapy for personal matters, not work issues." Or, "I don't want to upset or burden my therapist with this, he's such an upbeat guy." The best response to these kinds of statements is "I think you should share this with your therapist. You owe it to yourself and your therapist to be authentic and forthcoming."

If the supervisee is not in treatment, the supervisor should watch for the resident's reaction. If they are open to the idea of therapy, then the transition should be smooth. But despite the long history of trainees seeking personal psychotherapy during residency and the institutional acceptance (or recommendation) of such treatment, some residents are ambivalent. Losing a patient, even when there is no evidence of wrongdoing, can still be traumatic for residents, rendering them emotionally vulnerable and cognitively shaky. They may misread the psychotherapy supervisor as rejecting or avoiding them. It is good practice to reassure the supervisee that continuing to talk about the loss is perfectly acceptable, and educational, in ongoing supervision. And one might add that when residents take the time to think about the deaths of patients under their watch, they develop a professional maturity that not only serves them well but also benefits the students they teach.

When One's Patient Is Dying

Much of the discussion above also applies to situations in which the supervisee's patient is in the process of dying. The supervisor assists the supervisee with the reality of what is coming and tracks the content of what arises in psychotherapy with the patient. Not all dying patients can access their feelings in this journey, but some can. Residents will appreciate guidance from supervisors who can help normalize the process of dying and can also provide helpful suggestions that trainees might use in psychotherapy to assist their patients in verbalizing what they are facing. Transference and countertransference emotions can be intense and complicated in therapy with a dying patient, but again, wise counsel from sage supervisors can render this an educationally bountiful experience for residents— and also for supervisors, who can learn much by simply listening to their supervisees. Both the patient and the resident will need to examine all of their emotions, especially those around abandonment and protective defenses, which are a hallmark of this journey. Supervisors can help trainees maintain the focus of therapy and identify important topics that may have been avoided. One of the advantages of being the supervisor is having enough emotional distance from the therapy to notice what is not said by patients.

When the Supervisee Experiences the Death of a Loved One

Dr. B, a third-year resident, lost her 96-year-old grandfather in November 2020. He was in a nursing home and had contracted COVID-19. She had been close to him while growing up, as he did a lot of the child rearing. Dr. B's grandfather had suffered a major decline in his cognitive abilities over the past 5 years and was given a diagnosis of Alzheimer's. While discussing her loss with her supervisor, Dr. B lamented that she had not been able to visit her grandfather in the nursing home after March 2020, saying "Our grief has been colored by COVID." After her grandfather's death, because in-person funeral gatherings were prohibited, Dr. B's "family role" was to host a Zoom service, and she accepted this task with gratitude. All went smoothly, and she was comforted by having her partner, also a resident in psychiatry, by her side.

There is great variation in how much residents share personal losses in the psychotherapy supervision setting. There are no hard-and-fast rules. In the vignette above, this resident was positive about how much support she received from her psychotherapy supervisor, her clinical supervisor, and her personal therapist.

Dr. Natalie Gluck (2005), in a first-person account of losing her father in the early weeks of her third postgraduate year (PGY3), described her experience:

> "I noticed a kind of self-consciousness about being a person in mourning, unsure of what others expected of me. I worried that supervisors would restrain their questions in an effort to avoid the dangerous territory where supervision becomes individual therapy. I worried that my colleagues might interpret a bright affect as pathological. I even scanned the DSM-IV (American Psychiatric Association 1994) criteria for 'abnormal grief reaction' for fear of confirming their suspicions." She expresses gratitude to her fellow residents and her patients. Especially relevant to this chapter is this sentence: "I am grateful for the supervisors who acknowledged my sorrow but respected the work enough to keep me from drowning in it."

When the Supervisor Experiences the Death of a Loved One

> I lost my father when I was an early-career psychiatrist. When I returned to work, I told the residents about my loss, two of whom I was supervising on the inpatient unit of our teaching hospital and two who were in psychotherapy supervision with me. I didn't give a lot of detail, but I did give them a heads-up that I was "a bit wobbly" and not my usual self. I found that this simple disclosure of my vulnerability worked wonders. Not having to "pretend" put me at ease, and to my knowledge, my teaching was fine. In the early weeks, when an occasional wave of sorrow would suddenly wash over me, I could allow that to happen without panic or apology. I remember very clearly an encounter that occurred during a psychotherapy supervisory session. The resident's patient was a college student whose parents were in the midst of a divorce. His father had met another woman, and he was not visiting the patient's family very often. I asked the resident what, if anything, he had said to the patient, to which he replied, "Yes, I used a clarification technique, something like 'It sounds like you really miss him.'" My eyes filled with tears. Seeing my involuntary reaction to those words, the resident understandably looked a bit ill at ease. Without missing a beat, I asked him how his patient reacted to his gesture. He said that his patient got kind of teary. We both started laughing. I complimented him with the affirmation "You're good at this."

I share this personal story as simply one option for supervisors to consider. Not all supervisors will share personal losses with their supervisees. As supervisors, we have a responsibility to take care of ourselves so that we will be able to provide objective and professional supervision of trainees under our tutelage. But ultimately, of course, we are human, and are subject to life's vagaries (Kaplan 1993). Caring for ourselves may mean requesting and availing ourselves of the support of our families and friends, close colleagues (peers) at work, personal psychotherapy, grief counseling, and so forth. And in situations in which the loss is particularly stressful or extreme (e.g., a child, a family member to suicide or homicide, multiple loved ones through an accident or disaster), a leave of absence may be necessary.

When One's Patient Dies by Suicide (or Makes a Serious Suicide Attempt)

> Dr. E, a third-year resident, spoke in detail to the author about the suicide death of his patient, a 59-year-old man with severe polysubstance abuse (cocaine, cannabis, benzodiazepines, alcohol) comorbid with unspecified depression and anxiety. Dr. E was seeing the patient biweekly, but after three or four visits (all virtual), the patient began to pull away. At their last visit, the patient was vague, evasive, and drug-seeking, with passive suicidal ideation but no expressed plan or intent. One week later, he failed to show up for his session and did not respond to telephone calls. A family member called Dr. E and told him that the patient had died, and that suicide was suspected. "I was in shock, but I offered my condolences," Dr. E said. He spoke candidly to the author about his attempts to process the death, which included second-guessing himself, coping with guilty ruminations, obsessively reviewing the medical record, feeling self-consciousness and shame, and having a "paranoid feeling" that everyone knew about his patient. Dr. E then expressed gratitude for the support of his partner, the diligence of his attending psychiatrist and peers, the kindness of his training director, and the value of talking about his feelings in the resident process group. A huge weight was lifted from his shoulders when the internal quality assurance chart review concluded. He said "I felt much less certain that I did something wrong."

In this vignette, the resident felt completely supported from the very beginning, literally within minutes of learning of his patient's demise. He is grateful to his attending psychiatrist, his psychotherapy supervisor (who listened carefully, refrained from interrupting, spoke little, and met with him semi-weekly for the first month), another psychiatrist with expertise in suicide loss, the chief residents, all of the other PGY3 residents, his training director, his partner, and his family. He also found it comforting "in a dark way" when he was told that other residents in the program had lost patients to suicide as well. This information helped diminish his sense of isolation and shame.

Another situation that arises in psychotherapy supervision is when a supervisee's patient attempts suicide but does not die. Although the magnitude of the supervisee's reaction usually correlates with the severity of the patient's attempt, it does not always. Some residents are severely traumatized by the event; they feel responsible, and that they have failed the patient or the family. Some are angry, but they often seem more cross with themselves than with the patient. Because supervisors have more clinical experience than trainees, they can perceive the broader context of the attempt and its dynamic underpinnings. The good news that the patient did not die may fail to reassure or relieve the guilt of the resident. The next step in psychotherapy supervision would be for the supervisor and the resident to examine and explore the conscious and unconscious meanings of the attempt. This might include discussing specific details about the therapy, such as the therapeutic alliance and any misalliances or ruptures; acting out as a defense; resistance, separation anxiety, and problems of attachment; and so forth. For the psychotherapy supervisor, paying attention to and respecting the trainee's hunches and musings are key.

Guidance and metaphorical hand-holding by supervisors will assist greatly, because residents may be fearful that their patient will make another attempt. Trainees often will obsess about this possibility, both for the particular patient who has attempted suicide and for others under their care. Again, the supervisor can assist the resident in creating an enhanced reporting and access-to-care protocol with their patient. Having such a protocol in place will help reassure the trainee therapist.

When the Supervisee Attempts Suicide

A rare but not unheard of event is a suicide attempt by a resident one is supervising. Such an event calls for an empathic and humanistic response on the part of the supervisor, which will be far more helpful to the resident than if the situation were to be handled in an impersonal, purely pragmatic way by the supervisor, the training director, or both. Medical leave may or may not be necessary. In some settings, the supervisor will take over the care of the supervisee's patient; in others, the patient may be transferred to another resident. If the trainee continues in supervision, there will need to be an explicit discussion about the boundaries of supervision and how supervision differs from personal psychotherapy. The focus in supervision will remain on assisting the trainee with their work and education. The health and functioning of the resident must be left to their treating clinician.

Conclusion

It is not unusual for residents to talk about patients other than the ones that the supervisor is actually overseeing. When a patient dies suddenly or they lose a patient to suicide, trainees may welcome the opportunity to use a portion of their time with the psychotherapy supervisor to talk about the loss. However, because the magnitude of such a loss will eclipse the weekly discussion of the trainee's regular patient or patients, supervisees who feel overwhelmed with emotional distress may not feel quite as safe talking with the actual supervisor of the deceased patient, the program director, or their peers. It is advised that the supervisor try to determine how much of the supervisee's distress is reality based (i.e., due to the magnitude of the loss and varying faculty availability) and how much is transferential—although both may apply. If the resident's distress does not appear to be diminishing with the passage of time, it would be prudent for the supervisor to bring up the possibility of individual therapy, but with sensitivity and care, to alleviate any thoughts of rejection that the resident might be harboring. When such discussions are handled well, the transition into personal therapy will be respectful and seamless.

Additional Resources

Association for Death Education and Counseling. The Thanatology Association (www.adec.org)

The Center for Complicated Grief (https://complicatedgrief.columbia.edu/professionals/complicated-grief-professionals/overview)

Clinicians as Survivors: After a Suicide Loss. Suicide Prevention Resource Center (https://www.sprc.org/resources-programs/clinicians-survivors-after-suicide-loss); also Coalition of Clinician-Survivors (https://cinnamon-begonia-rsxy.squarespace.com)

Gutin NJ: Losing a patient to suicide: what we know. Current Psychiatry 18(10):15–22, 30–32, 2019

Gutin NJ, McGann VL, Jordan JR: The impact of suicide on professional caregivers, in Grief After Suicide: Understanding the Consequences and Caring for the Survivors. Edited by Jordan JR, McIntosh JL. New York, Routledge, 2011, pp 93–111

Halifax J: Being With Dying: Cultivating Compassion and Fearlessness in the Presence of Death. New York, Penguin Random House, 2009

Kay J, Myers MF: Current state of psychotherapy training: preparing for the future. Psychodynamic Psychiatry 42(3):545–561, 2014

Myers MF, Fine C: Touched by Suicide: Hope and Healing After Loss. New York, Gotham/Penguin, 2006

Zambrano SC, Chur-Hansen A, Crawford GB: Attending patient funerals: practices and attitudes of Australian medical practitioners. Death Studies 41(2):78–86, 2017

References

Agrawal A, Gitlin M, Melancon SNT, et al: Responding to a tragedy: evaluation of a postvention protocol among adult psychiatry residents. Acad Psychiatry 45(3):262–271, 2021 33686537

American Psychiatric Association: Diagnostic and Statistical Manual of Mental Disorders, 4th Edition. Washington, DC, American Psychiatric Association, 1994

Appelbaum PS: Patients' responsibility for their suicidal behavior. Psychiatr Serv 51(1):15–16, 2000 10647130

Bishara J.: Making peace with patient suicide. Psychiatric News 51(11):1–3, 2016. Available at: https://psychnews.psychiatryonline.org/doi/full/10.1176/appi.pn.2016.6a19. Accessed March 9, 2022.

Caldwell D, Mishara BL: Research on attitudes of medical doctors toward the dying patient: a methodological problem. Omega (Westport) 3(4):341–346, 1973

Cazares PT, Santiago P, Moulton D, et al: Suicide response guidelines for residency trainees: a novel postvention response for the care and teaching of psychiatry residents who encounter suicide in their patients. Acad Psychiatry 39(4):393–397, 2015 26063679

Dickinson GE, Tournier RE, Still BJ: Twenty years beyond medical school: physicians' attitudes toward death and terminally ill patients. Arch Intern Med 159(15):1741–1744, 1999 10448777

DiMaggio JR: Educating psychiatry residents about death and dying. A national survey. Gen Hosp Psychiatry 15(3):166–170, 1993 8325498

Gitlin MJ: A psychiatrist's reaction to a patient's suicide. Am J Psychiatry 156(10):1630–1634, 1999 10518176

Gluck N: Death and life in residency. Psychiatric News 40(15):32, 2005. Available at: https://psychnews.psychiatryonline.org/doi/full/10.1176/pn.40.15.00400032. Accessed March 9, 2022.

Kane AC, Hogan JD: Death anxiety in physicians: defensive style, medical specialty, and exposure to death. Omega (Westport) 16(1):11–22, 1985–1986

Kaplan AH: The aging and dying psychotherapist: death and illness in the life of the aging psychotherapist, in Beyond Transference: When the Therapist's Real Life Intrudes. Edited by Gold JH, Nemiah JC. Washington, DC, American Psychiatric Press, 1993, pp 51–70

Lyss-Lerman P: Grief process following the sudden death of a patient. Am J Psychiatry 174(6):512, 2017 28565959

Tsai A, Moran S, Shoemaker R, Bradley J: Patient suicides in psychiatric residencies and post-vention responses: a national survey of psychiatry chief residents and program directors. Acad Psychiatry 36(1):34–38, 2012 22362434

Viswanathan R: Death anxiety, locus of control, and purpose in life of physicians: their relationship to patient death notification. Psychosomatics 37(4):339–345, 1996 8701011

23

When Lines Get Blurred

Cecil R. Webster Jr., M.D.

KEY LEARNING GOALS

- Understand that the asymmetrical supervisor–supervisee relationship requires a nimble framework of continual self-reflection and attention to maintaining mutual trust for it to be useful for the supervisee's professional and educational development.

- Manage receptivity to criticism, especially when related to emotionally laden areas such as race or sexuality, to ensure a healthy supervisory relationship.

- Recognize the importance of continually assessing your on-line presence, especially if you believe that you *have* no online presence.

- In responding to unanticipated missteps, always lean toward being human and open to feedback, in the same manner that is expected of trainees with their patients.

PSYCHOTHERAPY HAS traditionally relied on well-developed frameworks to protect and promote the work of therapy. These frameworks require careful ongoing observation and reflection by the therapist.

Supervision of psychotherapy similarly has a number of tasks and frameworks. Supervision often takes place between a more-experienced practitioner of psychotherapy and a trainee charged with attaining those skills. Supervision serves complementary and essential functions including the professional development and support of the supervisee, and the cultivation of the supervisee's observation and self-evaluative capacities.

Within the supervisor–supervisee relationship, inherent asymmetries of power converge with the attainment of skill. The area where they meet may seem blurred and contradictory. Understanding common and often overlooked areas of conflict and keeping a supple frame adaptable to real-time critical needs are essential jobs of the supervisor. Embracing the impossibility, for the psychotherapy supervisor and the supervisee, of anticipating or foreseeing every challenge that may arise from their unique relationship is a wise approach. With these important caveats in mind, this chapter will use fictional vignettes to exemplify the complexity of the issues at hand and the potential paradoxes that may arise.

Supervisory Missteps

Dr. Arya Hakim is a fourth-year psychiatry resident who recently inherited a small psychotherapy caseload in the safety-net hospital clinic of his training program. Dr. Hakim received comprehensive sign-outs from the outgoing resident at this clinic and has been assigned a psychotherapy supervisor, Dr. Veronica Williamson, who shares Dr. Hakim's interest in psychodynamic psychotherapy. Dr. Williamson welcomes Dr. Hakim to her office, states her preference for feminine pronouns, and invites Dr. Hakim to offer his preferred ways of being addressed. Dr. Hakim has not previously had an instructor begin a meeting with pronouns, and he is pleased and hopeful that this practice may indicate that his new supervisor will be an excellent resource for insight into his transgender psychotherapy patients. Drs. Williamson and Hakim outline their respective times for meeting weekly, broadly review Dr. Hakim's psychotherapy interests and caseload, and discuss Dr. Hakim's childhood in Los Angeles and their shared love of Korean barbecue. Dr. Williamson is aware that the residency program had suffered the unexpected death of a co-resident and inquires how Dr. Hakim has adjusted and felt about the loss. Dr. Williamson, recognizing Dr. Hakim's last name as Arabic, then says, *"Eid Mubarak*, Arya." Dr. Hakim is initially perplexed; his family is Persian and Jewish and emigrated to the United States before he was born. He was raised in an agnostic household in California. He thanks Dr. Williamson for her salutation but clarifies that he is not Muslim.

What do supervisors do when they inevitably encounter a potentially awkward moment like this? We may understand this interaction and its importance on a number of paradoxical levels. The first major paradox involves the realities within which the supervisor and supervisee operate. It may be prudent for both to acknowledge that they share a reality but also to consider that their respective realities may differ significantly. Dr. Williamson assumes that Dr. Hakim is Arab and Muslim and offers a timely, common holiday greeting. Although her greeting was well intentioned, her assumptions regarding Dr. Hakim's ethnic and religious origins were incorrect, an error that presents a number of challenges. Dr. Williamson has several options for recovering from this misstep, but let us first consider the framework of what has occurred.

The first consideration is the power asymmetry. Dr. Hakim, a trainee, felt trusting and empowered enough to politely correct his supervisor around aspects of closely held identities. In this case, he told her that he was not a part of the Muslim religious community. Other closely held identities besides religion may include national origin, ethnicity, gender, sexuality, ability/disability, or present or past poverty. The exchange between Drs. Hakim and Williamson may be considered a healthy sign.

However, if Dr. Williamson is like many, this reversal of the usual direction of critique, which is in fact a reversal of the difference in power between the supervisee and the supervisor, may create a sense of disruption within the supervisor. It may be prudent for the supervisor to respond in a way that prioritizes the development of trust and rapport with the supervisee rather than focusing on the supervisor's own internal turbulence or reflecting the supervisor's discomfort back onto the supervisee. For example, some individuals in Dr. Williamson's position might outwardly bristle. At worst, others might academically penalize the supervisee under the guise of professionalism. This range of responses may, in fact, simply represent a displacement of the supervisor's own discomfort, shame, or other negative emotions. It is essential that supervisors retain sufficient self-reflective capacity to ensure that their internal disruption does not damage the supervisor–supervisee relationship. Self-reflective capacity may be aided by, for example, consulting with colleagues, or by one's own psychotherapy.

Another possible reaction would be a profuse apology on the part of the supervisor. This response might represent an abreaction to shame in potentially having offended another person in a sensitive area. An ardent, lengthy apology may ironically burden the supervisee with the task of lightening the perceived guilt or brittleness of the supervisor, an outcome likely to result in erosion of the trust and rapport necessary to the shared task of supervision. Such missteps often occur around areas of significant cultural energy, such as race or racial difference, sexual and gender identities, or matters of money. The psychoanalyst Anton Hart (personal communication, July 2021) noted that clinicians routinely listen to a patient's complaints about the clinician with some distance. Complaints about the therapist being dismissive may be solely attributable to a paternal transference, for example, rather than to the therapist's being, in reality, possibly dismissive. Overinvestment in being recognized as good can hamper therapists' ability to explore the ways in which they may, in fact, be having a negative impact.

Therefore, the mere discussion of race, with its difficult and emotion-rich cultural history, may inherently represent a threat to a personal sense of "goodness." A nimble clinician may prioritize providing skilled clinical work even at the cost of personal discomfort, which may include the risk of offense and a momentary loss of "goodness." By extension, we can consider that a good supervisor may prioritize good supervision, creating a sense of trust, rapport, and openness to feedback, over the risk of getting something wrong or the risk of losing their personal "goodness."

In short, correction by supervisees of aspects of their supervisors' understanding of their identities may reflect a healthy and useful level of comfort, connection, or confidence; supervisors must prioritize openness. Dr. Williamson, in this case, may communicate this openness in her response to Dr. Hakim:

> Dr. Williamson straightens herself and replies, embarrassed, "Oh, my apologies, Arya. Thanks for clarifying. I'm happy you could tell me that. Please enjoy the rest of your day."

Dr. Williamson's reply is succinct, starts with a light apology, does not center on her own discomfort, implicitly encourages future corrections, and provides ample room for the flow of their interaction to continue. She might also consider an adroit apology at their next meeting, when the confusion of the moment will have passed. She may even consider a brief email communication to Dr. Hakim as an invitation to discuss her erroneous assumption further at a future time (Table 23–1 offers useful questions for initiating discussion of potentially charged topics in supervision). Although Dr. Hakim felt comfortable correcting his supervisor in the vignette above, many supervisees might have found it impossible to risk the overt or subtle rejection that could result from disrupting the internal world of the supervisor.

Charged Topics in Supervision

Besides the formal psychotherapy curricula offered by training programs, and the informal teaching provided in settings such as supervision, a

Table 23–1. Useful questions and prompts for inviting discussion of difficult elements of supervision

Mutual trust, collaboration, openness to criticism

"It may be helpful to get to know one another. I'd love to hear more about you, and I'd be happy to share a bit about myself."

"Please know that I will get things wrong from time to time. I hope you will feel comfortable enough to bring up differences of opinion here."

"I'd like us to be able to freely express differing views. Perhaps we may have something to offer one another."

Emotionally laden identities

"Some supervisees feel uncomfortable at first talking about things like race or sexuality in supervision. Let's make sure we prioritize those things as best we can."

"What is it like to have a supervisor who is [specific identity (e.g., white, female, Muslim)]?"

"For some people, having a supervisor who is [specific identity] may make it feel easier or more difficult to talk about certain psychotherapy experiences."

"Are there lines of identity that you hold that you feel are important to our work here?"

"Some people encounter difficulties in training with people with $\underline{X}$ identities. Has that affected your experiences?"

Support

"You know, that sounds similar to a dilemma I faced in residency. This is how I thought of it; how do you think about it?"

"I've noticed $\underline{X}$ recently. Is that reflective of something else? How do you imagine I may be best supportive?"

supervisor's behavior may tacitly but powerfully convey a set of expectations, values, rules, and assumptions also known as the "hidden curriculum" originally described by Hafferty and Franks (1994) in psychiatric education. While initially conceived as an ethical framework for the medical education of students, it has since been applied outside of ethics as a tool for providing positive identifications for residents and other learners (Gabbard et al. 2011; Webster et al. 2015). In part due to the asymmetrical power dynamic, the supervisor is responsible for continually offering invitations to keenly observe aspects of personhood that are inadvertently overlooked, charged, or incorrect. This position may potently impart messages about what is important to a skilled clinician in today's world—including charged topics such as race and its frequent avoidance in the consulting room.

Aspects of identity, such as race, are particularly vulnerable to remaining unarticulated. Psychoanalyst Kimberlyn Leary first coined the clinical concept of "racial enactments" to refer to interactive sequences that express (through action or inaction) our cultural attitudes toward race and racial differences. She postulated that America's most significant racial enactment has been its relative silence about race (Leary 2000). Supervisors whose actions imply that discussions of race or racial differences evoke apprehension or shame may come across as defensive or discomfited (which they may or may not notice in themselves). This defensiveness or discomfort may arise between supervisor and supervisee and/or between supervisee and patient. A sense of unease, which may be a result of this defensiveness, may be shared by both the supervisor and the supervisee, regardless of their own racial identifications. In addition, this unease may suggest implicitly or explicitly that the supervisor has a limited capacity to elicit (in themselves or in others) feelings and meanings surrounding race as an important issue in psychotherapy, or a limited ability to examine or tolerate the lived experiences of their supervisees. For example, Black supervisees might note that their white supervisors find it difficult to think or speak about historical racialized violence in America. Similarly, a Japanese American therapist might have difficulty asking about and exploring the parts of a Korean patient's ancestral history that center on Japan's violent Korean occupation.

For supervisees of color, who may routinely experience verbal, behavioral, and environmental marginalization, frequently described as microaggressions (Sue et al. 2007), this misidentification or avoidance of race and its significance may suggest a lack of safety with the supervisor and may also serve to limit the trust and rapport that should form the foundation of their work. Conversely, a supervisor who demonstrates ease in or an aptitude for discussing racial themes may help expand a trainee's clinical capacities or at least help create a greater sense of ease between the supervisor and the supervisee around discussion of potentially charged topics. Many training programs make an effort to pair clinical trainees and supervisors with similar underrepresented racial identities. However, such pairing can lead to another overlooked constellation of misassumptions.

> For the past several months, Dr. Williamson has enjoyed working with another resident in the same program, Dr. Sandy Haynes. Dr. Williamson admires Dr. Haynes's general clinical acumen and practical experiences as a high school teacher before medical school. The two Black women live in the same leafy neighborhood, and their children attend the same small private middle school. Dr. Haynes reminds Dr. Williamson of her younger

self. Over the past several weeks, Dr. Williamson has noted that the normally engaged Dr. Haynes has appeared tired during their noontime supervision sessions. In addition, Dr. Haynes seems surprisingly irritated and subtly brittle in her psychotherapy interactions with her patient, a challenging older law professional. Dr. Williams is aware that Dr. Haynes is the only Black woman in her class and has felt an urge to protect her from the more abrasive elements of the program. Today, Dr. Williamson observes that Dr. Haynes has arrived 20 minutes late to their session and is wearing subtly but distinctly mismatched shoes. She feels uncertain about how to proceed.

One gray area in the supervisor–supervisee relationship involves the paradoxical demands inherent in the supervisor's role. Supervisors are responsible for supporting the personhood of their supervisees (in the service of their professional development) but are also tasked with ensuring that supervisees meet the basic standards of clinical work. This is often complicated by our human nature. Significantly, Drs. Williamson and Haynes share many experiences and identities. Dr. Williamson holds Dr. Haynes in high regard generally and empathizes with her position in her training program. While Dr. Williamson is not certain about the cause of the recent distinct shifts in Dr. Haynes's timeliness and appearance, she might reasonably speculate that Dr. Haynes's Black identity in the program is an important element. Dr. Williamson, in her shared identity as a Black woman, may accurately perceive a punitive environment that may not reach the level of perception by others. She might provide a much-needed resource during challenging periods of training. On the other hand, the identities and experiences Dr. Williamson shares with Dr. Haynes may cause her to misinterpret the significance of the changes she has observed in Dr. Haynes. It is important to note that while more attention is generally placed on easily identifiable and marginalized identities such as race or gender, less attention is placed on privileged identities. It may be far more common for supervisors to lower scrutiny for trainees who share similarly privileged alma maters, languages, socioeconomic statuses, family constellations, or regional origins. Regardless of shared or differing identities, it may be helpful for the supervisor to regularly ask the supervisee about important lines of identity that they both hold that may either facilitate or hinder aspects of their work (see Table 23–1).

What happens in the moment that a supervisor notices details suggesting that her supervisee may be struggling to keep up with her work? As mentioned earlier, Dr. Williamson may prioritize being a good *person* who would like to avoid offending Dr. Haynes, versus being a good *supervisor* who must provide clinical and personal observations, even at the cost of the comfort and camaraderie that the two share. Like those in similar positions, Dr. Williamson may explicitly hold any number of common concerns; for example, she may worry about misjudging or inadvertently exposing Dr. Haynes to academic consequences, or about creating awkwardness in their ease with one another. In contrast, the supervisory relationship, which depends on trust, requires supervisors to provide assistance to supervisees if needed and may also require supervisors to attend to personal aspects of the supervisor and the supervisee. For example, offering vital human connection by congratulating a supervisee on a new child, consoling them after a hard night of call, or even recommending a place where one may get one's hair braided may reinforce a healthy supervisory foundation in which educational attainment may be optimally realized.

However, supervisors are not immune from experiencing tension between the responsibility to nourish their connection with trainees to facilitate growth in trainees' clinical capacities and the responsibility to address important aspects of trainees' clinical capacities that may require improvement. Again, this is especially important when a trainee's capacities have observably eroded. The supervisor's responsibility to attend to the supervisee's clinical performance may prove especially difficult when clouded by an especially personal or personally identified relationship.

Consider specifically that Drs. Haynes and Williamson share marginalized identities. Although Dr. Williamson, as the psychotherapy supervisor, inherently holds greater power, their shared background does not carry a power imbalance in ways that other aspects of their roles and identities might. If supervisors happen to embody historically privileged identities (e.g., white identity, male gender, heterosexual orientation, high academic status), those supervisors would be wise to consider how the additional imbalances carried by these privileged social categories may tint any needed critical messages expressed to their supervisees. In short, the more privileged social categories that a supervisor embodies and the more significantly these categories differ from those of the supervisee, the greater care a supervisor must take when offering critique, criticism, and support. Comments must come from a place of care and ideally should be anchored in a solid and trusting supervisor–supervisee relationship (see Table 23–1).

How might Dr. Williamson tactfully respond to the signs of stress she has noticed in Dr. Haynes? She has a number of options, all of which necessitate tolerating some discomfort. Although such discomfort may be mitigated with approaches such as appropriate self-disclosure or humor, the supervisee's well-being and education must be consistently prioritized.

> Dr. Williamson leans over Dr. Haynes's chair and says, "Sandy, I'm not sure how to say this, but I believe your shoes are mismatched. I remember

all those mornings getting ready before dawn in residency. My first psychotherapy patient pointed out that my heels weren't the same color one morning! I was *so* embarrassed but I was even *more* tired. My attending that day let out a huge laugh when he noticed, patted me on the back, told me, 'We all have those sorts of mornings,' and told me to go home to get some rest. Sandy, is it that sort of morning?"

Dr. Williamson takes a light tone, providing a direct invitation to Dr. Haynes to explore what she has noticed recently and offering a conclusion that Dr. Haynes may politely correct if necessary. This may lower Dr. Haynes's burden to share. Drs. Williamson and Haynes have previously established a trusting relationship. However, supervisors who have a less stable supervisory base may need to take the time to emphasize their desire to care for the supervisee and their receptivity to being corrected.

Self-Disclosure

In work with patients in psychotherapy, use of self-disclosure needs to be considered carefully. In supervision, by contrast, there is less need to limit self-disclosure, and in fact, such communications may often be fruitful. Many supervisees idealize their supervisors in ways that may not take into account the supervisor's humanity and clinical fallibility. Dr. Williamson's offering a story about her own distresses in residency may signal her openness to imperfection (her own and that of others) and provide a warm invitation for Dr. Haynes to elaborate on a shared problem. When used, self-disclosure should be focused on assisting supervisees in their professional development and is most useful when it is reflective of the lived experience of the supervisor. If Dr. Williamson were to witness a shift in their relationship in which Dr. Haynes begins to discuss in more detail their children's shared school, that shift might signal a number of possibilities, including defensiveness around as-yet-unexplored or difficult clinical matters. Conversely, such a shift could reflect a deepening personal connection. In other words, a continual appraisal of the supervisor–supervisee relationship and its shifts is imperative and may open up a wide array of possibilities.

In response to Dr. Williamson's query, Dr. Haynes admits that she has recently been struggling, both with being a new mother and with having the added responsibilities of training. She has noted that her clinical work has suffered slightly but feels that her workload is manageable, especially because her wife has been spending more time at home recently. Dr. Haynes adds that her program hasn't been as flexible as she would like and wonders whether she should finally engage in therapy for herself.

It is not uncommon for supervisors to help supervisees find a therapist for personal psychotherapy. Practically speaking, a supervisor may be in an excellent position to assist a trainee in finding a compatible therapist and starting personal psychotherapy. Supervisors may be familiar with the interpersonal style, disposition, demographic information, and other preferences of a supervisee. Especially when the supervisee requests assistance, the supervisor may aptly identify those who may be a good fit for the supervisee and those best to avoid. However, given the small worlds of psychotherapy clinicians, there may be risks of social overlaps (e.g., next-door neighbors, future instructors, close friends of a fellowship director). A conscientious supervisor may outline potential conflicts and review what types of information may be reasonably kept in confidence. For example, instead of referring Dr. Haynes to her own therapist, Dr. Williamson might recommend a close colleague whom she believes would be a good match for Dr. Haynes. Outlining psychotherapy confidentiality and a general disposition toward tact and privacy may be essential for such a referral. Again, these efforts are best centered on the needs of the supervisee to expand their psychotherapy capacities.

Supervisors sharing common identities and experiences with supervisees can be indispensable and enlivening to the collaborative tasks of developing clinical capacities and professional identities. Some degrees of connection, especially those that revolve around privileged versus marginalized identities, may covertly constrict a supervisor's ability to comprehensively evaluate a supervisee. When in doubt, supervisors should err in the direction of being human and open to criticism, in the same manner that is expected of trainees.

Social Media

There may be other aspects of Dr. Williamson's life that may intrude into the supervisory space. In addition to personal information supervisors may explicitly share, supervisees may indirectly gain a glimpse into the lives of supervisors through their manner of dress and speaking, the vehicles they drive, and the artwork or pictures in their offices.

> Dr. Will Garren has enjoyed his time in supervision with Dr. Williamson. As a fourth-year resident, he has especially appreciated her advice about starting a private practice and negotiating insurance contracts, and he finds her clinical knowledge of child development valuable for his child psychotherapy case. However, he recently followed Dr. Williamson's professional Twitter account and was distressed to discover a number of links to articles calling for greater psychiatric involvement in determining who is eligible for gender-affirming surgeries. Dr. Garren has heard many opin-

ions about gender-affirming surgeries in adolescents. After this discovery, he is not confident that Dr. Williamson is unbiased enough to discuss a request for a letter in support of gender-affirming surgery for his 17-year-old psychotherapy patient.

Social media presence offers an implicit and explicit reflection of a clinician. The advent of social media has played a tremendous role in expanding the observable world of clinical medicine and psychotherapy in general. Many clinicians utilize social media to disseminate useful information about common mental health concerns, lower stigma about what mental health care clinicians do, help make sense of an increasingly complex world, or simply to show a lighter more human side of themselves to friends and colleagues.

Broadly speaking, for younger clinicians who are native to the digital landscape, the difference between online and offline worlds might appear indistinct, with both experienced as ever-present. As educational institutions and training programs increasingly endorse the value of an online presence, it may be impossible for clinicians to avoid social media or consider it a separate, well-circumscribed entity. For many clinicians who have not grown up with the presence of social media accounts and their broad reach, the boundary between the two may feel distinctly different. References to one's online posts in an offline setting, for example, may feel jarring or like a deep intrusion.

Dr. Garren's reluctance to bring up Dr. Williamson's posts may relate to this perception. Perhaps issues of power imbalance and risk of reprisal also linger. The specific issues surrounding adolescent trans identities and gender-affirming health care are outside the scope of this chapter but represent a timely example of a broad, emotionally laden topic in which clinical consensus is currently lacking. These topics are ripe for powerful, expansive, and elucidative discussions under the best circumstances. The power imbalances inherent within the supervisory relationship may work counter to the potential for an enriching exchange of ideas when not attended to by those with higher status. In most cases, this is incumbent upon the supervisor.

One should consider that a supervisor may be unaware of the impact of their words broadly. By extension, we may consider a supervisor's words to include social media posts and responses, or other online content. The reverse scenario, a supervisor discovering provocative online content posted by a supervisee, may allow feedback and discussion to occur within the expected supervisory framework. Again, it may be prudent for the supervisor to be conscientious of a wide imbalance in social categories between a supervisor and supervisee, that may allow feedback given to a trainee to come across more harshly than intended.

Although it is impossible to anticipate every scenario, a basic rule of thumb regarding social media may be constructive: be mindful of your online content, especially if you assume you have no online presence. Supervisors and supervisees would do well to periodically search their online presence. Many people overestimate how private and underestimate how publicly accessible online content may be. Examples of content clinicians should look for include online reviews of their clinical work, posts or tweets by family members or relatives that might refer to themselves, previous letters to the editor in their college newspaper, and real estate and divorce records, in addition to an array of erroneous or misleading information.

Dr. Garren's discovery of gender-related posts by Dr. Williamson may foreclose the dyad's ability to discuss important clinical material. However, if a trusting space has been deliberately established, Dr. Garren may have enough space to bring up this and other uncomfortable questions. Likewise, Dr. Williamson may be unaware of the posts, mistakenly attributed to her, from a similarly named clinician, or she may be prepared to contextualize and elaborate. In any such scenario, providing enough room for uncomfortable questions is at the heart of a healthy supervisory relationship.

Conclusion

Supervision relies on a light and supple framework built on mutual trust and self-reflection. By modeling receptivity to criticism, appropriately grounded self-disclosure, willingness to navigate difficult topics, and humility, supervisors transmit powerful messages about what is expected of clinicians in their professional capacities. Keeping rapport and trust at the core of actions toward the educational development of psychotherapy supervisees provides a compelling north star. Eschewing defensiveness and paying careful attention to areas often overlooked or scrutinized, such as privileged social categories, race, and social media, may enhance those efforts. Relatedly, being a good supervisor necessitates engagement in uncomfortable interactions in the service of the professional development of trainees. Continually assessing connection and the potential for difficult conversations is at the core of the many paradoxical tasks of the asymmetrical supervisory relationship. When these tasks are well attended to, exciting and mutually beneficial exchanges can occur in the muddled, blurred planes of this educationally focused and unique relationship.

References

Gabbard G, Roberts L, Crisp-Han H, et al: Professionalism in Psychiatry. Arlington, VA, American Psychiatric Publishing, 2011

Hafferty FW, Franks R: The hidden curriculum, ethics teaching, and the structure of medical education. Acad Med 69(11):861–871, 1994 7945681

Leary K: Racial enactments in dynamic treatment. Psychoanalytic Dialogues 10(4):639–653, 2000

Sue DW, Capodilupo CM, Torino GC, et al: Racial microaggressions in everyday life: implications for clinical practice. Am Psychol 62(4):271–286, 2007 17516773

Webster C, Valentine L, Gabbard G: Film clubs in psychiatric education: the hidden curriculum. Acad Psychiatry 39(5):601–604, 2015 25476226

24

Legal Considerations in Psychotherapy Supervision

Maya G. Prabhu, M.D., LL.B.

KEY LEARNING GOALS

- Understand the different types of liability to which supervisors are exposed, both because of their own actions and because of the actions of their trainees.

- Become familiar with the landscape of "legal considerations" for supervision, which is ever-changing and is shaped by institutional procedures, case law, statutes, and professional standards.

- Be aware of the circumstances in which outside consultation with a peer, legal expert, or member of the department's forensic faculty is advisable if dilemmas arise in supervision.

This work was funded in part by the State of Connecticut, Department of Mental Health and Addiction Services, but this publication does not express the views of the Department of Mental Health and Addiction Services or the State of Connecticut. The views and opinions expressed are those of the author.

THIS CHAPTER IS intended to provide a framework for legal considerations that may arise in the course of outpatient psychotherapy supervision of psychiatry residents. Because there are many permutations of supervision, this chapter will limit the focus to supervision that is removed from the clinical setting in which the trainee interacts with the patient. The scope of potential legal issues is vast, ranging from malpractice liability materializing from clinical situations to misunderstandings emerging from the supervisor–supervisee relationship to statutory obligations of supervisors. Because no single chapter can address every possible legal or risk management dilemma, further consultation should always be sought from local peers or legal experts.

Integration of Legal Considerations Into Supervision

Most psychotherapy supervisors are keenly aware that in addition to the educative, mentoring, and developmental roles they serve for trainees, they also serve a protective function for patients and third parties. Nonetheless, some psychotherapy practitioners view legal considerations and risk management strategies[1] with a jaundiced eye. Some of this skepticism relates to practice recommendations that have been described as "overly legalistic," "mechanistic," or frankly onerous to the busy practitioner (Kroll and Radden 2017). Other practitioners have pointed out that because there are relatively few examples of litigation involving psychotherapy supervisors, our understanding of risks for psychotherapy supervisors flows from "legal principles involving other medical and paramedical specialties" (Hall et al. 2007). The application of legal considerations and risk mitigation lessons from other settings can be an awkward fit due to the distinctive nature of outpatient psychotherapy supervision. More philosophically, risk mitigation can be seen as antithetical to "the humanistic heart of supervision." It is argued that focusing on legal considerations distracts from the supervisor's most important duty—to instill curiosity, empathy, and the "characterological virtues essential to functioning as an ethical therapist" (Kroll and Radden 2017).

This chapter takes the position that such a stark dichotomy is unnecessary. No practitioner can deny that appropriate risk management strategies and legal awareness are integral to the practice of modern psychiatry. Mistakes on the part of both trainees and supervisors "may have far-reaching repercussions" (Thomas 2014; see also Cobia and Pipes 2002) for all

---

[1] Throughout this chapter, the terms *legal considerations* and *risk management strategies* will be used interchangeably.

persons involved, including third parties who might be harmed (such as the identified potential victim of a homicidal plan). Risk management practices not only shield patients and others from trainee error but hold supervisors accountable. There is no reason to shield supervisees from knowing and discussing these legal obligations. On the contrary, good supervision *requires* both didactic education and the modeling of legal awareness integrated into ethical clinical formulation and management (Barnett 2011; Barnett and Molzon 2014). Ideally, supervisors will demonstrate that it is possible to balance the needs of supervisees, patients, and themselves as supervisors. Supervisors can model practices that go beyond "defensive" or "cynical" measures that merely meet the minimal standards of the profession (Barnett and Molzon 2014). Finally, because supervisees look to supervisors for guidance as they develop their own "inner supervisor" and transition into supervising others, an integrated perspective protects not only current patients but also future patients.

Authors who resist "forensically informed" recommendations about supervision have pointed to the limited published data on psychotherapy liability as evidence that additional precautions are not necessary. Mehrtens et al. (2017) surveyed all program directors of the Accreditation Council for Graduate Medical Education (ACGME)–approved adult psychiatry programs. None of the 64 respondents (out of a potential 189) reported "any knowledge of a lawsuit against a [psychotherapy] supervisor at their institution" (p. 413). This could indeed suggest that the base rate of litigation against supervisors is low, although it cannot be concluded that nonresponders were unaware of supervisor error, academic or licensure complaints, or other negative outcomes.

As outlined by Recupero and Rainey (2007), there are significant financial incentives to include a supervisor in any civil suit. Supervisors are more likely to have greater assets and more generous insurance than trainees themselves. This may secure a larger settlement in a complainant's successful lawsuit. Second, a supervisor's malpractice insurance may cover *supervision*-related negligence in a *separate* claim from that brought against a resident's or hospital's insurance, again, allowing for a larger settlement. Third, there may be circumstances in which neither the resident's nor the program's insurance will cover the damaging acts, such as in intentional torts or sexual misconduct; in these cases, supervision-related negligence may still be an available claim to the complainant.

Given the array of potential legal considerations and theories, one organizing approach is to consider the risk issues at different stages of supervision—before, during, and at termination. The following sections will take each stage in turn.

Legal Considerations at the Commencement of Supervision

Negligent Administration

It is a well-settled legal concept that supervisors are responsible not only for their own behavior with supervisees (*direct liability*) but also for the negligent actions of supervisees with their patients (*vicarious liability*) (Saccuzzo 1997). One form for direct supervisory liability is *negligent administration*. Negligent administration follows from a supervisor's failure to follow program requirements or expectations for supervision as well as any legally required standards. Because there is no uniform standard for supervision across all U.S. states (Riess 2009), supervisors should confirm the requirements of their own state's professional board. Examples of residency program expectations might include the frequency of meetings, the form and content of documentation, or obligations to report resident behavior (Recupero and Rainey 2007).

Surprisingly, despite the foreseeability of liability exposure, Schulte et al. (1997) found that 87% of the training director respondents ($N=118$) to a survey examining awareness of liability issues acknowledged that their psychotherapy supervisors received "no formal training in the risk of liability related to outpatient psychotherapy supervision" (p. 137). The study concluded that "the vast majority of psychotherapy supervisors may be teaching without clear guidelines from their academic institutions with reference to the extent and limits of their liability or about how to conduct supervision in a manner that minimizes potential lawsuits (and hopefully also minimizes risk of inadequate therapy and patient harm)" (Schulte et al. 1997, p. 137).

Well before formal supervision begins, supervisors are encouraged to fully understand the expectations of the residency program, including the evaluation criteria for residents. Inquiry should also be made about the extent of liability protection the program will provide; supervisors may be under the misapprehension that their supervisory activities are wholly protected by the academic program or trainee insurance. Ideally, supervisors would receive program policies in writing. Supervisor documentation of "compliance with those practices" may minimize supervisor risk (Recupero and Rainey 2007). In the absence of up-to-date or comprehensive program guidelines, supervisors should review the most recent recommendations from the Accreditation Council for Graduate Medical Education (ACGME) and the American Psychiatric Association. A published training program for psychotherapy supervisors at Massachusetts General Hospital also identifies core topics for supervisors (Riess and Herman 2008).

Supervision Contracts

Parallel to the formal receipt and acknowledgment of residency policy, some scholars have suggested that supervisors themselves develop a formal "supervision contract" with trainees (some residency programs may provide a template) (Thomas 2007, 2010). Many trainees will be unaware that their supervisors have independent legal obligations arising from supervision, not just potential liability extending from trainees' treatment of patients (Schulte et al. 1997). A supervision contract would enumerate the program's and supervisor's expectations and document the trainee's agreement to the terms. Barnett and Molzon (2014) provided an exhaustive list of supervision contract items, including fees, emergency contact information, the use of audio and video recording, expectations for and limitations on confidentiality, mandatory reporting obligations, evaluation criteria, and policies surrounding termination of the supervisory relationship.

Supervision contracts have been criticized by those who feel that it places the supervisor–trainee relationship on a foundation of mistrust. A more collaborative approach is to frame the contract as an *informed consent agreement*. Viewed in this way, the participation and consent of the competent supervisee is given voluntarily and is understood as an exchange of risks (such as the limits of confidentiality and ongoing evaluations) and benefits (such as the ability to hone clinical skills).

Patient–Trainee Contracts

Many have suggested that residents in turn should obtain the patient's consent to being treated by a trainee, disclose the supervisor's identity, and describe the manner in which patient information will be exchanged. There is some debate about whether supervisors should meet with psychotherapy patients in part to confirm the disclosure. Recupero and Rainey (2007) argued that greater contact can be construed as having greater control over the treatment and therefore opens the door to greater liability; Hall et al. (2007) argued that greater distance cannot be assumed to be protective unless supervisory duties are met. Supervisors could explore this question for themselves by determining the expectations of their residency programs and the practices of their peer supervisors. Patients themselves may assert their right to meet the supervisor (Saccuzzo 1997).

Telesupervision

At the beginning of the COVID-19 pandemic, many states relaxed restrictions on telehealth practice, including "geographic location" requirements, to allow medical practitioners to continue to provide health care services. Psychotherapy supervision similarly moved online, with telesupervision becoming the "predominant way to deliver supervision…as the pandemic has evolved and lengthened" (Phillips et al. 2021, p. 285). A likely legacy of the pandemic will be the continuation of synchronous audio and video supervision, in part for health and safety reasons, but also because of the obvious flexibilities it offers for busy treaters.

Even before the COVID-19 pandemic, numerous legal issues had been raised in connection with telesupervision. Supervision usually involves the transmission of a patient's protected health information (PHI) and therefore falls under the purview of Health Insurance Portability and Accountability Act (HIPAA) regulations, which require protection of the confidentiality of all electronic health information. Not all modalities of video or teleconnection will be considered HIPAA-compatible either by professional organizations or by training programs. Other legal issues include "the lack of consensus regarding who regulates services when the client and therapist reside in different legal jurisdictions, the duty of care owed to the client…, liability risks, and client privacy/confidentiality" (Dever Fitzgerald et al. 2010, p. 181).

Supervisors should inquire whether video supervision will continue to be allowed in their jurisdiction and by their residency programs, either routinely or intermittently. Up-to-date guidelines and state regulations for telemedicine and telepsychiatry can be found on the American Psychiatric Association's Telepsychiatry Toolkit web page (www.psychiatry.org/psychiatrists/practice/telepsychiatry/toolkit) and the Federation of State Medical Boards website (www.fsmb.org). Supervisors should also consult with their state psychiatric societies. Rousmaniere et al. (2014) recommended that supervisors ask which jurisdiction has legal accountability if supervision is conducted across state or international lines; whether their jurisdiction has confidentiality or privacy rules beyond HIPAA; and whether their liability insurance policies cover telesupervision. Practical issues such as note review and co-signing must also be anticipated.

Process Notes

Many supervisors encourage residents to create "process notes" or "psychotherapy notes"; supervisors may create these as well. In order for process notes to qualify for the limited protections allowed under HIPAA, they must be separated from clinical progress notes. HIPAA defines process notes (which it refers to as "psychotherapy notes") as "notes recorded in any medium by a healthcare provider who is a mental health professional, documenting or analyzing the contents of conversation during a private counseling session, group, joint or family counseling session" (45 C.F.R. §164.501). Process notes *must* be kept separate from the patient's medical record. Per HIPAA, these notes may not include information about "medication prescription and monitoring, modalities and frequencies of treatment furnished, [or] results of clinical tests"; or summaries of diagnoses, functioning, treatment plans, symptoms, prognoses, or progress. Process notes are not immune from disclosure by a court order or with a client's authorization (American Psychological Association 2016). Because each state licensing board promulgates its own rules about record keeping and disclosures, providers should review their home state's requirements.

Supervision Under Remedial or Disciplinary Circumstances

Vignette 1

You have been asked to provide additional supervision for a senior resident who has been struggling to meet the expectations of the residency program. The program director is vague on the details, but you are aware that concerns have been raised about the resident's fund of knowledge, timeliness of documentation, and boundaries. When you meet the supervisee, he is eager to leave a good impression and, given the proximity to graduation, eager to ensure that there is a positive evaluation. The resident explains that his anxiety has contributed to the difficulties he is experiencing in the program and asks whether supervision with you could be "more like individual coaching or mentoring."

Riess and Herman (2008), considering Sherry (1991), described supervision as being inherently fragile because of "the power differential of the participants; the 'therapylike' quality of the relationship; and the conflicting roles of the supervisor as educator, overseeing patient welfare, and evaluating the trainee" (Riess and Herman 2008, pp. 261–262). Supervision in remedial or disciplinary cases is particularly complex, ethically and legally. There is considerable evidence that trainee nondisclosure of clinical, personal, and supervision-related issues is a frequent aspect of supervision (Mehr et al. 2010). Supervisees may self-censor for many reasons, including fear of personal criticism or a negative evaluation, which jeopardizes both supervision and treatment (Barnett and Molzon 2014; Ladany et al. 2013). Although the creation of a trusting and safe environment is essential for supervision, a remedial or disciplinary supervision will necessarily be evaluative. The expectations and standards to be met should be thoroughly explored in the supervisory contract/informed consent process.

Clear documentation of the supervision provided may be one step in risk management. Readers may refer to Falender and Shafranske (2004). Both supervisors and trainees would benefit from documenting each supervision session; such records "serve an important risk management role in providing a tangible record of what has transpired in supervision and the supervisor's reasonable good faith efforts to provide high-quality clinical supervision" (Falender and Shafranske 2004 [quoted in Barnett and Molzon 2014, p. 1057]).

Another risk management step may be to provide supervisees with a list of specific critical events about which the supervisor requires swift notification; examples might be disputes with patients, allegations of unethical behavior, threats of a complaint or lawsuit, trainee or patient mental health emergencies, or contact with the patient outside of appointment hours (Thomas 2014). Such required reports may prompt disclosures in supervision; failure to inform the supervisor about one of these critical events could have clear consequences for supervision, the program, or the disciplinary board. Unfortunately, such supervisory cases might be considered potentially higher risk if the trainee has already demonstrated skill gaps. There is no immunity from licensure or board complaints or malpractice claims for supervision of these cases.

Legal Considerations During Supervision

As previously noted, supervisors are considered to be ultimately responsible for the care of the resident's patient. Under theories of "vicarious liability" (sometimes referred to as *respondeat superior*), supervisors are responsible for the actions of their trainees, even actions that are not sanctioned by the supervisor. This responsibility is based on the premise that the trainee acts as an agent of the supervisor or that the supervisor has authority or control over the trainee (Saccuzzo 1997). In the context of outpatient psychotherapy supervision, particularly in the absence of an employment relationship or fee arrangement between the resident and the supervisor, an "agency" relationship can be difficult to prove.

Direct liability, however, represents a much broader set of exposures for the supervisor. In *negligent supervision*, any number of acts or omissions on the part of the supervisor that lead to harm to a patient could be the basis of a claim. Recupero and Rainey (2007) identified numerous pitfalls for supervisors, including lack of awareness of a resident's actions, failure to provide oversight, recommending a contraindicated intervention (e.g., prescribing an addictive controlled substance to a patient with a substance history without adequate assessment), or failure to identify worrisome patterns of behavior to the residency program.

Supervisors who rely solely on the "self-report" method limit their ability to monitor and direct the supervisory relationship and the treatment (Saccuzzo 1997). Resident reports may not disclose deliberate or careless conduct (Recupero and Rainey 2007). Therefore, supervisors are encouraged to undertake multiple efforts to monitor treatment, including chart reviews or taped or live supervision. Documentation of care and the supervision process itself is the best defense against negligence claims.

Other risks that require mitigation may arise due to a supervisee's inexperience. Because supervisees are not yet practicing independently, it is essential that they do not experience any lapses in supervision coverage. If supervisors know in advance that they will be unavailable to supervisees, alternative arrangements or consultative resources should be identified.

Finally, a frequent cause of litigation against psychiatrists is sexual misconduct. Monitoring for dual relationships of supervisees with patients is vital. Although such relationships are not limited to sexual relationships, all such relationships are suspect because of their potential to impair professional judgment and enable exploitation (Saccuzzo 1997). Riess (2009) advocated that residents be taught to avoid dual relationships and learn how to "recognize, formulate, and respond appropriately to sexual feelings and other intense affects."

Vignette 2

Your trainee reports to you that his outpatient psychiatry patient described homicidal ideation during a session; the patient then pulled out a weapon and identified the potential victims with whom the patient had a long-standing grudge. The supervisee, though frightened, sought advice from an on-site clinical supervisor and arranged for the transfer of the patient to a psychiatric emergency room for an evaluation. The patient is currently hospitalized. As you and the supervisee discuss the case, you wonder about what your own reporting obligations are and to whom.

Few scenarios provoke more anxiety for both trainees and supervisors than a patient who expresses an imminent and specific threat and seems to demonstrate an ability to carry it out.

Most residents will be aware of a *"Tarasoff* duty" toward potential victims of homicidal ideation but may not know how to fulfill it. This duty derives from a series of landmark court rulings following the murder of a University of California (UC) Berkeley student, Tatiana Tarasoff. Another graduate student had told his therapist that he intended to kill her; the therapist wrote to the campus police about the threat, but neither the police nor the therapist directly warned Tarasoff. In the civil litigation brought by Tarasoff's parents, the court articulated, first, a therapist's duty to *warn* a potential victim, and then, in a later ruling, a duty to "use reasonable care to protect the intended victim against such danger" (*Tarasoff v. Regents of University of California* 1974, 1976). Since then, states have evolved their own specific duties to warn or protect. There is "substantial state-by-state variation in whether and how the duties are defined and codified" (Johnson et al. 2014, p. 470). Critically, there is no overriding federal duty to warn or protect.

In Vignette 2 above, it is very likely that the resident will have many supervisors or faculty directing them or communicating with them from different parts of the residency program. Liability and risk may be obscured when several supervisors give differing advice about the same patient. These circumstances require careful collaboration with the inpatient team to ensure that the team has full details about the nature of the ideation. The resident should be aware of the inpatient team's discharge planning, including whether the hospital administration's legal advice was sought and whether other notifications (e.g., to police) had been made. Outpatient clinics in training programs frequently have a risk management committee informed by forensic expertise, which provides risk assessment and/or risk management functions; the resident should be advised to notify this committee of the case before discharge from the inpatient setting occurs. There should be comprehensive documentation of all steps taken to notify all parties who will be involved in the patient's ongoing care. Whether there is an independent obligation on the part of the outpatient supervisor to take protective measures may depend on statutory language.

Vignette 3

You are supervising a new resident who has expressed a great deal of interest in social justice issues and health disparities. You think the resident's interests are related in part to the resident's own family migration story and ask with great interest about the resident's personal history. You notice that the resident becomes more withdrawn over the course of the supervision session. Over the next few weeks, you try to explore the resident's interest in cross-cultural issues as they relate to their patients but have difficulty engaging the resident, despite their stated interest in these topics. A few months into the supervision, you are invited to a meeting with the psychotherapy program director where you are advised that the resident has requested a transfer of supervisors, which has been granted. You are dismayed to learn that the resident has reported that you have engaged in a series of "cultural microaggressions"; the resident feels that you have expressed racial bias. You have never faced such allegations before and are wondering what implications they could have. You would like to meet with the resident and "smooth out" any misunderstandings. You had thought you were appropriately drawing attention to issues of cultural identity and cultural competence.

Supervisors should be aware that the norms and language surrounding cultural and racial identity are changing rapidly, especially in academic settings. The value of a multiculturally informed supervision that attends to culture and diversity issues "cannot be overestimated in contemporary practice" (Hook et al. 2016, pp. 150–151). Such an approach has been found to have a positive impact on supervisee development and the supervisory alliance (Hook et al. 2016).

However, the empirical literature also indicates that supervisors may lack knowledge about important identity variables, such as gender, race, sexual orientation, ability/disability status, social class, culture, and religion (Ladany 2014). Racial microaggressions have been highlighted as problematic in supervision (Dressel et al. 2007) especially for trainees of color. These microaggressions are compounded by the power dynamics inherent in the supervisory relationship.

There has also been heightened attention paid to issues of mistreatment, harassment, and bullying in medical education (Hill et al. 2020). The ACGME has mandated that training programs "provide a professional, respectful, and civil environment that is free from mistreatment, abuse, or coercion of students, residents, faculty and staff" (Accreditation Council for Graduate Medical Education 2020). In response, academic institutions have developed comprehensive harassment policy statements and reporting protocols. These documents and procedures generally provide examples and definitions of harassing behavior, outline informal and formal resolution processes, and emphasize the protection of the trainee's confidentiality and sense of safety. Information can usually be found in multiple locations on institutional websites, such as the offices of the Dean of Students, Title IX (Education Amendments of 1972) and DEI (Diversity, Equity, and Inclusion) coordinators, legal counsel, and ombudspersons. In the scenario described in Vignette 3, it is possible that the trainee voiced concerns not only to the psychotherapy program director but also to many other "entry points" into the university grievance process.

Supervisors are encouraged to avail themselves annually of any diversity, equity, and inclusion training that may be offered through the academic institution affiliated with the residency program. Such training often includes institution-specific information about the complaints/incident reporting process, data-gathering procedures, mediation options, and settlement decisions. The pathway to resolution is often determined by the trainee's preferences regarding whether to resolve matters informally or to seek more formal redress.

"Interventions" proposed by the academic department may begin with a "quiet conversation" with the faculty member and may progress to additional training and education, individual coaching, or supervision. Serious cases may be referred to human resources, the campus police, and/ or licensure boards. The question of when and how to seek legal counsel will depend on the complexity of the allegations and the financial means of the supervisor.

Legal Considerations at the End of Supervision

Supervisors and residents will recognize the event of psychotherapy termination as a potentially fraught scenario for all parties. Consensus studies have attempted to identify the elements of "successful termination" (Norcross et al. 2017). In addition to wanting to avoid the patient's internal experience of feeling abandoned, treaters need to avoid the malpractice allegations of legal abandonment of a patient. This is particularly important in situations involving "forced termination," as when a resident is completing training or switching program sites.

A patient abandonment claim in a medical malpractice action involves three elements: "1) the unilateral severance of the doctor–patient relationship by the doctor; 2) without reasonable notice or without providing adequate alternative medical care; and 3) at a time when there is a necessity of continuing medical attention" (PMRS 2021; Van Susteran 2001). The likelihood of a claim of legal abandonment can be reduced if the resident takes the sufficient precautions and documents them in a follow-up letter to the patient. A copy of the letter should be filed in the patient's record. These precautions include reasonable notice that is consistent with state requirements, communication about the risks and benefits of remaining in treatment, resources for alternative treatment, and clarity about when medication prescribing by the resident will cease. There is some case law that suggests it would be advisable to identify a specific next treater and facilitate a meeting or first appointment.

Some state medical boards have additional requirements in the termination process.

Conclusion

The landscape of legal and risk issues relevant to psychotherapy supervision is ever-changing, with case law, licensing board rules, statutes, academic practices, and professional guidelines all shaping the regulatory context. Supervisors are encouraged to think of legal awareness as a core supervision competency that can be developed longitudinally and flexibly in response to changing practice. The consistent implementation of basic principles of supervision outlined by Recupero and Rainey (2007), Saccuzzo (1997), Mehrtens et al. (2017), and the other authors (see References) is likely to assist in mitigation of many liabilities and risks. Supervisors can then model practical and reflective implementation of those principles for trainees in a manner that enhances their supervisory experience. Above all, when in doubt, supervisors are reminded to seek out guidance from peers, legal counsel, risk managers, and program administrators and to act in a manner that upholds their primary obligation to protect the welfare of the patient.

References

Accreditation Council for Graduate Medical Education: Section VI: Background and Intent. Common Program Requirements (Residency). 2020, p 35. Available at: www.acgme.org/Portals/0/PFAssets/ProgramRequirements/CPRResidency2021.pdf. Accessed May 5, 2022.

American Psychological Association: Protecting patient privacy when the court calls. Monitor on Psychology 47(7):64, 2016

Barnett JE: Ethics issues in clinical supervision. The Clinical Psychologist 64(1):14, 19–20, 2011. Available at: https://www.div12.org/wp-content/uploads/2014/01/2011.64.1.pdf. Accessed February 17, 2022.

Barnett JE, Molzon CH: Clinical supervision of psychotherapy: essential ethics issues for supervisors and supervisees. J Clin Psychol 70(11):1051–1061, 2014 25220636

Cobia D, Pipes R: Mandated supervision: an intervention for disciplined professionals. Journal of Counseling and Development 80(2):140–144, 2002

Dever Fitzgerald T, Hunter PV, Hadjistavropoulos T, Koocher GP: Ethical and legal considerations for internet-based psychotherapy. Cogn Behav Ther 39(3):173–187, 2010 20485997

Dressel JL, Consoli AJ, Kim BSK, Atkinson DR: Successful and unsuccessful multicultural supervisory behaviors: a Delphi poll. Journal of Multicultural Counseling and Development 35(1):51–64, 2007

Falender CA, Shafranske EP: Clinical Supervision: A Competency-Based Approach. Washington, DC, American Psychological Association, 2004

Hall RC, Macvaugh GS 3rd, Merideth P, Montgomery J: Commentary: delving further into liability for psychotherapy supervision. J Am Acad Psychiatry Law 35(2):196–199, 2007 17592165

Hill KA, Samuels EA, Gross CP, et al: Assessment of the prevalence of medical student mistreatment by sex, race/ethnicity, and sexual orientation. JAMA Intern Med 180(5):653–665, 2020 32091540

Hook JN, Watkins CE Jr, Davis DE, et al: Cultural humility in psychotherapy supervision. Am J Psychother 70(2):149–166, 2016 27329404

Johnson R, Persad G, Sisti D: The Tarasoff rule: the implications of interstate variation and gaps in professional training. J Am Acad Psychiatry Law 42(4):469–477, 2014 25492073

Kroll J, Radden J: Deconstructing risk management in psychotherapy supervision. J Am Acad Psychiatry Law 45(4):415–418, 2017 29282230

Ladany N: The ingredients of supervisor failure. J Clin Psychol 70(11):1094–1103, 2014 25220894

Ladany N, Mori Y, Mehr KE: Effective and ineffective supervision. The Counseling Psychologist 41(1):28–47, 2013

Mehr KE, Ladany N, Caskie GIL: Trainee nondisclosure in supervision: what are they not telling you? Counselling & Psychotherapy Research 10(2):103–113, 2010

Mehrtens IK, Crapanzano K, Tynes LL: Current risk management practices in psychotherapy supervision. J Am Acad Psychiatry Law 45(4):409–414, 2017 29282229

Norcross JC, Zimmerman BE, Greenberg RP, Swift JK: Do all therapists do that when saying goodbye? A study of commonalities in termination behaviors. Psychotherapy (Chic) 54(1):66–75, 2017 28263653

Phillips LA, Logan JN, Mather DB: COVID-19 and beyond: telesupervision training within the supervision competency. Training and Education in Professional Psychology 15(4):284–289, 2021

PMRS (Professional Risk Management Services): Psychiatric abandonment? But there was no treatment relationship! 2021. Available at: www.prms.com/services/risk-management/abandonment. Accessed May 5, 2022.

Recupero PR, Rainey SE: Liability and risk management in outpatient psychotherapy supervision. J Am Acad Psychiatry Law 35(2):188–195, 2007 17592164

Riess H: Risk management for the supervising psychiatrist. Psychiatric Times 26(9), 2009. Available at: https://www.psychiatrictimes.com/view/risk-management-supervising-psychiatrist. Accessed July 17, 2022.

Riess H, Herman JB: Teaching the teachers: a model course for psychodynamic psychotherapy supervisors. Acad Psychiatry 32(3):259–264, 2008 18467486

Rousmaniere T, Abbass A, Frederickson J: New developments in technology-assisted supervision and training: a practical overview. J Clin Psychol 70(11):1082–1093, 2014 25230920

Saccuzzo DP: Liability for failure to supervise adequately mental health assistants, unlicensed practitioners and students. California Western Law Review 34(1):115–150, 1997

Schulte HM, Hall MJ, Bienenfeld D: Liability and accountability in psychotherapy supervision: a review, survey, and proposal. Acad Psychiatry 21(3):133–140, 1997 24442898

Sherry P: Ethical issues in the conduct of supervision. The Counseling Psychologist 19(4):566–584, 1991

Sturm C: Record keeping for practitioners. Monitor on Psychology 43(2):70, 2012

Tarasoff v Regents of University of California, 529 P.2d 553 (Cal. 1974)

Tarasoff v Regents of University of California, 551 P.2d 334 (Cal. 1976)

Thomas JT: Informed consent through contracting for supervision: minimizing risks, enhancing benefits. Professional Psychology: Research and Practice 38(3):221–231, 2007

Thomas JT: The Ethics of Supervision and Consultation: Practical Guidance for Mental Health Professionals. Washington, DC, American Psychological Association, 2010

Thomas JT: Disciplinary supervision following ethics complaints: goals, tasks, and ethical dimensions. J Clin Psychol 70(11):1104–1114, 2014 25220953

Van Susteran L: Psychiatric abandonment: pitfalls and prevention. Psychiatric Times 18(8), 2001

25

Addressing Exhaustion and Burnout in Psychotherapy Supervision

Randon S. Welton, M.D.
Katherine G. Kennedy, M.D.
Mary C. Vance, M.D., M.Sc.

KEY LEARNING GOALS

- Recognize that exhaustion and burnout may impair therapeutic and supervisory alliances and hinder the quality of psychotherapy and supervision.

- Recognize that supervisors are in a unique position to help supervisees identify and address exhaustion through exploration of factors that contribute to exhaustion and burnout (such as microaggressions, moral injury, and systemic issues).

- Understand that discussing exhaustion and burnout during supervision may help to strengthen the supervisory alliance, decrease stigma around this highly prevalent experience, and help supervisees to monitor themselves for signs of burnout.

- Recognize that supervisors need to self-monitor for signs of their own burnout and/or exhaustion and address these when possible and necessary.

HEALTH CARE within the United States has been impacted by the related issues of physician wellness, exhaustion, and burnout. Over the past three decades, physicians have been increasingly burdened by productivity demands, managed care bureaucracy, and the implementation of the electronic health record. More recently, stress from the COVID-19 pandemic, and society's response to the pandemic, have added to the existing strain. During the pandemic, many physicians faced record numbers of ill and dying patients, struggled to find child care as daycare facilities closed and schools went online, and could not count on the usual social support from family and friends. Most psychiatrists rapidly shifted models of health care and supervision to virtual platforms, despite wariness about differences between virtual and in-person interactions, and concerns about the diminished quality of physician–patient and trainee–supervisor relationships. Many reported feelings of exhaustion and burnout.

Although definitions of burnout vary, the most common describes a triad of symptoms: emotional exhaustion, depersonalization, and a reduced sense of personal accomplishment. *Emotional exhaustion* includes feelings of physical fatigue accompanied by a sense of emotional emptiness and a feeling of being "drained." *Depersonalization* involves a change of attitude toward others: rather than viewing each person as a singular and unique individual, people are dehumanized and classified as objects. For example, patients may be referred to by their diagnosis (e.g., "the schizophrenic in bed five"). Physicians who use depersonalization may present as callous, cynical, and uncompassionate. A *reduced sense of personal accomplishment* relates to the internal belief that one's work is not consequential and that one has little of value to offer one's patients (Maslach et al. 1996; West et al. 2018). Although the prevalence of burnout among physicians has been found to vary, many studies have found that rates of burnout among medical students, residents, and attending physicians are at or above 50% (Rotenstein et al. 2018; Walsh et al. 2019; West et al. 2018).

Factors Contributing to Burnout in Physicians

Case Vignette 1

The supervisee, Dr. I, started working at a community mental health care center shortly after graduating from residency. Although he entered public psychiatry deeply motivated to help underserved populations, the last 4 years have been a disillusioning experience. He consistently falls behind his organization's productivity demands, and because his patients are often "no show," he is frequently double-booked and asked to see walk-ins. Dr. I is assigned to a treatment team but rarely meets with team members because he is scrambling to complete his electronic documentation. As part of his initial contract negotiation, he had requested time for supervision and to see a few patients for long-term psychotherapy. However, these activities require him to stay into the evening several days per week.

In the following conversation, Dr. I is meeting with his psychotherapy supervisor, Dr. Z, for their weekly 1-hour supervision.

> SUPERVISOR: Before we move on to the next patient, I want to check in with you. You seem especially quiet today, perhaps even a bit upset. Is everything OK? How are you doing?
>
> SUPERVISEE (*looking down, voice cracking*): I'm fine.
>
> SUPERVISOR: Are you? I'm not so sure. What's going on?
>
> SUPERVISEE: I'm just so tired.
>
> SUPERVISOR: Were you on call?
>
> SUPERVISEE: No. That's not it. I feel tired all the time. Today is especially bad.
>
> SUPERVISEE: Why today?
>
> SUPERVISEE: I'm so far behind. I can't keep up with my charting. I'm seeing so many new patients, and the new system's intake requirements are ridiculous. I used to be able to file my initial assessment in 20 minutes, and now I have to scroll through and check so many boxes that it takes me more than 40 minutes. I can't keep up this pace. Also, I got married last year and my husband wants to adopt a child. I barely have anything left for my husband, and certainly no available time or energy for a child. What's worse is that I almost don't care what happens to my patients—or to my marriage. I just feel so overwhelmed and tired. I don't know what to do.

Burnout has a negative impact on patient care and health care systems and deprives physicians of a healthy satisfaction from their work and personal life. Burnout is associated with reduced quality of patient care, impaired professionalism, and an increased rate of medical errors. The impact of burnout extends beyond the individual who is suffering. Patients whose physicians are burned out experience longer delays in recovery and lower satisfaction with their care. Burned-out providers are less efficient and more likely to quit their jobs. There is also a personal cost. These clinicians are at increased risk for poor self-care, depression, substance misuse, and motor vehicle accidents (Abedini et al. 2018; Walsh et al. 2019; West et al. 2018).

A variety of occupational and personal factors add to the risk of physician exhaustion/burnout. Burnout escalates with excessive workloads, inefficient work processes, and increased documentation requirements, which are worsened by inefficient electronic health record systems. Additional external demands placed on clinicians or interpersonal or inner conflicts make exhaustion and/or burnout more likely. The risk of burnout is elevated for physicians who are women and younger, and for those with heavy external responsibilities such as children or dependent elders. All of these factors are amplified by isolation or by a lack or loss of administrative or social support. The risk is further increased by factors that contribute to an inability to experience a sense of control, autonomy, or meaning at work (West et al. 2018), such as being unable to control one's schedule or workload. Supervisees often fall into many of these categories.

Notably, psychiatrists and psychotherapists may be at greater risk than other types of clinicians for exhaustion and burnout. Because psychotherapy and psychiatric treatments typically require extra reservoirs of empathy and an enduring capacity to humanize patients, these clinicians may be at higher risk for depletion of their emotional resources and a subsequent onset of exhaustion, depersonalization, and burnout. A self-selected survey of more than 2,000 psychiatrists found that 78% had scores suggestive of high levels of burnout (Summers et al. 2020). In a systematic review of almost 9,000 therapists, moderate to high burnout was found in 54.5% (Simionato and Simpson 2018). The decrease in empathy, attention, and connectedness associated with burnout may lead to errors in treatment, and these may worsen patient outcome measures (Simionato et al. 2019).

For psychotherapy supervisors and supervisees whose identities overlap with those of racial, ethnic, or sexual/gender minoritized groups, experiences of discrimination and marginalization within and outside of the workplace may also contribute to exhaustion and burnout. The accumulation of microaggressions can negatively affect clinician mental health; in fact, the experience of microaggressions has been shown to have a dose-dependent effect on subsequent depression and other mental illness diagnoses (Torino et al. 2019). These experiences may be additional contributors to exhaustion, burnout, and clinician depression.

Interventions for Preventing and Mitigating Burnout

The literature on preventing or mitigating burnout in physicians is less robust than that establishing the existence of burnout (Walsh et al. 2019). Most interventions have shown some success in decreasing burnout, but the effect size is usually small to moderate. A review of 15 randomized controlled trials (N=716 physicians) and 37 cohort studies (N=2,914 physicians) found that interventions with physicians decreased the rate of burnout from 54% to 44% (West et al. 2016).

Interventions that target organizations and systems of care may be more effective than those dealing exclusively with personal change (Panagioti et al. 2017). Occupational interventions involve manipulating the workplace or dealing with organizational factors. Strategies can include reducing workloads, improving the efficiency of work processes, increasing administrative support, or strengthening physicians' technical skills. Providers who feel powerless can be included in decision making and be granted more autonomy (e.g., more control over their schedules) (Abedini et al. 2018; Panagioti et al. 2017; West et al. 2018). Studies have found that providers who are permitted to spend 20% of their time at work doing something they find personally meaningful are less likely to burn out (Shanafelt and Noseworthy 2017).

Personal interventions are among the most frequently recommended strategies for addressing physician burnout; such interventions commonly include mindfulness exercises, stress management training, and assertiveness training. However, very often the instruction to "do more to make yourself well" strikes exhausted physicians as an additional burden rather than a useful strategy for feeling better. Individuals facing personal stresses (e.g., financial challenges, problems at home) may benefit from counseling or psychotherapy. Many physicians show improvement when meaning is added back to the work they do. Ways of regaining meaning can involve reengagement with the local community or simply increasing the time spent with patients as opposed to time spent on computers. Being able to take time for reflection and enhanced self-awareness has also been shown to be helpful (Abedini et al. 2018; West et al. 2018).

Some personal stresses are existential in nature and challenge physicians' views of themselves as effective and competent providers. Physicians facing these types of stressors can be aided by being helped to recognize and acknowledge their fatigue. Once they understand that their perceived failings are in actuality a predictable response to their situation, they can be encouraged to seek professional help or to make changes in their situations. Receiving support from fellow physicians can also help them restore connections with their patients and profession. Finding role models who support their personal and professional development as physicians can provide an effective antidote to feeling alone and adrift (Abedini et al. 2018). Residents in supervision who are helped to recognize that they are attaining meaningful developmental goals are often better able to manage the stressors they experience (Raj 2016). Figure 25–1 depicts how mood and energy levels may be impacted by the strength of various factors in one's work and personal life.

Role of Psychotherapy Supervision in Alleviating Trainee Burnout

Psychiatry trainees and early-career psychiatrists are often in clinical positions that place the highest demands on and allow the least control over

Social support   Excessive workload
Administrative support   Inefficient systems
Finding meaning in work   Administrative burden
Time for family, friends, hobbies   Health problems
Increasing competence   Family issues
Adaptive coping skills   Financial issues
Appropriate assertiveness   Interpersonal conflicts

Energized/   Exhausted/
Excited   Defeated

Figure 25-1.   Finding a healthy balance.

their professional lives. This stage of adult development (typically covering the late twenties through the middle thirties), during which professional identities are in the process of being established and personal lives often involve life-changing decisions about marriage and children, as well as additional stressors such as moving and caring for aging parental figures, carries particularly high risks for exhaustion and burnout. In addition, the psychotherapy relationship asks more of the psychiatrist than many other clinical roles. Psychotherapists are expected to be engaged, empathic, and focused on the nuances of patients' verbal and nonverbal expressions. These abilities are among the first to be degraded by exhaustion and burnout. Maintaining an open, nonjudgmental, and compassionate attitude and tolerating a patient's negative transference are difficult, if not impossible, when a therapist is feeling emotionally depleted.

Supervision may help to identify, name, and perhaps even address supervisee experiences of exhaustion and burnout (Summers et al. 2020). In fact, lack of supervision has been identified as a significant contributor to burnout (Jovanović et al. 2016). The emotional bond formed in the supervisory alliance can help create a safe and supportive environment that may mitigate a supervisee's experience of burnout (Brenner et al. 2019). It is believed, but not firmly established, that a virtual presence is as effective as an in-person interaction between supervisor and trainee when it comes to providing this safety and support (see Chapter 10, "When Psychotherapy Supervision Is Virtual"). Supervisors can assist their trainees by nurturing this supervisory alliance and by exploring with supervisees potential strategies or changes that may help support and empower them. Supervisors can also monitor their trainees for signs of exhaustion by listening for reports or descriptions of uncharacteristic interpersonal responses and interactions from supervisees during discussions of patient sessions. These uncharacteristic interpersonal interactions could include displays of abruptness, disdain, inattentiveness, pessimism, dismissiveness, anger, or frustration. Monitoring the strength of the supervisee's therapeutic alliances can also provide clues suggestive of incipient exhaustion or burnout; for example, a string of ruptured alliances might suggest that a trainee is no longer able to generate the compassion and emotional energy to work closely with patients.

If signs of burnout and/or exhaustion should appear, supervisors will want to consider a range of different causes, including work-related problems such as workplace discrimination, microaggressions, and other negative workplace dynamics. Personal stressors, mental health problems, and substance use issues should be considered in the differential as well. Supervisors can encourage trainees to discuss their situations, while being careful to maintain appropriate boundaries and avoiding excessive probing into supervisees' personal affairs. Using empathy, validation, and normalization, supervisors can provide support. In general, supervisors should do more listening than instructing. Helping trainees to feel heard and understood should be the first step. In addition to providing space for supervisees to explore their experiences, supervisors can share times in their own professional careers when they have felt overwhelmed and/or exhausted, thereby offering hope to trainees that "things will get better." However, when sharing personal experiences, supervisors should avoid reminiscences about how much harder things were "back in the day," as such recollections are unlikely to be helpful to trainees.

Supervisors can encourage supervisees to explore how their occupational and personal life affects their ability to conduct psychotherapy. If supervisors have concerns about potential adverse impacts on supervisees' work with patients, they should discuss these concerns in a tactful and empathic manner and offer specific suggestions about possible next steps.

Case Vignette 1 (continued)

As they continue to talk, Dr. Z helps Dr. I identify the sources of his stress and the impact exhaustion is having on his life and clinical performance. They begin to explore how Dr. I might improve his situation.

> SUPERVISOR: In addition to making you miserable, I worry that your exhaustion might be affecting the care you are providing. Your clinic workload sounds extreme and unsustainable, and you mentioned that you missed an appointment with one of your patients, Mr. J, this week. What are your thoughts about that, and also about your work in general?

SUPERVISEE: I know. I completely forgot about that appointment with Mr. J. He is so demanding and critical. I think that, unconsciously, I just did not want to meet with him. I know I really messed up.

SUPERVISOR: How are you feeling about meeting with him this coming week?

SUPERVISEE: We don't have an appointment—I mean, I called him and left a message, but he never responded.

SUPERVISOR: Have you called back?

SUPERVISEE: No. I have to admit that I feel relieved not to have an appointment with him. I have so little reserve, and I think if I meet with him, I won't have anything left for other patients—or for myself.

SUPERVISOR: It sounds like you are having a harder time then I realized. How about if we figure out together what to do next? Maybe Mr. J needs to be transferred to another clinician for now, and you and I can work on getting your clinic load lightened? Maybe even consider some time off for you? How do you feel about considering some of those actions?

SUPERVISEE: I want to keep working, so I like your idea of lightening my load. But I don't know how. Do you think you can help me with that?

When discussing these experiences, supervisors will want to be aware that trainees experiencing burnout may be more sensitive to feedback from those with whom they have developed a strong relationship, such as the supervisor, and those in positions of authority (Simionato et al. 2019). Supervisors will want to err on the side of being as supportive and tactful as possible.

Even if no signs of burnout or exhaustion have been detected, supervisors can use the strength of a positive supervisory alliance to check in regularly on their supervisees' work experiences.

Case Vignette 2

In the following conversation, a supervisee is meeting with her supervisor for their weekly supervision session.

SUPERVISOR: It sounds like your psychotherapy patients help you get a chance to step back and take a breath.

SUPERVISEE: Yes, I feel like I can treat my psychotherapy patients the way they should be treated. Actually, I think my psychotherapy work with patients, and my meetings with you, are my only safe havens.

SUPERVISOR: Your only safe havens? How so?

SUPERVISEE: I mean those are the only two places where I feel valued, where I don't feel ignored and criticized.

SUPERVISOR: What about your three other days on the C-L [consultation-liaison] service? How is that going?

SUPERVISOR: It's been so hard on that service. My chief resident constantly interrupts and talks over me. He lets patients call me "nurse," and laughs when they do. He takes my suggestions and states them as his own. When I try to point out what is happening, he stares at me and walks away.

When learning that trainees are experiencing ongoing stress from a demoralizing interpersonal situation, supervisors will want to support and empower them by validating their experience, offering specific suggestions, and even considering engaging in role-play to explore ways to manage the difficult situation. The Microaggressions Triangle Model, a framework for understanding and dealing with microaggressions from the perspectives of recipient, source, and bystanders, has been shown to be helpful in addressing these types of encounters (Ackerman-Barger and Jacobs 2020).

Supervisor Self-Monitoring and Self-Care

Finally, supervisors should be aware that they too are at elevated risk for burnout and exhaustion, often for the same reasons as trainees. Supervisors need to be alert to and monitor themselves for any signs of burnout and exhaustion, and to reflect on any recent changes in their own interpersonal relationships with patients, supervisees, colleagues, friends, and family members. If such signs are detected, the next steps would include efforts to break through their own self-stigmatizing, forgive themselves, share their feelings with colleagues, and seek supervision or personal psychotherapy. During this phase, supervisors should exercise caution in regard to sharing their feelings of being overwhelmed or exhausted with their trainees, because these types of exchanges may unfairly burden or stress supervisees. However, after resolving a situation of exhaustion and burnout, supervisors can feel free to share these experiences with supervisees as a way to decrease stigma around burnout and to encourage supervisees to speak more openly about their feelings and concerns.

Conclusion

The experience of being listened to, understood, and valued by their supervisors can help alleviate the distress of supervisees who feel exhausted or burned out. In general, supervisors can help their supervisees by 1) maintaining a strong positive supervisory alliance, 2) listening to them and validating their experiences, and 3) helping them to identify a path forward that addresses their symptoms and situation. This assistance can include a range of responses, such as helping supervisees to confront a difficult workplace situation, encouraging them to begin personal therapy, and/or facilitating time off or a medical leave. Throughout this process, the needs of the patients whom supervisees are treating need to be constantly considered and attended to. Although these responsibilities have not typically been considered to be part of the psychotherapy supervisor's traditional mission, supervisors have a unique opportunity to detect and address exhaustion and burnout in trainees. We believe that helping one's supervisees in this way should become an integral part of the role of the psychotherapy supervisor.

References

Abedini NC, Stack SW, Goodman JL, Steinberg KP: "It's not just time off": a framework for understanding factors promoting recovery from burnout among internal medicine residents. J Grad Med Educ 10(1):26–32, 2018 29467969

Ackerman-Barger K, Jacobs NN: The microaggressions triangle model: a humanistic approach to navigating microaggressions in health professions schools. Acad Med 95 (12S [Addressing Harmful Bias and Eliminating Discrimination in Health Professions Learning Environments]):S28–S32, 2020 32889926

Brenner AM, Coverdale J, Guerrero APS, et al: An update on trainee wellness: some progress and a long way to go. Acad Psychiatry 43(4):357–360, 2019 31236856

Jovanović N, Podlesek A, Volpe U, et al: Burnout syndrome among psychiatric trainees in 22 countries: risk increased by long working hours, lack of supervision, and psychiatry not being first career choice. Eur Psychiatry 32:34–41, 2016 26802982

Maslach C, Jackson SE, Leiter MP: Maslach Burnout Inventory Manual, 3rd Edition. Palo Alto, CA, Consulting Psychologists Press, 1996

Panagioti M, Panagopoulou E, Bower P, et al: Controlled interventions to reduce burnout in physicians: a systematic review and meta-analysis. JAMA Intern Med 177(2):195–205, 2017 27918798

Raj KS: Well-being in residency: a systematic review. J Grad Med Educ 8(5):674–684, 2016 28018531

Rotenstein LS, Torre M, Ramos MA, et al: Prevalence of burnout among physicians: a systematic review. JAMA 320(11):1131–1150, 2018 30326495

Shanafelt TD, Noseworthy JH: Executive leadership and physician well-being: nine organizational strategies to promote engagement and reduce burnout. Mayo Clin Proc 92(1):129–146, 2017 27871627

Simionato GK, Simpson S: Personal risk factors associated with burnout among psychotherapists: a systematic review of the literature. J Clin Psychol 74(9):1431–1456, 2018 29574725

Simionato G, Simpson S, Reid C: Burnout as an ethical issue in psychotherapy. Psychotherapy (Chic) 56(4):470–482, 2019 31815507

Summers RF, Gorrindo T, Hwang S, et al: Well-being, burnout, and depression among North American psychiatrists: the state of our profession. Am J Psychiatry 177(10):955–964, 2020 32660300

Torino G, Rivera D, Capadilupa C, et al: Microaggression Theory: Influence and Implication. Hoboken, NJ, John Wiley & Sons, 2019

Walsh AL, Lehmann S, Zabinski J, et al: Interventions to prevent and reduce burnout among undergraduate and graduate medical education trainees: a systematic review. Acad Psychiatry 43(4):386–395, 2019 30710229

West CP, Dyrbye LN, Erwin PJ, Shanafelt TD: Interventions to prevent and reduce physician burnout: a systematic review and meta-analysis. Lancet 388(10057):2272–2281, 2016 27692469

West CP, Dyrbye LN, Shanafelt TD: Physician burnout: contributors, consequences and solutions. J Intern Med 283(6):516–529, 2018 29505159

Index

Page numbers printed in **boldface** *type refer to tables or figures.*